Healing the Masses

Healing the Masses

Cuban Health Politics at Home and Abroad

Julie Margot Feinsilver

with a Foreword by David E. Apter

UNIVERSITY OF CALIFORNIA PRESS

Berkeley / Los Angeles / London

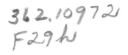

362.10972
F29h

University of California Press
Berkeley and Los Angeles, California

University of California Press, Ltd.
London, England

© 1993 by
The Regents of the University of California

Library of Congress Cataloging-in-Publication Data

Feinsilver, Julie Margot.
    Healing the masses : Cuban health politics at home and abroad /
Julie Margot Feinsilver.
        p.   cm.
    Includes bibliographical references and index.
        ISBN 0-520-08218-4 (alk. paper). — ISBN 0-520-08298-2
(pbk. : alk. paper)
        1. Medical policy—Cuba.   2. Medical care—Political aspects—
Cuba.   3. Medical assistance, Cuban—Political aspects.
4. Symbolism in politics—Cuba.   I. Title.
RA395.C9F45 1993
362.1'097291—dc20   92–31124
Printed in the United States of America   CIP

9 8 7 6 5 4 3 2 1

The paper used in this publication meets the minimum requirements
of American National Standard for Information Sciences—Permanence
of Paper for Printed Library Materials, ANSI Z39.48–1984.

To the memory of
Ethel Marcus Feinsilver
and to
Jacob Monroe Feinsilver

Contents

Tables

Foreword

David E. Apter
Yale University

This study of Cuba as a "world-class" health power is particularly interesting because it concerns what is fast becoming the lone socialist bureaucratic state. Whatever the difficulties and problems of socialist transitions, everywhere except in Cuba the conceptual basis of the state is changing from the centrist principles of a Marxist ideology to a logic of open, more "econocentric" alternatives. In Cuba, however, market has yet to displace plan, and the need for democratization has yet to be recognized. Democratization is still explicitly denied in both principle and practice. Cuba, then, continues to go its own way, the last state in which national goals remain specified by the regime as an expression of a socialist worldview. It continues to regard the party as the sole repository of wisdom, with Fidel Castro as its Agent.

One of the characteristics of the Cuban model is the special significance attached to moral rather than material exchanges and reciprocities. Symbolic capital takes priority over economic. The future is overvalued at the expense of the present. It is necessary to transform the "symbolic capital" the regime earns into economic capital in order to exchange moral symbolism for pragmatic realism. The continued reliance on highly valued symbolism in the face of eroding material practices leaves an emptiness at the center, an emptiness which not only bodes ill for the regime in power, but also makes the Agent appear more and more absurd as the last hold out in a universe which has largely disappeared.

Putting matters in this light, however, has led many to shortchange the regime and to overlook its more remarkable accomplishments. The two areas in which the symbolic and the practical have come together with considerable success are education and health. Public education and public health, as powerful symbols of egalitarian values, were given the highest priority in the earliest years of the Cuban revolution, and health care, in particular, because it symbolized "science," became a form of empowerment. Health care and medical practices have become the touchstone for the allegedly superior virtues of the Cuban revolution and the signal virtue of Cuban socialism.

Such priorities have not been unique to Cuba, of course. In all the erstwhile socialist systems education and public health became centerpieces, the signifiers of an improved body politic. But in virtually all such systems, health care programs were overwhelmed and bureaucratized. While experiences varied, not only among countries but also within each country, the overall record of socialist medicine is hardly salutary.

In Cuba, as Julie Feinsilver so powerfully demonstrates, the story has been different. Symbolic factors aside, achieving an exceptionally high level of medical research and health care has become the central focus of the regime, an emphasis which represents a very shrewd policy. For a small country like Cuba, concentrating on health care is one way of maximizing rewards from minimal resources (resources diminished further by the U.S. economic embargo). The regime recognized early on that it had to accomplish something remarkable in its own eyes as well as in the eyes of outside beholders. Hence by putting most of its eggs in this one basket, Cuba has become, in the field of health, an example more powerful countries might do well to consider. Indeed, if one used as a sole criterion the standard of health care provided all Cuban citizens, other governments might not appear as politically healthy. Notwithstanding Cuba's long distance from democratic grace, on this score at least it competes very well with states that may call themselves democratic but rank low on the scale of social welfare obligations and entitlements. Even if there is room for improvement in Cuba's medical sector, it still compares very well with American practice, which only now is being recognized for what it is: a monument to inefficiency, insufficiency, and discrimination.

Because Cuban health care is the best example of a Cuban "success," it is not surprising that Cuba has sought to extend that success abroad. Certain African countries have been made the beneficiaries of Cuban medical treatment and delivery services, with people living in some remote areas experiencing modern medicine for the first time. Indeed, it is widely acknowledged that the Cubans have practiced good medicine under difficult field conditions, so much so that health care as a form of political outreach has become one of the dominant narratives of the Cuban revolution.

Cuba's stated goal of becoming a world class medical power has proved to be an effective strategy at home and abroad. Indeed, good medical practice became part of the "historic and inversionary struggle" against imperialism in general and American instances of such imperialism in particular. One of the many virtues of Julie Feinsilver's book is its exacting analysis of how the Cuban strategy works at every level, from research to practice in the field. Moreover, her emphasis on the connection between the symbolic and economic aspects of health practice is unique. She describes the importance of medical *science* as a secular indicator of socialist accomplishment and shows how this accomplishment is realized in the practice of health care delivery, domestic and foreign.

Feinsilver's book is all the more remarkable if we remember how difficult it is to do field work in communist countries. It was only by great determination, the skeptical scrutiny of statistical information, and extensive interviewing, returning again and again over many years, that she was able to piece this story together. She also had to overcome a good many obstacles placed in her way by some local officials and resentful individuals, making this multifaceted study of medical science and practice in Cuba even more of an achievement.

As Feinsilver argues very convincingly, these medical accomplishments make the present regime more rather than less politically vulnerable. She gives us a remarkable lens through which to examine changes in Cuba, and with it a fresh way to view the theory and practice of politics in a socialist country. Her analysis of details also takes account of broader political and social concerns. She calls a spade a spade and gives credit where credit is due, without losing sight of the larger political picture in Cuba. And her work raises a haunting question. If the regime is overthrown or, less likely, if it can reform itself from within, will medical and health care benefits for ordinary citizens become socially skewed, and for many inadequate, or will the Cubans find innovative ways to respond and preserve their significant accomplishments? Feinsilver's study raises interesting questions not only for Cuba but for countries elsewhere—including our own.

Preface

The Cuban government's unusual concern for the health of its population is but one of many reasons why the regime has survived so long after the demise of communism in Eastern Europe and the Soviet Union. The provision of considerable social welfare benefits (health, education, social security, and subsidized housing, food, transportation, cultural and sporting events, and consumer goods) served to legitimize the regime for some time. When economic adversity made it impossible for the government to live up to its own standards in the provision of these social welfare benefits and to fulfill all of its citizens' basic needs, delegitimization began.

Other important factors that help explain the regime's survival against all odds are nationalism, tight domestic security, and more important, the lack of alternatives. Unlike the rise to power of communist regimes in Eastern Europe, the Cuban revolution was nationalistic and not imposed in the wake of the Red Army. Many Cubans still supported the goals of the revolution even when they no longer agreed with the leadership about its policies or wanted their government to survive. Castro's security forces, however, are still able to deter any potential opposition movement from expanding and mounting an insurrection.

In Cuba, the alternatives to socialism have not been very attractive. There appear to be no effective socioeconomic models in the east or west to fill the void left by socialist ideology and practice. The transition to democracy and economic privatization in both the former

Soviet bloc and Latin America has been no panacea for the majority of the people of those countries.

Cuban media coverage of the deleterious effects of these transitions has shown powerful images of increased economic chaos and hardship, material and psychological insecurity, government corruption and ineffectiveness, ethnic and racial violence, and increased crime. Even though Cuba's transition would be aided by investment from the Cuban community in exile, just as German reunification has made the transition easier for East Germany than for the others, social unrest, unemployment, racism, and the loss of many social welfare benefits have made life in the eastern German states quite difficult.

The Cuban media has always given considerable attention to increasing crime, homelessness, unemployment, and inequality in the U.S. These images paint an unpleasant picture of what might be in store for the Cuban people in a transition to a privatized economy.

Socialism, as the Cubans have known it, is a thing of the past, but capitalism and democracy in developing countries have been no beacons of hope either. Again, extensive Cuban media coverage of the negative effects of IMF structural adjustment programs, which disproportionately affect the poor of Latin America, depicts what might be in store for the Cubans. Nor have the political corruption and attempted coups in Latin America indicated a promising path for Cuba to follow.

Few Cubans in Cuba want to see the Miami Cubans return to take over the island's economy and government and reclaim their properties; they are the people who have tried to destroy the revolution and who have made life on the island hard for over three decades. Those seeking greater political freedom have little to hope for from that quarter; the most vociferous anti-Castro Miami Cubans are no more democratic than Castro.

Despite the lack of inspiring alternatives, the Cuban people desire a vast improvement in their standard of living, which recently has fallen to a very low level. Although the government still provides free medical care and education, there has been a tremendous deterioration in the quality and quantity of services available because of the collapse of trade relations and estrangement from former allies, and because of the three-decade U.S. economic embargo. With the absence of the Soviet Union, the same U.S. economic, political, and military pressure that persuaded the Nicaraguan people to vote for

Violeta Barrios de Chamorro is likely to persuade the Cuban people to seek an alternative to the Castro government.

Like all the Third World health officials and international organization officials I have interviewed since 1978, I believe that Cuba's health system, while no Garden of Eden, deserves considerable praise and can serve as an important example. Moreover, it is important to speak in defense of one of the few successes in a socialist country because these are quickly dismissed along with the more numerous failures. Nevertheless, problems in the Cuban health system will only get worse with the continuing economic deterioration that has followed change in Eastern Europe and the former Soviet Union. This study, therefore, shows the outcome of the politics of health in Cuba and the projection abroad of Cuban medical diplomacy in the heyday of the revolution, in the late 1970s and throughout the 1980s. By 1991 it was clear that irreversible change had occurred. Cuba's achievements in the 1980s, however, still offer valuable lessons to both developing and developed nations, and help explain why the Castro government survived so long after the demise of communism in Eastern Europe and the Soviet Union.

My interest in Cuba arose from my travels throughout Latin America in the late 1960s and early 1970s. At the time, I was struck by the disparity in income and wealth not just among people within a country but among countries as well. Cuba seemed to be undertaking a fascinating social experiment in improving life for the vast majority of its population, and it was considered by many Latin American intellectuals to offer an alternative path to development. It is this alternative path, the effort to provide equal access to goods and services, that distinguishes Cuba's social and economic development policies from those of its neighbors. In this time of global economic crisis and crisis in health-care systems, both developing and developed countries could learn from the Cuban experience in the health sector.

This study began as a doctoral dissertation at Yale University but has been revised and updated to 1992. I was fortunate to be one of the first U.S. social scientists in almost a decade to be allowed to do field research in Cuba on a contemporary subject as part of the limited rapprochement that occurred under the Carter administration. This first-hand observation proved invaluable not only for the collection of data but also for its interpretation. Thus many of the data for the present study were collected during nine research trips to Cuba in 1978, 1979, 1980, 1980–81, 1988, 1990 (two), 1991, and 1992. Except for one seven-month stay, the trips ranged from five days (one trip) to three to four weeks each. Other data are from sources available at libraries in the United States, particularly the Yale University libraries, the library of the Pan American Health Organization in Washington, D.C., and the Library of Congress.

By the time I was able to spend an extended period in Cuba to do research, the 1980 U.S. presidential election was approaching, and Cuban officials, like most Americans, anticipated a Reagan victory. The Cuban Ministry of Health officials were therefore reluctant to allow me virtually any access to data, people, and places; doing research became extremely difficult. Persistence finally paid off, but only after months of minimal access and many obstacles. My information, then, has come perhaps as much from unofficial sources as from official sources. Although the latter may be cited more frequently herein, the former very much colored my interpretation of all data.

It has been said that researchers who go to Cuba for one week write a book. Those who go for two weeks write an article, and those who go for longer don't write anything. Given the length of my stay in Cuba and the gestation period for this manuscript, perhaps it would be more accurate to say that the longer one stays in Cuba, the longer it takes to write about it.

Acknowledgments

My greatest intellectual debt is to two men who in their own ways stimulated and encouraged my work and offered cogent critiques over the years: David E. Apter and George A. Silver. Apter's work on symbolic politics inspired my own. George Silver kindled my interest in international health and inspired me to analyze it politically. The keen intellects and the advice of both men have been invaluable to me.

The following people also kindly provided significant comments on one or more chapters of this or earlier manuscripts: Marta Cehelsky, Jorge I. Domínguez, Susan Eckstein, Kai Erikson, Miguel A. Figueras, Robert Fishman, Daniel J. Goldstein, Tamar Gordon, Günther Handl, Lisandro Pérez, José Luis Rodríguez, Amy Saldinger, and Andy Zimbalist. Pan American Health Organization (PAHO) officials Daniel Joly (retired), César Vieira, Alberto Pellegrini, and Cristina Puentes provided strong encouragement for my research as well as important feedback.

Cubans who have provided encouragement, access to data, and their own perceptions of the Cuban health system and Cuban medical diplomacy are too numerous to mention. I would, nonetheless, like to thank two. I am indebted to Francisco Rojas Ochoa, vice rector of the Instituto Superior de Ciencias Médicas in Havana and former director of the Instituto de Desarrollo de la Salud (IDS) in Havana, for "sponsoring" my research locally in the period from 1978 through 1981 and for his continued friendship and insights into

Cuban health policy. Finally, I am very much obliged to the late Mario Escalona Reguera, former director of education at IDS and former vice minister of health, for his candid appraisals of the Cuban health system and Cuban politics in general as well as his encouragement and support, even when these were unpopular.

All of these people have influenced this work in some way, although they may not recognize their contributions in the resulting product. The analyses and opinions stated here may not reflect their views nor those of the funding agencies. Any shortcomings, of course, rest with me.

Funding for field research in Cuba in 1980–81 and Puerto Rico in 1982–83 was provided through the generosity of the American Council of Learned Societies and the Social Science Research Council. Initial research trips to Cuba and Puerto Rico in 1978 were funded by the Yale University Concilium on International and Area Studies and the Yale University Department of Sociology Shell Grant, respectively. Jorge I. Domínguez provided a stimulating environment at the Center for International Affairs at Harvard (1981–1982) in which to write up my 1980–1981 field research. The Research Council of Colgate University provided partial funding for the two 1990 research trips to Cuba. An Asher B. Edelman Released-Time Fellowship from Bard College gave me a reduced teaching load to allow me to work on revising the book. The Pan American Health Organization provided funding for the 1991 trip. Jonah Gensler at Bard College and Kerry Reichs at Oberlin College provided assistance in preparing the final manuscript and thus have my gratitude.

Last but not least, I would like to thank my editors at the University of California Press, Erika Büky and Paul Michelson, without whom this would be a much less readable book, and Naomi Schneider, who brought this project to fruition. It has been a great pleasure to work with them.

Introduction

Most government leaders espouse the principle of health for all, yet few pay more than lip service to the ideal or allocate adequate resources for its development. In Cuba, by contrast, health care is seen as a basic human right and the responsibility of the state, and its leaders consider health indicators as measures of government efficacy.[1] Accordingly, health care has taken a prominent place in the Cuban government's domestic and foreign policies despite Cuba's economic vulnerability.

Although socialist ideology professes the goal of ameliorating the human condition, only Cuba has made health a defining characteristic of its "revolution" and has consistently given health such preeminence that daily operational issues are discussed at the highest level of government. As a result, many in Cuba say that the real minister of public health is Fidel Castro. Since 1978 Castro has made a number of declarations about the direction of Cuban medicine, indicating that Cuba would become "the bulwark of Third World Medicine," put a doctor on every block, become a "world medical power," and equal or surpass the United States on certain health indices.[2]

Why did Cuba, a small developing nation with scarce resources, a strong economic dependence on a distant benefactor (the Soviet Union), an economic embargo by its most natural trade partner (the United States), and the constant threat of destabilization from abroad, try to achieve such goals? Further, how could a developing country like Cuba even attempt to become a "world medical power"? How does becoming a "world medical power" fit in with the larger goal of societal transformation? Why and how does Cuba provide medical aid to other developing nations? Finally, can Cuba maintain its current commitment to health and medical diplomacy in the post–Cold War era? I address these questions and also consider whether Cuba's invocation of the term "world medical power" is credible; how the development of Cuba's domestic medical system provided a springboard for its medical diplomacy; what the symbolic significance might be of becoming a "world medical power"; what Cuban medical diplomacy means for Cuba, the Third World, and the developed nations; and, finally, what Cuba's prospects for the future may be in a unipolar world without Soviet aid.

Analysts of both the Cuban health system and Cuban foreign policy have tended to overlook Cuba's medical diplomacy; it is a phenomenon little known outside certain health and development circles, international organizations, and the recipient countries. Limited attention has been given to the larger political and economic forces behind Cuba's domestic and international medical programs. Nor has the relationship between health and medicine on the one hand and political economy on the other been studied. More important, no one has analyzed the symbolic political issues involved in Cuba's foreign and domestic health policies. I attempt to fill the gap by focusing on symbolic politics, political economy, and foreign policy in the Cuban health sphere and by analyzing the current domestic health system as part of the infrastructure for medical diplomacy and, thus, for material and symbolic capital accumulation.

Within the former socialist bloc the Cuban government's preoccupation with the provision of health care was unparalleled. All socialist countries, of course, sought to improve health by providing medical and public health services, generally with no direct charge to the patient.[3] Their efforts resulted in significant gains in life expectancy, infant mortality, and general morbidity and mortality, although some recent setbacks have been registered.[4] Cuba had not yet faced such setbacks by the end of 1991.

Economic difficulties and political choices about resource allocation have prevented some socialist countries from providing adequate health care for everyone.[5] For example, until 1965 China's health system served only the urban population, which represented about 15 percent of the total population.[6] In Cuba, however, the leadership began the public health service in the rural areas, where the need for medical attention was greatest. Even as late as 1989, the Soviet Union and the Eastern European countries experienced great difficulty in providing adequate, universal health care. Cuba, by contrast, has provided such a service for more than two decades. It has not achieved a perfect system, as any Miami Cuban who has had to send medicines to relatives on the island will attest; but not even defectors criticize the Cuban health system.

Until recently, Cuba was largely insulated from the present world economic crisis because of its integration into the Community for Mutual Economic Assistance (CMEA). The political and economic changes that swept Eastern Europe in the fall of 1989, however, have permanently altered economic relations among the former CMEA countries, particularly the nature, amount, and terms of trade. With economic decentralization and privatization, the CMEA became defunct. Trade relations among these countries, where they still exist, are no longer between states but rather between enterprises, with prices set in convertible currency at world market levels.

The need and desire for Western markets has become more critical as the former socialist countries seek hard-currency earnings, Western consumer goods, and access to advanced technology to modernize and bolster their floundering economies. These changes, along with political differences, have led to their curtailment of trade with Cuba. Preferential prices or subsidies by and large vanished by January 1991, when all payments of remaining intra-CMEA exchanges had to be made at world market prices and in convertible currency rather than in barter or nonconvertible currencies. Moreover, Soviet trade subsidies to Cuba, which were tied to world market prices, had been decreasing since 1985,[7] and largely ended in January 1991 as the Soviet Union faced its own domestic economic and political difficulties. The exceptions during 1991 were Soviet subsidies for Cuban sugar.[8] Although in 1991 Soviet-Cuban trade was denominated in hard currency, it was actually carried out through clearing accounts without the exchange of hard currency.

Cuba, of course, has always traded with capitalist countries and thus has long been affected by revaluations of hard currencies, fluctuations in interest rates and world market prices, and increasingly unfavorable terms of trade. The recent changes in Cuba's trade relations, however, pose a much more serious challenge to the Cuban economy and government. The early 1990s will be a trying time for Cuba as well as the former socialist countries as they adjust to the world market and short-term contracts.

By 1991 the Cuban economy was in dire straits and negative growth had been predicted for the foreseeable future. The Soviet Union, in a state of economic and political disintegration, shipped little of what the Cubans had contracted for 1991 except oil. By September 30, 1991, less than 50 percent of grain and most other contracted items had been shipped; most shipments, in fact, were less than 20 percent of the expected quantities.[9]

As a consequence, Cuban officials and trade representatives have been making greater efforts to increase trade with market economies, particularly in Latin America. Castro has stated that the Cuban economy is ripe for integration with the economies of the region, so much so that he will offer special advantages to Latin American investors interested in joint ventures in Cuba.[10] It seems unlikely, however, that investment, trade, and aid from international organizations will be sufficient to shore up the economy. It will not be the first time, however, that Cuba has faced adversity. Indeed, the past thirty-four years testify to Cuba's ability to overcome seemingly impossible odds.

Consider, for example, the 1980s. Elsewhere in the Third World this decade has been characterized as the "lost decade" because of the severe social and economic dislocations caused by the debt crisis. In most developing nations, massive external debt, coupled with International Monetary Fund austerity measures, precluded the expansion, or even the maintenance of current levels, of social expenditures. Economic constraints have led many countries, including the United States, to privatize public services and reduce social service expenditures.[11] The Soviet Union, which decreased health expenditures to levels below what would be expected at its stage of economic development more than two decades ago, continued this practice through the 1980s.[12] Cuba, in contrast, increased general social service expenditures until 1991 and continued even then to increase the public health budget in the face of economic adversity.[13]

Cuba's focus on health care projects an image of progress that other developing nations do not have. To gain international influence and prestige, Castro has chosen to represent Cuba as a country of increasing social development and scientific sophistication. This, of course, is difficult for a developing nation that relies on a single product (sugar) for the lion's share of its exports and has long depended on trade subsidies from a single, large market. For a variety of reasons, domestic inefficiency and the U.S. economic embargo among them, Cuba cannot compete in the economic sphere with the Asian newly industrialized countries (NICs), nor can it compete with the already developed world. Its potential for product diversification is limited because of a dearth of the hard currency and raw materials needed for manufacturing processes.

Where Cuba has been able to surpass other countries and approach the level of the developed world is in improving the health of its population and providing its medical expertise to other countries. This is not to say that the entire Cuban health system is on a par with that of the United States; but health outcomes in certain critical areas are. The improvement of the population's health initially required more political commitment than hard currency and scientific expertise. Once the obvious public health, health education, and sanitation measures were taken, however, further progress depended on other factors, such as the expenditure of considerable hard currency on a system of well-equipped medical institutions and the rapid incorporation of scientific advances.

In numerous speeches prior to the demise of the socialist bloc, Castro had claimed that Cuba would become a "world medical power." He has used this phrase to attempt to gain credibility for Cuba in much larger arenas than health and medicine alone. It connotes socioeconomic development, scientific achievement, a model health system, and international influence. Socioeconomic development is generally quantified by several indicators, but the most telling are infant mortality and life expectancy at birth; these figures include a whole range of other indicators as inputs, among which are sanitation, nutrition, medical services, education, housing, employment, equitable distribution of resources, and economic growth.[14] For Cuba to qualify as a "world medical power," moreover, its medical system should have an effect on other countries, and its health achievements should be admired and emulated by others.

I evaluate Cuba's success in achieving this goal first, and primarily, by Cuba's own standards. These criteria are: general health indicators, especially infant mortality rate and life expectancy at birth; the extent and distribution of human resources, particularly the physician-to-population ratio and the overall health personnel-to-population ratio; provision and expansion of universal primary and preventive care

and high-technology tertiary care; biotechnology research; and provision of medical aid to other developing nations. Later in this study
I also compare Cuban achievements with broader criteria.[15]

The provision of medical aid to other countries will be evaluated
in the context of its importance in Castro's diplomatic efforts with
the Third World and international organizations. Unable to offer monetary aid to nations, Cuba has instead offered what it excels at and
what is easily available. The international recognition of Cuba's health
expertise has made medical diplomacy an effective foreign policy
tool. What country would reject humanitarian aid that appears to be
purely altruistic, but has a payback rate of the type attributed significantly
to Cuba's claim to the status of world medical power, and vice versa?
Provision of medical aid is one of several of these more important criteria
because it transcends purely domestic and projects the country's capabilities in far-flung parts of the world. For this reason a rather extensive chapter is devoted to medical diplomacy, and its importance
is reiterated throughout the book.

Chapter 1 sets the stage on which Cuba acts in the international
arena and discusses theories of symbolic politics and symbolic capital
as they affect Cuban medical diplomacy. Chapter 2 provides the background to the health ideology and organization necessary to understand Cuba's domestic success in this sphere and its ability to export
medical assistance. Chapter 3 picks up the domestic thread of Chapter 2 and weaves an impression of how health education and popular
participation have made the Cuban model compelling to outsiders.
Chapter 4 evaluates Cuban health indicators and compares them with
those of the United States to ascertain whether Cuba was, in fact,
becoming a world medical power before the collapse of the socialist
bloc.

Cuba's medical diplomacy would have been all but impossible
without the development of its domestic health system and its considerable success in achieving First-World health statistics. Chapter 5
discusses Cuban biotechnology and medical exports, areas of considerable scientific sophistication and real and potential profits. Chapter
6 presents Cuban medical diplomacy in all of its forms and considers
the benefits to both the host country and Cuba. Chapter 7 concludes
with a discussion of the costs and applicability of the Cuban model
to other nations; problems and prospects for the domestic medical
system and medical diplomacy, particularly in the post–Cold War era;

and an analysis of the symbolic significance of Cuba's health system and medical diplomacy. Obviously, changes in the socialist world that occurred after the writing of this manuscript have made this into a historical work that tells a tale of what was (during the 1980s) and what could have been.

1

Cuba on the World Stage

Symbolic Politics

Geographically small states are presumed to have little ability to be major actors on the world stage.[1] This is particularly true of developing nations with scarce resources. Some small, albeit developed, states have held great power through military might, economic prowess, scientific and technical achievement, or political control over large territories (or colonies).[2] Among the developing nations, only Cuba and China have been influential in the global context, particularly as ideological beacons for Third World intellectuals and revolutionaries. However, no small developing country has been able to exert the power and influence characteristic of a major player in world politics except Cuba,[3] and "few [countries] with more resources, match the worldwide scope of Cuba's foreign policy."[4]

Cuba's behavior and power has [*sic*] come to influence virtually all other countries in the international system to some degree.... Cuba is a factor in many of the world's "hot spots" ranging from Central America to the Horn of Africa, from the western Sahara to Indochina, and from South Yemen to Southern Africa.[5]

What accounts for Cuba's disproportionate share of world power and visibility? Cuba has projected its influence beyond what would seem possible through extending its military might in Angola and

Ethiopia, through economic largesse as a purveyor of both military and civilian technical aid, as a mediator in regional conflicts, and as a forceful and persuasive advocate of Third World interests in international forums. Also, although Cuba's scientific achievements are limited, it shares them with other Third World countries, thereby furthering Cuban influence and prestige abroad.

The Cuban government explains its policy of proletarian internationalism (civilian and military aid) and solidarity as repayment of its debt to humanity for international assistance received, particularly in the early years of the revolution. Cuban leaders recognize that their revolution could not have withstood U.S.–sponsored threats, either military or economic, without the aid of the former Soviet Union and East European countries. Thus they strongly believe it is their duty to aid other developing countries and national liberation movements.[6] This ideological motivation is more than just socialist anti-imperialism; it also follows the Latin American tradition of Bolivar, San Martín, and Martí, all of whom sought independence for Latin American countries besides their own.

Some argue that Cuba has acted as a proxy for the Soviet Union, but this is not the case. Cuba has its own foreign policy, which at times has coincided but at other times has been at variance with Soviet policy. Cuba has even led the Soviet Union into commitments that it would not have made otherwise, such as in Angola, Nicaragua, and Grenada.[7] It has even been argued that in the mid to late 1980s Cuba was not the Soviet Union's proxy but rather its successor in the Third World.[8]

Soviet aid facilitated Cuba's international activism but did not determine it prior to mid 1991.[9] Policy was made by the Cubans, but Soviet aid in general allowed them to divert resources to their own foreign assistance programs. By 1991, the collapse of trade and aid relations made it impossible for Cuba to continue the level of aid that it had previously granted, not because of a lack of skilled workers to send abroad, but because of the government's inability to transport and support them there.

Soviet aid to Cuba for many years has been less per year, both in absolute terms and per capita, than U.S. aid to Puerto Rico. Cuba's population of ten million is three times the size of Puerto Rico's. Since Puerto Rico received anywhere from 1.2 to 3.8 times the absolute aid that Cuba received during the period from 1965 to 1983, this aid is equivalent to 3.6 to 11.4 times Cuba's per capita aid.[10]

Despite massive federal aid, Puerto Rico has accomplished less than Cuba both in general socioeconomic development and in the health sphere, and is not even attempting the sort of far-reaching health programs at home or abroad that Cuba has.[11] Despite the desires of various U.S. administrations, Puerto Rico has never been the showcase of the Americas.

Not only is Cuba's relationship with one superpower (the United States) a hostile one, but also its relations with the other former superpower and its longtime benefactor (the Soviet Union) have been problematic. During the 1960s the Cuban and Soviet leaderships disagreed on foreign and domestic policies, as well as on ideology.[12] Although these problems were largely resolved by 1970, some differences persisted and new, more serious ones arose in the 1980s and 1990s.

Already in 1986 Castro's domestic policies were at odds with Gorbachev's perestroika. Most notable was Cuba's virtual elimination of market mechanisms introduced in 1980 to stimulate productivity and improve the quality and quantity of goods and services, and Cuba's increased centralization of economic decision making.[13] Until October 1988 Cuba was alone among socialist countries in reversing economic reforms that allowed market mechanisms and local economic decision making. At that time China's overheated economy was slowed down and local economic autonomy was limited, but the market was not eliminated as in Cuba.[14]

Geopolitical changes and the opportunity to effectively aid revolutionary forces or progressive governments also partially determine Cuba's foreign policy. Castro's interest in and commitment to Central America and the Caribbean were not shared by the Soviets, who, since Yuri Andropov, sought to limit foreign entanglements to ones of mutual economic benefit. As the former Soviet Union focused on its internal economic, political, and social problems, it increasingly fostered economic ties with capitalist countries, developing and developed, rather than with revolutionary regimes requiring heavy subsidies.[15] In fact, before fragmentation of the Soviet Union, the Soviets had extricated themselves from aid relationships with Third World regimes, with the notable exception of Cuba and Vietnam.

Five incidents stand out as demonstrating the fragility of Soviet-Cuban relations over time. They clearly reveal that, without consulting Castro, the Soviet Union took actions perceived as detrimental to Cuba if these actions furthered Soviet objectives. For example, the

Soviet Union and the United States resolved the 1962 missile crisis without Cuba's participation and to the considerable ire of Castro.[16] Second, a similar event occurred almost twenty-five years later, after the Chernobyl nuclear accident, when the United States and the Soviet Union agreed to exchange information on the safety of Cuba's Soviet-origin nuclear reactors without Cuban participation, and once again to Castro's chagrin.[17]

Third, the Soviets indicated their willingness to use coercion in their dealings with Cuba when they had serious domestic and foreign policy disagreements in 1968 and withheld oil shipments critical to Cuba's economic survival.[18] Fourth, in a show of indifference to Cuba's strategic interests, the Soviet Union invaded Afghanistan while Cuba, as the chair of the Non-Aligned Movement, was seeking election to the United Nations Security Council in a highly contested and close race. The invasion doomed Cuba's chances, particularly because Cuba had long argued, without success, that the Soviet Union was the "natural ally" of the Third World. To make matters worse, Soviet officials neither consulted Castro before the invasion nor briefed him thereafter.[19] Fifth, Gorbachev did not apprise Castro in advance of his announcement on September 11, 1991, to withdraw a 2,800-member combat brigade from Cuba. The announcement, much to Castro's ire, was made in a press conference with U.S. Secretary of State James Baker.[20]

Other illustrations of their problematic relationship include a rift between the Soviets and Cubans that arose from the death of pro-Cuban Maurice Bishop of the New Jewel movement in Grenada at the hands of the more pro-Soviet Coard-Hudson faction. The Soviets blamed Cuba for losing Grenada. Although it was not clear which, if either, side was responsible, Havana's November 1983 celebration of the anniversary of the Soviet revolution was canceled because of the rift.[21]

Furthermore, after the U.S. invasion of Grenada, the Cubans realized that if invaded they would have to defend themselves without Soviet assistance. Worse yet, U.S. hostility toward Cuba since 1989 has equaled that during the worst times in the early days of the revolution over three decades ago. This hostility comes at a time when the crumbling of the socialist regimes in Eastern Europe and the disintegration of the Soviet Union has led to an end to all forms of solidarity with Cuba, and to outright hostility between Cuba and the former socialist countries. Castro has criticized them for their transition to capitalism and has proclaimed that Cuba will be the last bastion of socialism ("socialism or death").

Despite the signing of a 1990–91 trade agreement and the rhetoric of their leaders, relations between Cuba and the Soviet Union remained difficult in 1991. Because of their close economic integration, both economies suffered when each failed to meet its contractual obligations to the other. Political alliances between Cuba and the republics of the former Soviet Union were broken altogether because of the rapid pace of change in the East and disagreements over what was to be done. With these alliances ruptured, Cuba could no longer be assured of economic assistance. Thus, even prior to the emergence of a unipolar world, Cuba's security, both economic and military, and its prestige have been, in the last analysis, solely Cuban problems.

This situation has led the Cuban government to cultivate allies among the developing nations. Some observers note that Cuba's foreign policy initiatives have been geared toward ensuring Cuba's security in an adverse geopolitical situation through support of progressive governments and the creation of a Third World constituency,[22] to gain not just diplomatic support in international organizations but also economic or trade benefits. This is, in fact, what Cuba has been doing for many years, particularly as a fervent advocate of South-South trade and of creative economic relations not involving hard-currency transfers.

Nationalism, defined as political and economic self-determination and tempered by ideological considerations and Soviet aid, has been offered as another explanation for Cuba's global foreign policy. Another analyst cites as explanations both the strategic value of Angola and Ethiopia and the opportunity to provide a revolutionary experience for Cuban youth and thereby increase their commitment to the Cuban revolution.[23]

There is little doubt that the chance to do internationalist service and to see firsthand what colonialism, imperialism, and capitalism mean for Third World peoples, tends to increase the revolutionary zeal of Cuban youth, whose relative apathy worries Cuban leaders. This experience also makes the youth more appreciative of what the revolution has accomplished domestically. In medicine, internationalism has provided Cuban doctors with experience in tropical medicine and diseases of poverty long since eradicated in Cuba and has given them even greater pride in Cuba's own medical accomplishments. The impact on Cubans' revolutionary morale, however, may be more an unanticipated benefit of globalism than the motivation for launching these foreign policy initiatives.

Finally, economic factors, such as potential trade, actual foreign contracts for goods and services, and increased leverage with the Soviet Union, have also accounted for Cuba's global reach.[24] A large pool of young, underemployed, educated, and skilled workers who can be tapped for foreign policy purposes is a factor that has contributed significantly to Cuban international activism.[25] Economic integration into the CMEA limited Cuba's ability to diversify its exports and to earn the hard currency necessary to purchase goods unavailable from the former Eastern bloc. This too has impelled the Cuban government to develop its human capital as an export commodity.[26] Now the disintegration of the CMEA may only serve to reinforce the trend toward the export of services as primary-product exports lose their subsidies and as world market prices for Cuban commodities remain low.[27]

U.S.–Cuban Relations and Symbolic Politics

Demography and Soviet aid partially explain how Cuba was able to sustain its activist stance. Why Cuba played such a major role and why Cuba was relatively successful are more easily understood by considering the power of symbolism and U.S.–Cuban relations. Cuba's ideology prominently advocates the duty to fight against imperialism, colonialism, and racism and to assist others in their struggle for liberation. This effort is often translated into direct and indirect political competition with the United States. Although the Cuban threat to the United States has largely been a symbolic threat to U.S. hegemony in the hemisphere, it can be argued that for the purposes of creating social cohesion at home, it is necessary for Cuba to either maintain a hostile relationship with the United States or else invent another external threat.[28]

In some measure, Cuba owes its international success to the vehement opposition of the United States. The failure of U.S. policy to overthrow the Castro government (not just in the Bay of Pigs invasion),[29] or to force domestic and/or foreign policy changes has cast Cuba as a David confronting the Goliath of the North, a drama which, in turn, has helped convert this otherwise small, insignificant island nation into a Third World power.

Despite decades of hostility and mistrust between the two countries, Cubans consider their relationship with the United States to be
one of love and hate.[30] Although they admire the United States, Cubans hate its government for trying to overthrow and thwart their
own. Cuban leaders also greatly resent the historical role of the
United States in distorting Cuba's political and economic development. Fidel Castro wrote in 1958 that "when this war is over, I'll start
a much longer and bigger war of my own: the war I'm going to fight
against them [the Americans]. I realize that will be my true destiny."[31]
This early statement presages Cuba's global anti-imperialist activities
as well as its political competition with the United States in the
health sphere.

The "fraternal" Soviet relationship with Cuba notwithstanding, Cubans have always preferred that which is American (except the government).[32] As a result, the United States has been the ever-present,
unseen actor who, in the Foucauldian sense, has indirectly affected
Cuba's policies even when not directly affecting them.[33]

In Foucault's analysis of Velázquez's painting "Las Meninas," the
real subject of the painting is the two sovereigns, King Philip IV and
his wife Mariana, whose reflection one dimly sees in the mirror in
the background of the composition, and not the Princess Margarita
and various attendants who, in the foreground, appear to be the principal subjects. The royal couple is visible only as a reflection. But all
forward-gazing eyes within the painting are turned toward them.
Though absent from the group of models, the royal couple is, nonetheless, both the focal point of the painting within the painting and
the audience for whom the painting was created.[34] Cuba's actions on
the world stage can be viewed in the same manner: very much influenced by the United States, and often for the United States, even
though the United States may be elided from the scene. Although
seemingly looking elsewhere, such as to the Third World or the former socialist bloc, Cuba has really looked to the United States for
recognition.

Symbolism in the Revolution

Myth is both a binding agent of society and a catalyst
for social action. As such it is an important aspect of ideology,
the "symbol system that 'links particular actions and mundane prac-

tices with a wider set of meanings.'"[35] The core symbols of Cuban revolutionary myths and ideology, struggle and millennialism, have performed both functions over time and have remained constant since the beginning of the revolution.[36]

Although symbols and myths are pervasive in all societies, they are an integral part of everyday Cuban political consciousness. "Symbolism is the vehicle of significance, a means by which a people or a movement communicates to itself its most important experience and messages."[37] Castro astutely utilizes symbolism to educate and cajole, to praise and criticize the masses. He is a master creator, interpreter, and manipulator of symbol and myth. He developed new symbols and myths in the course of the insurrection and later during the evolution of Cuban socialism, and he has resuscitated Cuba's history.[38]

Castro has reframed Cuba's history with its pattern of liberation struggles and co-opted it into the present revolutionary society. He has symbolically collapsed all historical liberation struggles into the present one. This recasting of history bestows on the Cuban people a heightened awareness of the historical nature of social life and a sense of unilinear direction, progression, and achievement.

Using the socialist model, Castro has harnessed moral incentives to productivity through new symbols of documentation and collective achievement: flags, pennants, certificates, diplomas, and titles. Socialist emulation, the friendly competition among workers, workplaces, industries, towns, and provinces to achieve or overachieve a particular goal, is frequently rewarded by these symbolic means. People are encouraged to become "vanguard workers." Along with the title, they receive a certificate recognizing their achievement. Their pictures and names appear on the bulletin board at work. Enterprises may win pennants for producing more than others in their sector. During the literacy campaign in 1961, towns received flags indicating that they had eliminated illiteracy. Although moral incentives have frequently been coupled with material incentives during the past thirty-four years, they were the only incentive at times in the 1960s and were very important again after 1985 because of economic necessity.[39]

Both domestic and international events have come to symbolize Cuban national prowess in a number of fields. For example, Cuba's victories at the Bay of Pigs and in Angola and Ethiopia symbolize Cuban military might. Cuba's successful literacy campaign and public health campaigns symbolize the country's humanitarian values. The conversion of barracks into schools symbolizes the moral superiority of the revolution to the previous capitalist regime of Batista.[40] Cuba's provision of civilian technical aid to other developing nations symbolizes Cuba's social development and technical capacity as well as its humanitarianism.

Cuban revolutionary symbolism provides continuity between the present and Cuban and Latin American historical figures such as the Indian chief Hatuey, who fought the Spanish conquest; nineteenth-century Cuban independence leaders Antonio Maceo, Carlos Manuel de Céspedes, and José Martí; Simon Bolivar, the Latin American liberator; and Marx and Lenin. Thus those Cubans who defend the revolution and perform internationalist service are continuing in this tradition of fulfilling Cuba's duty (*el deber cubano*) to fight imperialism, colonialism, and capitalism.[41]

Individuals too have come to symbolize revolutionary values. Che Guevara, one of the more important symbols of the revolution, represents both the "new person" and internationalist solidarity. The Cubans who died during the invasion of Grenada are, according to Castro, symbols, not corpses.[42] And Castro himself has been seen in the past as a symbol of revolution and social justice by many in the Third World.

Most important for my analysis is the notion that

gains of the revolution are seen as symbolic of the contrast between socialism and capitalism with aspects of U.S. society and dependent capitalist societies symbolic of capitalism's inherent inequality and failure to provide Martí's goal, that is, *"una vida de decoro"* ("a life of dignity").[43]

One therefore finds comparisons of life in the United States with that of Cuba in Castro's speeches and in the Cuban media. Since news reports from capitalist countries tend to focus on the negative and those in communist countries generally report the positive—as exemplified in production quotas and related items—these comparisons are skewed. Nonetheless, the political competition between Cuba and the United States both produces symbols and is itself a symbol of anti-imperialist struggle, class warfare, and socialism versus capitalism.

Symbolism in Domestic and International Politics

The sensitivity aroused by the manipulation and interpretation of symbols, which are an important aspect of both domestic and international politics, testifies to the power of symbolism. This fact is demonstrated by the following example from U.S.–Cuban relations. The U.S. government chose to affront Cuba both politically and symbolically by creating an anti-Castro radio station (1985), and later a television station (1990), named after the man revered in Cuba as the intellectual author of the revolution, José Martí. This deliberate symbolic attack added insult to injury. The political effect of Radio Martí was limited because Cubans can easily receive foreign broadcasts by the Voice of America, the British Broadcasting Corporation, Radio Deutsche Welle, and Radio Exterior de España, as well as some radio stations from Miami, the Dominican Republic, and Puerto Rico.

On the other hand, the symbolism of using Martí's name struck a raw nerve. In fact the creation of Radio Martí in 1985 so enraged Castro that he broke off the December 1984 immigration agreement with the United States and temporarily foreclosed on the opportunity to reduce tensions between the two countries. The agreement was not reinstated for almost three years, during which time U.S.–Cuban relations were the worst they had been since the Bay of Pigs and the Cuban missile crisis in 1961 and 1962 respectively.

Responding to the initial broadcasts of Television Martí in April 1990, Castro equated the U.S. decision to name the station after José Martí with naming a whorehouse or garbage dump after George Washington. By the same token, Cuban officials refer to their ability to jam Television Martí signals within ninety seconds of broadcasting as an "electronic Bay of Pigs."[44]

Symbols serve political ends in all countries, but as we have seen, they are particularly important in U.S.–Cuban relations. When the Cubans triumphed over the U.S.–sponsored invasion by Cuban exiles at the Bay of Pigs, they symbolically triumphed again when they knocked the eagle atop the monument to the battleship *Maine* off its pedestal. The eagle-less column remains as a symbol of Cuba's victory over the United States.[45] Because of its symbolism and because it is located diagonally across the Malecón from the U.S. Interests Section (formerly the embassy), it has often been the site of anti–U.S. rallies.

At the 1988 meetings of the United Nations Human Rights Commission, the United States launched a major campaign against Cuba, first by appointing as head of its delegation Armando Valladares, a former Cuban political prisoner renowned for his book about life in Castro's prisons,[46] and second by focusing solely on Cuban human rights abuses.[47] Despite other cases of rights abuses that were more severe than Cuba's in both magnitude and deprivation, the United States dealt only with the Cuban case.

The choice of Valladares as ambassador is curious unless one considers the power of symbolism. Valladares, a powerful symbol of anti-Castroism who lives in Spain rather than in the United States, was made a U.S. citizen expressly to represent the U.S. at the U.N. Human Rights Commission (to assail Cuba). His original appointment and his service in this capacity throughout 1990 illustrate once again the U.S. government's keen awareness of the force of symbolism, and the government's willingness to exploit this force in its campaign against Cuba.

In both politics and political analysis, much is made of the symbolism of nuances and changes, whether of form or substance. When Khrushchev gave Castro a bear hug at the United Nations, for example, the embrace was interpreted to mean that the Soviets accepted Cuba into their camp. Likewise, almost two decades later when Maurice Bishop embraced Castro in the same forum, this too was interpreted as showing Grenada's allegiance to Cuba. That Angola was called Cuba's Vietnam,[48] just as Afghanistan was considered the Soviet Union's Vietnam, implicitly places Cuba in the role of superpower. A major difference, of course, is that Cuba, unlike the two superpowers, left its Vietnam as a winner. This too is symbolically important.

Symbolism and substance may be opposed but may also be intertwined, as when the Berlin Wall opened and later fell, when the lone man fended off a column of tanks in Tiananmen Square, when statues of Lenin were toppled across Eastern Europe and the former Soviet Union, and when Nelson Mandela was released from a South African prison. On the one hand, the 1988 U.S. presidential election campaign is a prime example of the triumph of symbolism over substance in politics. On the other hand, while the Reagan-Gorbachev summit meeting in Moscow resulted in the signing of an arms-limitation treaty, the symbolism of the meeting and of Reagan's change of heart about the Soviet Union was its real substance.[49]

Political analysts have paid particular attention to symbolic acts in closed societies because access to data has varied between difficult and impossible. As a result, when a Communist party politburo member failed to appear in a group photograph, analysts speculated on that person's fate and on what it meant for governmental organization and policy.[50] The situation is similar in international relations:

when a head of state or of the party is absent from an international gathering, the nature of relations between that country and the others is questioned. Thus when Castro failed to attend Konstantin Chernenko's funeral, Reagan administration officials interpreted his absence as a symbol of friction between Cuba and the Soviet Union and a demonstration of Castro's "periodic urge to show his independence."[51]

When Zhao Ziyang wanted to convey, both at home and abroad, a radical departure from his predecessor's policies, he and four other members of the Chinese politburo's standing committee wore western suits to a news conference. These suits were considered symbolic of "new leaders, aggressive new policies and increased openness."[52] Zhao's point was made more effective by the symbolic change of clothes.

Likewise in China, when an evening television news reporter wore a Mao suit to read the news two nights in a row, China-watchers assumed that a major policy change was in the wind. But it turned out that the newsman had worn the Mao suit simply because he had not had time to get his western suit ironed.[53] Although these public acts had unintended consequences, they form part of a text of public rituals that are not only read and interpreted from different perspectives by the actors involved, but also acted upon. The symbolic meaning given these texts shapes the discourse among the participants in the narrative-in-process that is the essence of political activity.

Semiotics and Symbolic Politics

In one of the more cogent demonstrations of the power of semiotics and symbolic politics to explain the deeper meaning of political events, David E. Apter and Nagayo Sawa conclude in their analysis of the Sanrizuka airport protest movement that the resistance was more than just a protest against the construction of the airport; it was fundamentally a protest against the Japanese state.[54] Various events were interpreted by the participants as symbolic of larger issues and grievances and imbued with mythic significance. For the state, the airport was "a symbol of the new role Japan would play in the world."[55] For the protesters, "the airport [stood] for the state, the state in turn became the symbol of imperialism, militarism, and nuclear holocaust."[56]

Apter and Sawa illustrate the complexity of the protest by analyzing Sanrizuka as a "semiotic space" and as a mobilization space wherein the events provide the "narrative of struggle" that is interpreted by the participants as a series of metaphors that establish the "moral architecture." For example, the land survey was a metaphor for rape and a metonym for state capitalism. The physical landscape controlled by the protesters around the airport became the moral architecture, delimiting the space between good and evil.[57]

Each event became part of a radical text. Violation of local and private space, illegitimate conveyance [of land], polarization of society and the state, the creation of an industrial army, and the legitimization of struggle together formed a logic of necessity—the necessity for extra-institutional struggle against the parliamentary state.[58]

Only by assessing the semiotic and symbolic elements in the protest does one ultimately understand its true nature.

Apter and Sawa's approach, when applied to Cuba, unfolds a radical text in which the major domestic and international events of the Cuban revolution can be seen as the narrative of struggle against imperialism (read "the United States") and its legacy of underdevelopment. As the narrative of events is recounted, it takes on a mythic symbolic significance. The metaphors that these events elicit form the core of revolutionary symbolism, which in turn is the basis for political education.[59]

Military metaphors connoting revolutionary struggle are used to describe nonmilitary events such as the "war" against illiteracy. The symbolism of these events is paramount in creating revolutionary consciousness. For example, Castro stated that while Cuban exiles were planning to attack the island, the people of Cuba were planning to wage war against illiteracy and by implication demonstrate the moral superiority of socialism.[60]

There were also battles and wars against communicable diseases, low levels of schooling (the battle for the sixth grade, and then the ninth grade), absenteeism, low productivity, waste, cronyism, bureaucratism, and formalism, battles for production and defense and for a ten-million-ton sugar harvest, and in the health sphere, battles against obesity, sedentarism, and smoking. All of these campaigns strengthened Cuba's position in the real and symbolic war against its imperialist legacy.

As Castro has stated in a 1990 interview with foreign journalists, the symbolic war goes on: "What is Cuba today? Cuba is the symbol of resistance; Cuba is the symbol of the firm and intransigent defense of revolutionary ideas; Cuba is the symbol of the defense of revolutionary principles; Cuba is the symbol of the defense of socialism."[61] Since the crumbling of the socialist world, Castro has ended his speeches with "Socialism or death" and "Fatherland or death" to exhort the masses to forge ahead in the symbolic war against the United States.

The central metaphor in Cuba's anti-imperialist struggle as recounted in this analysis is that of health. The health of the individual is a metaphor for and symbol of the health of the "body politic," and in which the achievement of the status of "world medical power" is synonymous with victory over the imperialists. Medical doctors are the protagonists in this war both at home and abroad. They are warriors in the battle against disease, which is largely considered a legacy of imperialism and underdevelopment. Cuba, a David fighting Goliath (the United States), seeks to slay the giant in the battle for international prestige in health care.

The island and its health institutions become the moral architecture, dividing the world into us and them, good and evil, healthy and diseased. The radical text that evolves becomes a major ingredient in the ideology of the revolution. Apter states that

modern ideologies consist of various mixtures of myth and theory, which, over time, have a tendency to be transformed into each other.... The combination, a mytho/logics synthesized as doctrine and represented by the state, forms out of disjunctive moments. Such moments represent one way exceptional meaning is created out of events and exceptional political events out of meaning.[62]

The mytho/logics then determines the use of language and how signs are ordered.[63]

Language and signs must be interpreted. The interpretation of the social world produces objective and subjective meanings. The former are properties likely to be interpreted in the same manner by all, while the latter are "the product of previous symbolic struggles and express the state of the symbolic power relations"[64] that reflect objective power relations. As Marx has said, the ruling ideas are those of the ruling class.[65]

Symbolic struggles to interpret the present social world, "to impose the legitimate world-view," often refer to a reconstructed past or to the future.[66] In Cuba, history has been reinterpreted and re-written in light of current ideology and political ends, the future forecast in millennial terms, and history combined with future goals in the presentation of self on the world stage as a major actor and a "world medical power."

As Pierre Bourdieu writes,

> Knowledge of the social world and, more precisely the categories that make it possible, are the stakes, par excellence, of political struggle, the inextricably theoretical and practical struggle for the power to conserve or transform the social word [sic] by conserving or transforming the categories through which it is perceived. . . . It becomes clear why one of the elementary forms of political power, in many archaic societies, consisted in the quasi-magical power to *name* and to make-exist by virtue of naming.[67]

Although Bourdieu refers to social groups within a given nation, this concept can be extended to relations among states, where, for example, the United States has attempted to exclude Cuba from most international forums by symbolically denying Cuba's existence (refusing to name Cuba or, in international legal parlance, de-recognizing Cuba). Conversely, Cuba seeks to name and to reinterpret the social world in order to improve its own status.

Karl Marx stated that "the philosophers have only *interpreted* the world, in various ways; the point, however, is to *change* it."[68] Apter reminds us that "the way to change the world is to reinterpret it."[69] Apter discusses the power of myth and theory in ideologies and how they shape our conception of the world, particularly at the disjunctive moment when conflict leads to a new beginning and thus a new mytho/logics.[70]

Castro's assertion that Cuba was becoming a world medical power can be seen as part of a larger effort to project Cuba's influence abroad, an effort that began as an attempt to redefine the criteria by which Cuba, and by implication other countries, should be judged. Because the Cuban government measures its efficacy by the country's health indicators and because the health of the individual is a metaphor for the health of the "body politic," Cuban officials consider most other countries to be "diseased"—that is, to have poorer health indicators and less commitment to improving their population's health than Cuba. The Cubans endeavor to reinterpret and thereby change a portion of the world by creating a new mytho/logics from the disjunctive moment of the revolution and from the fierce postrevolutionary political competition with the United States, particularly on the semiotic and symbolic levels.

Symbolic Capital

Symbols may also function as a currency. As Pierre Bourdieu demonstrates, for example, symbolic capital (goodwill, prestige, influence, power, and credit), like material capital, can be accumulated, invested, and spent. In fact, symbolic capital is created by investing material capital and time in a project. The short-term benefits, which are symbolic, appear to be noneconomic and therefore disinterested. However, the mode of circulation of symbolic capital indicates that material capital is invested to produce symbolic capital, which ultimately is converted back into material capital ($mc \rightarrow sc \rightarrow mc$). Thus, symbolic and material capital become interconvertible.[71]

Bourdieu's concept of the accumulation of symbolic capital can be applied to Cuban foreign policy. The acquisition of allies or a clientele requires the investment of both material and symbolic capital in the form of economic, technical, and/or security aid as well as political or moral support. Although the outlay of symbolic capital is always very expensive in economic terms, and in the short term may be even more costly than the material capital gained, it is necessary in the long term in order to accumulate capital in its various forms.[72]

Symbolic capital cannot be converted into material capital immediately, for it is a long-term investment in better relations with another party and in more generalized prestige and influence. Poor countries have difficulty accumulating it because they have neither the material capital for the initial investment nor the time necessary for its conversion. Cuba, which has had a foreign policy more befitting a major power than a developing country, had both money and time to invest before the disintegration of the socialist world. This investment in the accumulation of goodwill has paid off to some extent in the flow of aid from international organizations that have supported one aspect or another of Cuba's development policies. For example, aid from various United Nations agencies totaled $210 million from 1976 to 1991, and these agencies have made available another $92 million for the period from 1992 to 1996.[73] Symbolic capital also can be converted when trade relations are established with an aid recipient. Although aid Cuba has given to an ally may initially have been disinterested, when the chips are down there is an expectation of trade or, at a minimum, diplomatic support. This too has paid off in a number of cases, but not all.

Bourdieu states that

the homologies established between . . . the different forms of capital and the corresponding modes of circulation, oblige us to abandon the dichotomy of the economic and non-economic which stands in the way of seeing the science of economic practices as a particular case of a *general science of the economy of practices,* capable of treating all practices, including those purporting to be disinterested or gratuitous, and hence non-economic, as economic practices directed towards the maximizing of material or symbolic profit.[74]

As this book shows, Cuba's medical diplomacy and efforts to become a world medical power can be seen in part as a drive to accumulate symbolic capital (prestige, influence, goodwill) that the Cuban leaders hope to convert into material capital (trade and aid).

2

Ideology and Organization of the Cuban Health System

To fully understand Cuba's drive to become a world medical power and Cuban medical diplomacy, one must look first at Cuban health ideology and the organizational infrastructure (moral architecture) developed to translate ideology into practice. It is on this base that the Cuban government has built its health system at home, projected its medical services abroad, and presented itself on the world stage as becoming a world medical power. Because in Cuba the health of the individual is a metaphor for the health of the "body politic," the method of providing health care is symbolically important.

Ideology

Since the 1959 revolution, Cuban health ideology has been based on the fundamental principle codified in the 1975 constitution that health protection and care is a right of all and a responsibility of the state.[1] In Cuba, health is considered indispensable not only in and of itself but also "to achieve a high level of education and culture, intellectual and physical development and optimal work capacity."[2] The Cuban leadership thus adopted the World Health Organization's definition of health as not just the absence of disease, but as the state of complete physical, mental, and social well-being. Hence, the state assumed responsibility for the "bio-psycho-social" well-being of its subjects. Cuban health ideology goes even beyond a holistic approach to health: health and well-being must be directly linked to a person's material environment.

As early as 1961, the Cuban Ministry of Public Health manifested its interest in providing a model for other developing nations. It suggested that the true eradication of misery and real improvement in health would occur only through revolution, that a band-aid approach would not eliminate disease (either real or metaphorical).[3] By the early 1970s, when the Cuban government changed its foreign policy from the attempt to export revolution to diplomacy and state-to-state relations, the Ministry of Public Health also changed its philosophy and recognized as worthy, but not sufficient, any effort to improve the health of a people, including health efforts that did not directly affect other economic sectors. Nonetheless, throughout the first three decades of revolution, the Cuban government has remained committed to showing other Third World countries how to improve the health of their peoples.

The roots of the Cuban revolutionary government's health ideology can be found in Fidel Castro's 1953 defense of himself before the Batista government's magistrate, later published as *History Will Absolve Me,* where he states that "no child should die for want of medical attention,"[4] and that

Only death can liberate one from so much misery.... Ninety per cent of rural children are consumed by parasites which filter through their bare feet from the earth. Society is moved to compassion upon hearing of the kidnapping or murder of one child, but they are criminally indifferent to the mass murder of so many thousands of children who die every year from lack of facilities, agonizing with pain.... They will grow up with rickets, with not a single good tooth in their mouths by the time they reach thirty;... and will finally die of misery and deception. Public hospitals, which are always full, accept only patients recommended by some powerful politician who, in turn, demands the electoral votes of the unfortunate one and his family so that Cuba may continue forever in the same or worse condition.[5]

Since he made this statement, Castro has repeatedly decried the misery of a large majority of the world's children and denounced the developed nations for their indifference.

Underpinning Cuba's health ideology is the notion that medicine alone will not improve the overall health of the population. What will improve it, Cubans believe, is embedding medicine within a significant transformation of the socioeconomic structure to eliminate the problems of underdevelopment:[6] the legacy of hunger, illiteracy, inadequate housing, discrimination, and the exploitation of labor.[7] The Cuban government set as its task just such a societal transformation, attempting to break the cycle of underdevelopment through a diversified economic program,[8] and to improve the standard of living through universal free education and medical care, a guaranteed minimum amount of food per month through rationing, heavily subsidized, low-cost housing, full employment before 1980,[9] the introduction of social security, an end to institutionalized discrimination, and other measures.[10] Because this task is multifaceted, the Cuban approach links health actions with efforts in other, related sectors.[11] In other words, socioeconomic development is integral to health.

Apart from this overriding concern for general socioeconomic development, Cuban health ideology includes three guiding principles to achieve health for all: (1) equal access to services, (2) an integral approach to health care, and (3) popular participation in health initiatives.[12] These principles underlie all health policies, programs, and organization, but, inevitably, there is some disjunction between ideology and practice, particularly with respect to the second and third principles.

Equality of access in Cuba entails legal, economic, geographic, and cultural access to health care. All health care is free regardless of its level of sophistication. A regionalized, hierarchically organized national health system, with referral from one level of care to the next, provides universal coverage, equitable geographic distribution of facilities, and standardization of services.

None of the other socialist or formerly socialist countries went as far as Cuba in providing equal access to health care despite regionalization of health-care services. Glasnost made very clear how deficient both the Soviet and Eastern European health systems had been and how poor the health conditions in some countries were. In fact, in 1984, life expectancy was longer in Cuba than in any of the Warsaw Pact nations, and the infant mortality rate in 1988 was the second lowest (after East Germany).[13]

Cuba's commitment to cultural access decreases the educational and class differences between medical practitioners and patients. People are educated to promote understanding of health and illness and encouraged to use the health services. Also, doctors are no longer the scions of the upper class but primarily the daughters and sons of agricultural and of blue- and white-collar workers. To further improve cultural accessibility, doctors are generally trained and stationed in their home provinces, except when there are not yet enough local doctors to fill the posts. Cultural access to health care as an ideal represents the homogenization of social classes at best and a narrowing of the gap between classes at a minimum.

An integral approach to health care combines prevention with cure, and treats the individual as a bio-psycho-social being, living and working or studying in a given environment.[14] This is, of course, a materialist approach in which the individual is viewed as a social being (worker) in harmony with the physical environment. Thus all aspects of individuals should be considered in order to maintain, protect, or restore their health in the broadest sense of the word. This approach signifies concern for the individual as a whole rather than for just a body part in need of repair.

Health professionals of all types work together in multidisciplinary teams to prevent and cure disease and to ensure continuity of care, consultation, and cooperation among the various health-care practitioners dealing with the same patient. Since 1984 many of the teams have come to consist of a family doctor and nurse. Working in teams is common in socialist health systems, but generally there is little time for preventive work. Cuba was no exception until the Family Doctor Program was introduced in 1984.

Popular participation in health activities was conceived of as allowing the general public, through their mass-organization representatives, a role in health planning, administration, evaluation, and implementation through monthly meetings with both the polyclinic administration and the municipal health director.[15] Despite the good intentions, however, popular participation has been primarily a means of mobilizing the Cuban people in order to implement health programs and policies devised by the Ministry of Public Health and the party leadership.[16]

Popular participation has greatly extended the health system's reach into the community and has also served an educative function, allowing people to observe health-policy deliberations and to see that they can resolve many problems themselves. These efforts are best exemplified by the campaign to eradicate dengue, which is discussed in Chapter 3. Popular participation demonstrates the government's desire to allow the individual to take some responsibility for social change in general and for improved individual and community health in particular. This role for the masses, a hallmark of the Cuban system, was less important in every socialist health system except China's, which is less organized and institutionalized than Cuba's.

Popular participation defined as popular implementation is mirrored in the health system itself, where government policy has been to delegate very little authority to nonphysician health workers. Unlike the Soviet Union, which has paramedics known as *feldshers,* China, which has "barefoot doctors" and "red medical workers" (a cross between a paramedic and a traditional healer), and other Third World countries where paramedics are prevalent in primary care, particularly in rural areas, Cuba's health system is physician-based.

It has been argued in both the developed and developing countries that there is no need for physicians to carry out all diagnostic and treatment tasks because many primary-care problems can be handled just as well and less expensively by paramedical personnel. Castro and the Cuban health planners believe, however, that only the physician should be allowed to diagnose, and that other health workers should assist the physician and carry out preventive measures and treatments. Correct or not, their decision was to provide what they considered to be First World rather than Third World medicine: physicians rather than paramedical personnel. As a result, the policy regarding the education of physicians has, until 1989, been one of producing an ever-increasing quantity with greater specialization. A gradual reduction in the number of first-year medical students was implemented in 1989, while the number of university-trained nurses increased because of the imbalance in the ratio between them and the already large pool of physicians.[17]

With the reorganization of primary health care in the mid 1980s in accordance with Cuba's changed structure of morbidity and mortality, all medical graduates except surgeons, nonclinical specialists, and future medical school professors have had to complete a residency in comprehensive general medicine (family medicine) before completing a second residency in one of the traditional medical specialties.[18] The aim is to have specialist-generalists at the point of entry into the health system and to provide health care equal to or better than that available in the United States (in the limited areas in which this is possible). By doing so, Cubans hope to accumulate symbolic capital (prestige) in the symbolic struggle against the United States in the health field.

Antecedents of Socialized Medicine in Cuba

Cuba's health ideology and organization are not purely the result of the socialist nature of the revolution. Important precursors can be found in prerevolutionary medical organization and ideology. Perhaps the most important prerevolutionary organization was mutualism,[19] a prepaid health plan much like the health maintenance organizations that became prevalent in the United States in the 1970s.

These mutual-aid societies in Cuba were established around the turn of the century by Spanish ethnic societies, such as the Asturians and the Galicians, in order to provide comprehensive medical services for their members. In 1938, the Transport Workers Union of Havana founded its own mutualist clinic to serve its members and others willing to pay the low fees. For the first time, blacks were included in a mutualist plan. Mutualist practice later spread to private group practices because of the overabundance of physicians in Havana. By 1958, mutualist clinics provided service to approximately half of the population of Havana.[20] Only a few mutualist societies, however, had facilities in some of the provincial capitals. No such services existed in the rural areas.

Among the factors influencing the development of postrevolutionary health ideology, the single most important was the guerrillas' confrontation with the abject poverty and enormous health problems of the rural population.[21] Many physicians participated in the insurrection, some as military leaders (such as Che Guevara). From 1948, the Cuban Medical Federation, one of the two Cuban medical associations, espoused social medicine under the leadership of progressive and leftist physicians, some of whom were communists.[22]

Contact with rural conditions and progressive physicians, plus familiarity with the practice of mutualism, radicalized the revolutionary leadership and led them to adopt a broad, even socialist approach to health. After the revolution and the later declaration of its socialist nature, socialist ideology became a further justification for health policy decisions already made.

Organizational Evolution

Unlike other socialist countries, whose health services were intended initially for the urban industrial labor force, the Cuban Revolution's provision of health services to the population began in the periphery,[23] addressing the traditional imbalance between urban and rural resources and services. This approach was followed in other sectors such as education, housing, and employment. Development projects were channeled to the rural areas while urban areas were allowed to languish, and in some cases decay.

During the insurrectionary period, from 1956 until January 1, 1959, the guerrillas provided free medical care to peasants in areas under their control.[24] After the revolution this experience in the sierra led to the establishment on January 23, 1960, of the Rural Health Service. This service required all medical school graduates to serve for one year in the rural areas upon graduation and provided for the creation of rural health facilities. In 1961 a rural dental service was added.[25]

After an earthquake in Chile in March 1960, Cuba sent a group of doctors on a temporary assignment to that country despite great need for them domestically.[26] This act presaged Cuba's first long-term medical-aid program abroad in 1963, a program which is generally considered the beginning of Cuba's medical diplomacy.

The old Ministry of Health and Welfare was disbanded on August 1, 1961, and replaced by the Ministry of Public Health, whose role was to guide the three types of organization that existed in the health arena: the public health system, the mutualist clinics and hospitals, and the private practice facilities.[27] During the same year, the People's Health Commissions were created to coordinate the liaison between personnel from the unions and various mass organizations, such as block committees—known as Committees for the Defense of the Revolution (CDRs)—and the Federation of Cuban Women (FMC), and the public health officials and to provide a means by which to mobilize the people for health tasks.[28]

The government organized its first mass vaccination campaign in 1962 with assistance from the CDRs and the organizational advice of Czechoslovak public health advisors.[29] This began the long, active involvement of mass organizations in health initiatives. In 1963 the public health subsystem embarked on the process of regionalization to provide coverage for the total population, while continuing to exist parallel to the mutualist and private practice subsystems.[30]

These health initiatives and ideological differences between the revolutionary government and the medical profession led to the exodus of about three thousand doctors or approximately half of the physician population.[31] In 1963, despite this medical brain drain and the great need for physicians on the island, Cuba sent its first internationalist medical brigade on a long-term mission to Algeria,[32] creating a pattern that was important in Cuban health policy from the mid-1970s on.

Beginning in 1964, health centers were transformed into polyclinics, with the population divided into sectors for health care and the basic-area health programs.[33] After a period of intense ideological antagonism between the old-guard physicians and the new revolutionary government and its medical supporters, the medical school graduates of 1965 renounced private practice, a policy that continued thereafter.[34] The last mutualist clinics were taken over by the state in 1967 to form part of its public health system, finally making the Cuban health system a socialized one.[35] Decentralized medical-school teaching began in 1968, reaffirming the commitment to regionalization and the amelioration of rural-urban differences.[36]

The 1970 political and economic reforms resulting from the failure of the ten-million-ton sugar harvest led to self-evaluation in the health sector as well.[37] Experimentation culminated in the gradual implementation of "medicine in the community" after 1975.[38]

With Cuba's heavy involvement in Africa, particularly in Angola and Ethiopia, from 1975 on, medical diplomacy ("proletarian internationalism" in Cuba's lexicon) came to the fore, draining resources from the domestic system.[39] Although Cuba has maintained a reasonably good physician-to-population ratio since 1976,[40] the internationalist commitment meant that high enrollments in medical schools would have to continue.[41] The commitment to Africa also resulted in the reestablishment of the Institute of Tropical Medicine and the study of tropical diseases no longer known in Cuba but important in the rest of the Third World.[42]

The 1980s marked another period of change within the health system as well as within the larger society. The goal of becoming a world medical power meant that the entire medical system and its educational institutions would be reassessed to determine what type of practitioner and system would best serve that goal.[43] Greater decentralization of administration led to somewhat better accountability for errors, inefficiencies, deficiencies, and insufficient services. The reassessment and decentralization helped spur the creation in 1984 of the Family Doctor Program, which attempted to put a doctor and nurse team on every block, the implementation of a major curricular change in medical education, and the creation of a comprehensive general medicine residency that almost all doctors would have to complete.[44]

Most recently, the economic crisis of the early 1990s resulting from the disintegration of the communist world led to the increased use of herbal medicines by family doctors. The crisis did not deter the government from its plans to continue producing family doctors and to deploy them in factories, schools, and communities even though they would have little more than herbal medicines with which to work.[45] At the same time, medicine became one of the two most important potential sources of foreign exchange earnings. Thus great stimulus has been given to biomedical, pharmaceutical, and biotechnology research that results in either import substitution or internationally marketable products.[46]

Organization of the Health Services: Regionalization

The regionalization of health services, following the Soviet model,[47] afforded patients equal access to these services and allowed the Cuban government central control over the health system, and therefore over economies of scale, and permitted the elimination of redundant services. The division of the country into geographic service areas also facilitated rational planning and organization of facilities. The hierarchical organization of services with referral from one level of care to the next and the formation of a clear authority structure to coordinate activities underpinned the regionalization scheme.[48]

The link between the various levels of care was designed to ensure that patients be treated by the facility with the least specialization necessary to provide adequate care. In other words, all patients are supposed to be seen first by their family doctor or by a doctor at their local polyclinic rather than by a doctor at a hospital, unless there is an emergency. This system works only if there are clearly established and enforced norms about what each level can and will do and if patients are educated to seek the appropriate level of attention.

The norms are well established, but because no health facility refuses care to anyone, patients often choose to go to a hospital emergency room rather than to their polyclinics for routine care because they know that the hospital has all the facilities necessary for complete diagnostic testing and because they believe, sometimes rightly, that the best doctors work at the hospitals.[49] To improve service to the population and to dissuade them from overburdening the hospitals, the government established the Family Doctor Program, which is discussed later in this chapter.

In the regionalism scheme, each province is treated as a self-contained region providing all levels of care within its borders except the type of care that, because of its enormous cost and high technological specialization, must be concentrated in an area of high population density. Provinces are divided into municipalities, which in turn are divided into health areas. These are the basic service areas for the polyclinics, or primary health-care facilities.[50] The polyclinic's health area is subdivided into sectors in order to create manageable geographic areas for the health teams.

At the primary-care level, routine preventive and curative care is offered in internal medicine, pediatrics, obstetrics and gynecology, and dentistry, along with environmental sanitation and hygiene services and psychological services. Other, more specialized, care is provided by specialists from the secondary level, the level of municipal and provincial hospitals, who visit these primary-care facilities regularly to treat patients in consultation with their primary-care physician.

At the municipal level, secondary or hospital care and specialized services are available. At the provincial level, tertiary or superspecialty care is provided. Superspecialty care is also provided at the national level, where it is more cost-effective to provide certain equipment such as CAT scanners and to conduct complex procedures. These superspecialty services are also often available on a regional rather than a provincial basis.

THE POLYCLINIC

Prior to the establishment of the Family Doctor Program, the polyclinic was the basic unit of an integrated network of health facilities. Until the Family Doctor Program is fully implemented in around 1995 (if the socialist regime survives until then), the polyclinic will remain the point of entry into the health system in many places. Where family doctors work, the polyclinic is now the backup institution that provides more specialized diagnostic techniques and consultation with specialists and is the site of medical education for students, interns, and residents, and of continuing education for family doctors. In fact, the polyclinic has become a true medical school that features community-oriented medical education.[51]

Understanding how the polyclinic functioned prior to the Family Doctor Program is important because it has been the laboratory, however imperfect, of much experimentation in the delivery of health services and in medical education. The polyclinic has provided services for a predefined population of 25,000 to 30,000 people in a health area divided into sectors with one internist for every 3,000 to 5,000 adults, one obstetrician/gynecologist for every 3,000 to 4,000 women over the age of fifteen, and one pediatrician for every 2,000 to 3,000 children under fifteen.[52] There is a nurse trained in the same discipline as the physician, so that the two form a horizontal (specialty) team for a specific sector. When working on psychological, social, or environmental issues within the sector, the horizontal team is joined by a vertical, or interdisciplinary, team including the social psychologist, hygiene and sanitation workers, a social worker, and community-health liaison activists.[53]

Because the team treats all people within a given sector, all adults within that sector have the same internist, and all children the same pediatrician. Continuity of care by the same health team promotes better understanding of patients and their environment. It is assumed, for example, that if adults in the same household or neighborhood are treated by the same physician and nurse team, any health problem with an environmental or psychosocial component will be more understandable and easier to treat because of the team's knowledge of the patient's physical and social environment. This team approach formed part of the general restructuring of the polyclinic's operations in 1976 and an integral part of "medicine in the community."

MEDICINE IN THE COMMUNITY

The strategy of providing medicine in the community is unlike the community medicine concept popular in capitalist countries in the mid-1970s where it simply implied the placement of public-health clinics in poor neighborhoods. The Cuban system uses the team approach to provide preventive and curative health care through an integrated national health system with the active participation of the communities served.

Most important, medicine in the community projects the polyclinic's services into the neighborhood. Not only do the physician-nurse teams attend patients in the polyclinic, but they also visit patients in their everyday environment: the home, school, day-care center, and workplace.[54] This contact with their patients' environment is believed to give the medical staff a fuller understanding of patients' needs.

Medicine in the community was meant to be the ultimate realization of the principle that the individual is to be treated as a bio-psycho-social being in a specific environment. The program also extends the government's reach into the people's everyday environment and symbolizes on a daily basis the humanitarian values the revolutionary leadership promotes. Critics might fear its potential as a form of social control.

In an effort to guarantee standardized universal coverage, the Ministry of Public Health supplied each polyclinic with what is known as the "red book," *Programas básicos del área de salud y su evaluación* (Basic Health Area Programs and Their Evaluation), now computerized in many polyclinics. As the name implies, the red book provides the norms, methods, and evaluation forms to be used as the basic work plan for each year in every polyclinic. The procedures are established by panels of experts from each primary-care discipline: general medicine, pediatrics, obstetrics and gynecology, and stomatology or dentistry.[55]

As the forms are completed, a statistical portrait of the community results, providing very detailed census information about the type and number of work centers: industrial, commercial, agricultural, and service; the number of workers and their gender; the type and number of schools and day-care centers and the age distribution of those attending them; the number of health facilities and health workers and the number of mass organization members; and a census of the general population by health sector. The red book also contains detailed statistical information about the state of hygiene and sanitation in the health area, the general health of the population, the morbidity and mortality rates, and immunization and other data.[56] Every effort is made to develop a complete community portrait. The data are considered very reliable because of this careful statistical accounting.[57]

The computerized version of the red book known as the "system of patient control" (SCP) was tested at the Policlínico Docente Lawton in 1988 and was to be introduced in the rest of the country as the computer equipment and staff became available. Because of the economic crisis brought on by the disintegration of the CMEA, full implementation of this plan seems unlikely in the near future despite some funding for automation by international organizations and Cuban production of microcomputer equipment from imported materials.[58] Thus in many polyclinics and in all family doctors' offices, data are still recorded by hand.

Where it is in use, the SCP provides doctors with instantaneous information on all of their patients, both individually and grouped by risk factor, disease, and preventive measure to be performed, along with information such as the date it should be carried out. The inclusion of risk factors in this community portrait reflects the current priority of encouraging healthier lifestyles as a method of disease prevention.

Family doctors or polyclinic doctors, for example, can quickly get a printout on smokers among their patients by the number of cigarettes smoked per day for different age groups and genders and then get a list of the patients.[59] While this technology may not seem especially impressive to those in the developed countries, it is unusual in many developing countries that still do not have many automated systems in the public sector. The commitment of resources to the computerization of health statistics at the local level symbolizes the Cuban government's efforts to function at the First World level in the health sphere by providing easily retrievable, reliable information on which to base plans of action.

Accordingly, the concept of medicine in the community requires that the first task of the polyclinic health team or the family doctor is to study the community it serves,

to discover the health status of the population, to select the at-risk population groups for various health programs, to define the environmental, biological, social, and psychological factors that interrelate as determining variables in the health-illness process, and to analyze the needs and resources available.[60]

Before the Family Doctor Program began, this study, called the diagnosis of the health sector, was supposed to be performed by the polyclinic's vertical and horizontal health teams every two months in order to update their data and assess the results of various health measures taken during the interval.[61] Discussion of the diagnosis theoretically included all members of both teams in order to get the broadest possible perspective on the problems faced. But in practice this often was not the case.

The disjunction between policy and implementation was evident as early as 1978 when a study conducted in a teaching polyclinic that was frequently used as a model for new procedures indicated that the health teams did not function as such; the individual members were not motivated to work in teams because they came from different educational backgrounds. Further, it was found that rather than presenting an integrated picture of the health sector, the team members each presented a purely medical view from the perspective of their own specialty. The reports and graphs were read without an objective analysis, there were no community representatives present, and the extent of popular participation was not appraised.[62]

Although medicine in the community was supposed to focus on prevention—the seeking out of risk factors in the environment before they become health problems—generally there was too little time devoted to noncurative medicine.[63] Problems that this program was to solve, such as continuity of care, the inadequacy of prevention, failure to treat the patient as a bio-psycho-social being in a specific environment, and unnecessary use of emergency rooms, had not been remedied. The medical teams did not know their patient population well, did not have time for much preventive work, and did not always obtain follow-up on their patients.[64]

Exacerbating this situation, patients often went directly to emergency rooms at hospitals where they thought they would get better treatment, thereby making it harder for the polyclinic to offer continuity of care.[65] In an effort to solve these longstanding problems and "revolutionize" primary care, the Cuban government established the Family Doctor Program as the cornerstone of its medical system.

INNOVATIVE PRIMARY CARE:
THE FAMILY DOCTOR PROGRAM

The Family Doctor Program, conceived by Fidel Castro himself, was designed to project the health system's resources further into the community than the previous system of "medicine in the community" had been able to do, by putting a doctor and nurse team literally on every city block and in the remotest rural communities. The fundamental task of the family doctor is to aggressively investigate and monitor the health of the entire population, not just the diseased. This is an extraordinary effort to assess the health of all people, promote their physical fitness, detect risk factors for disease, prevent and cure disease, and provide rehabilitation services. Because the structure of morbidity and mortality in Cuba had long since changed from diseases of poverty (parasitic and infectious diseases) to diseases of development (heart disease and cancer), this greater emphasis on prevention and chronic degenerative-disease management was needed.

Since the 1984 pilot project, each family doctor and nurse team has cared for 120 to 150 families, or about 600 to 700 people, in newly established three-room dispensaries consisting of a waiting room, a doctor's office, and an examination and treatment room.[66] Consultations in the dispensary are scheduled from 8 A.M. until noon and in patients' homes in the afternoons. One Sunday per month the health facility is open from 7 A.M. until 7 P.M. for those unable to see their physician during normal working hours. If patients are hospitalized, the family physician sees them in the hospital to act as the patient's advocate and to assure continuity of care, even though they are being treated by a hospital-based physician.[67]

Most family doctors and nurses live in apartments above their offices to immerse themselves in the environment and in the psycho-social-biological problems of their patients and to provide immediate and continuous care.[68] This geographic proximity to their patients allows the family doctors to be available at any time for emergency treatment and to work flexible hours. Although the Ministry has established norms for operating hours, the family doctors are allowed to adjust their schedules to maximize contact with their patients. For example, the family doctor attending the rural villages of Cagüeibaje and Palma Clara in Baracoa municipality, Guantánamo province, said that if she had no patients by 9:00 A.M., she would go out looking for them in the community and that her schedule was determined by her patients' needs rather than by a timetable established by the ministry.[69] This new flexibility was reiterated at the national level by a ministry official who said that the more work the family doctor does outside of the office and in the patient's natural environment, the better.[70] It was also codified in the *Programa de trabajo del médico y enfermera de la familia, el policlínico y el hospital* (The Work Program of the Family Doctor and Nurse, Polyclinic, and Hospital), which replaced the red book in areas where family doctors serve.[71]

Since family doctors are trained in social and comprehensive general medicine, they focus on both cure and prevention. The latter includes health education to alter unhealthy lifestyle practices such as sedentarism, smoking, and poor nutrition resulting from traditionally unhealthy food preferences. One of the tasks of the family doctors is to organize exercise classes for adults, particularly the elderly.[72] Every weekday morning at 8:00 A.M., one can see numerous senior citizens exercising in the parks, plazas, and other open spaces of Cuba. For the elderly, Cuban doctors claim, this daily exercise routine has resulted in decreased illness, less medication, and better psychological health because of their renewed interaction with others.[73]

The family doctor and nurse also provide daily care to the elderly and to patients who are chronically ill, recovering from operations, or suffering from acute episodic illness that might previously have required hospitalization. Castro has suggested that this policy will make every bed in Cuba a hospital bed. This care may be excessive, but it provides a sense of security for the patients as well as their families.[74]

Morbidity data from the initial experiment in 1984 that covered 1,200 families (approximately 5,000 persons) in a sector of Lawton in Havana indicated that 53 percent of the adults were healthy but that the rest suffered from the following illnesses in the following percentages: 13.9 percent had hypertension, 9.8 percent were obese, 6.7 percent had asthma, 5.8 percent had arthritis, 5.3 percent had diabetes, 4.4 percent had ischemic heart disease, and 2.6 percent had gastroduodenal ulcers. All of the children had received all of their immunizations and 83.6 percent were healthy, but 10.3 percent had asthma and 2.2 percent were obese.[75] Data for 1988 for all areas in which family doctors worked indicated the following disease rates among all age groups: diabetes, 18.8 per 1,000 inhabitants; asthma, 41.1 per 1,000; and arterial hypertension, 60.0 per 1,000.[76] These data demonstrated to the government the need for more preventive work and chronic disease management.

The Family Doctor Program had already served 1.3 million people as of 1985.[77] By the end of 1986, 13.8 percent of the Cuban population was under the care of 2,473 family doctors, including the dispersed rural population of the mountains of Guantánamo province, one of the more remote areas of the island.[78] There were 4,021 family doctors in 1987, of whom approximately 22 percent worked in rural areas, agricultural cooperatives, and remote mountainous regions.[79] By 1988 over 40 percent of the population (4.2 million people) were attended by 6,057 family doctors, by September 1990, with the addition of another 2,917 recent medical school graduates to the program, 50 percent were attended by a total of 8,965 family doctors,[80] and at the close of 1990, almost 60 percent were attended by 11,915 family doctors.[81] Of the 1990 figure, 71.8 percent worked on city blocks or in rural communities, 6.1 percent in factories, 5.4 percent in schools, 2.7 percent in day-care centers, and 14 percent on fishing or merchant marine ships or with construction brigades or homes for the aged. Also by 1990, all rural hospitals and 305 out of 420 polyclinics (73 percent) oversaw and supported the work of family doctors.[82] All of the mountainous areas were inhabited by family doctors, and nowhere was the distance greater than ten kilometers to a well-equipped health center.[83] The 1991 graduating class (September–October) will add another 3,244 family doctors to the program, bringing the total to 15,159.[84] (See tables 1 and 2.)

Prior to the changes that swept the socialist world, plans called for 20,000 doctors and 20,000 nurses to provide entry-level primary care on each city block and in the mountainous rural areas by the year 2000 and another 5,000 each to work in factories, schools, ships, and homes for the aged.[85] At the current rate of graduation, those

Table 1: Family Doctors by Province and Location of Practice, 1989

Province	Urban	Rural	Mountain	Agri-cult. Coop.	Schools	Work Centers	Homes for Aged	Day Care Centers	Reserve	Int'l	Others	Total
Pinar del Río	370	46	59	15	71	31	2	20	90	13	20	737
La Habana	306	21	–	3	34	52	1	5	53	2	8	485
Cd. de La Habana	2,399	–	–	–	80	256	7	125	284	22	208	3,381
Matanzas	261	75	–	3	86	41	4	15	42	4	26	557
Cienfuegos	244	17	17	10	17	34	–	11	19	3	13	385
Villa Clara	547	153	19	4	67	86	3	28	99	13	37	1,056
Sancti Spíritus	159	65	50	14	8	15	2	4	23	5	12	357
Ciego de Avila	115	115	–	8	13	12	1	4	14	1	14	297
Camagüey	342	165	–	11	54	46	5	23	57	16	23	742
Las Tunas	116	164	–	–	20	18	–	14	25	7	7	364
Holguín	326	179	87	10	26	29	6	8	52	7	31	761
Granma	230	99	156	1	43	34	2	16	67	8	7	663
Santiago de Cuba	460	192	379	2	54	48	–	33	155	44	75	1,442
Guantánamo	168	29	227	2	12	22	–	10	16	4	9	499
Isla de la Juventud	100	–	–	1	53	5	–	1	15	–	–	175
Totals	6,143	1,320	994	84	638	729	33	317	1,011	142	490	11,901

SOURCE: Percentages calculated and data reproduced from República de Cuba, Ministerio de Salud Pública, *Informe anual 1989* (La Habana: MINSAP, 1990), 1.

Table 2: Population Attended by Family Doctors by Province,
          September 1990

Province	Total Population	Pop. Attended by Family M.D.s	Percent
Pinar del Río	691,800	343,000	49.58
La Habana	646,000	231,000	33.75
Cd. de La Habana	2,109,000	1,679,300	79.62
Matanzas	611,100	237,300	38.83
Villa Clara	807,200	506,100	62.69
Cienfuegos	363,800	201,600	55.41
Sancti Spíritus	428,300	201,600	47.06
Ciego de Avila	366,000	166,600	45.51
Camagüey	745,600	362,600	48.63
Las Tunas	495,900	196,000	39.52
Holguín	993,200	421,400	42.42
Granma	788,900	340,200	43.12
Santiago de Cuba	990,000	723,100	73.04
Guantánamo	491,500	298,200	60.70
Isla de la Juventud	74,900	74,900	100.00
Totals	10,603,200	5,982,900	56.43

SOURCE: Reproduced from UNICEF, UNFPA, OPS/OMS, MINSAP, *El plan del médico de la familia en Cuba* (La Habana: UNICEF, 1991), 14.

numbers of physicians and nurses would be met before 1995, but the economic crisis will render virtually impossible the construction of new family doctors' offices, although space in existing buildings may be adapted.[86] It is highly unlikely, however, that the Castro government will be able to implement these plans.

By the year 2000 it had been expected that 7,000 comprehensive general medicine specialists would have completed a second residency and that another 2,000 would be performing their second residencies.[87] Already in 1990 there were 1,500 comprehensive general medicine specialists and 5,700 residents.[88] As each graduating class of doctors enters the Family Doctor Program, another group will be completing their comprehensive general medicine residencies and embarking on another specialization. In this manner, all doctors, with very few exceptions, will have had practical experience and postgraduate training in primary care through comprehensive general medicine. Most will have performed their residencies while working and doing research on primary health-care issues in their family doctors' offices and while attending seminars at the neighborhood polyclinic. Even those family doctors who work in remote areas will be able to complete their residencies with professors going to them (groups of neighboring family doctors) rather than the reverse.[89] As part of their continuing education, all family doctors must work one night a week in the nearest polyclinic or hospital, and this work is to coincide with periods when their professors are also on call there.[90]

Preliminary results indicate that the Family Doctor Program has cut medical costs through decreased hospitalization and emergency room use,[91] better patient compliance because of improved monitoring, improved patient fitness through the promotion of exercise and proper diet, and more effective prevention.[92] The rate of hospitalization, which between 1965 and 1985 had increased steadily each year, began to decrease gradually from 16.0 per 100 inhabitants in 1985 to 15.2 per 100 in 1990.[93] The slight decrease is not surprising because family doctors have detected a substantial number of health problems in the population but have remitted only those cases too complex to handle. The number of nonprimary-care medical visits (much more costly than primary-care attention) also decreased in that period.[94] The percentage of hospital emergency room visits compared to polyclinic emergency room visits decreased between 1980 and 1989 from 80.2 to 75.8 percent.[95] This decrease would seem to be the result of the Family Doctor Program, but it is not certain that it is.

Although the Cuban government denics that cost containment was a motive for this program, it is nonetheless an important benefit.[96] According to Castro, however, the most important goal is to improve the people's health.[97] The family doctors, therefore, are held ultimately responsible for the health of the population they serve. Their work program (*programa del trabajo*) stipulates a series of activities to be carried out, but unlike the policy specified in the red book used previously in the polyclinics, the Family Doctor Program does not stipulate numerical norms to be achieved, and their work is not measured simply by quantitative means but rather by qualitative results. Also in contrast with the red book Basic Health Area Programs, the family doctors' health activities are not divided by patients' age and gender but by categories of activities such as health promotion, prevention, medical care, rehabilitation, environmental hygiene, social cohesion of the community, education, and research.[98] Although many of the specific activities in both programs are the same, the family doctors' work plan places considerably greater emphasis on health promotion and disease prevention.

The Family Doctor Program has extended the real and symbolic reach of the revolution into the farthest reaches of the mountains and shores. The close medical surveillance this program provides has led to an enormous reduction in the infant mortality rate in rural areas, has improved health indices, and has increased patient satisfaction (as verified by surveys).[99] Reduced infant mortality in areas served by family doctors is exemplified by El Pedrero, a town high in the Escambray Mountains, where the rate decreased from 20 per 1,000 live births when the Family Doctor Program began there to 6 per 1,000 by the end of 1990. Similarly, in Párraga, an outlying Havana suburb, the infant mortality rate declined from 15 per 1,000 live births in 1985 to 7 per 1,000 in 1990.[100]

All the evidence suggests that the family doctors are having a significant effect on rural health and that the cost of the program is probably justified there.[101] In the urban areas, on the other hand, it may not be cost-effective because of the already well-established network of polyclinics, but it does provide security for the populace and thereby increases governmental legitimacy and enhances Cuba's prestige (symbolic capital).[102]

Nonetheless, one must question the need for a doctor on every block. The Family Doctor Program has been criticized in the First World for leading to the trivialization of medical practice and for failing to provide doctors with sufficient variety and complexity of cases to maintain their medical knowledge. These critics also claim the program fosters patient dependency and is not cost-effective.[103] Proponents of the program argue that it provides true universal preventive and curative care, with emphasis on prevention, something most Third World and international health officials can only dream about.[104] Whatever the facts might be, putting a doctor on every block is symbolically significant.

Although family medicine is not new,[105] the way the Cubans practice it is. More importantly, this is the first concerted effort to provide such care universally, without charge, on the national level, and as part of an integrated national health system. The entire health system is at the disposal of the family doctors and is obligated to respond to their needs and demands.[106] Most governments are either unable or unwilling to attend to all of their ill, and the prospect of providing regular preventive care to everyone is not on the horizon. For this reason, Cuba's Family Doctor Program has impressed health officials, researchers, international organization personnel, and politicians from developing countries who have seen it firsthand, and it has contributed significantly to Cuba's symbolic capital.[107]

The experience of being a family doctor translates revolutionary theory into practice for a generation born after the triumph of the revolution. It links the guerrilla experience of the older generation in the Sierra Maestra with a "health guerrilla" experience for the youth. Although in remote areas life has improved considerably since the revolution, it still poses challenges that can inspire young doctors and nurses from urban areas. This experience is really domestic "internationalism," or solidarity with those in less developed areas.

Basic Health Area Programs

Medical practice at the primary-care level has followed specific norms established at the ministerial level but adapted to local circumstances. The basic programs have changed over time to suit the changing health needs of the population. The focus has shifted from treating the diseases of poverty to preventing them, then from treating diseases of development to preventing them. Where they exist, the family doctors carry out the basic primary-care programs that have been implemented by the polyclinic staff. Irrespective of who carries out the programs, they are executed once the initial diagnosis of each health sector is completed.

Under the polyclinic guidelines, there have been ten programs: five for treating people, three for improving the health environment, and two for health administration. Those programs addressed to the care of the individual include integral care of women (age fifteen and above), integral care of children (under fifteen), and integral care of adults (over fifteen), dental care, and epidemiology. Programs dealing with the environment include urban and rural hygiene, food hygiene, and occupational health. The administrative programs include basic administration and "optimization" of the treatment of patients and their families or quality of care.[108]

As in the Soviet model and following Thomas McKeown's recommendation for Great Britain,[109] primary care was originally divided among specialists who treated a population divided into groups by age and gender to better integrate specialist care at the primary, secondary, and tertiary levels. The Family Doctor Program, however, has returned primary care to the generalists whom the Cubans intend to make into comprehensive general medicine specialists.

Analysis of a few salient examples of those programs continued by family doctors demonstrates the organizational development and ability of the Cuban health system and some positive and negative aspects of Cuba's primary health-care programs. Because Cuba recognizes that women are important as instruments of societal reproduction, one of the most important programs for individual care is that for women. Most governments, including that of the United States, do not consider women's reproductive role important, and consequently few adequately fund programs for prenatal care.

PROGRAM FOR THE INTEGRAL CARE OF WOMEN

Priority is given to maternal and infant-care programs beginning with pregnancy in order to inculcate good health habits in the mother-to-be and ultimately to produce healthy children. Of the thirteen stated objectives of the program for women, nine deal with pregnancy and the remaining four deal with contraception, early detection of uterine or cervical cancer, venereal disease, and other gynecological pathologies.[110]

In 1977, in order to assure healthy future generations, the Ministry of Public Health established a series of norms to be followed by all primary health-care centers: early detection of pregnancy (before the third month); early consultation with the obstetrical health team (also before the third month); provision of at least nine prenatal examinations and consultations for women in urban areas and six for women in rural areas; education about hygiene, health during pregnancy, childbirth, and child care, among other topics; special prenatal attention to women considered at high obstetrical risk; psychological counseling with regard to childbirth; instruction in birth exercises; and finally, provision that all childbirth take place in hospitals.[111] Although the norms changed in 1984 and 1988 in regard to the number of prenatal visits expected (an average of 15.1 in 1989 for both urban and rural women), their content did not.[112]

In addition to educational lectures in the polyclinic and discussions with the medical staff and the family doctors, new mothers are given a six-page pamphlet with precise and complete instructions as to what, when, and how much to feed an infant from birth through the twelfth month. Breast-feeding is stressed at the outset, with an explanation of its health benefits for the infant, the frequency with which it should be done, and how to do it. The back cover expresses Cuba's concern for children: "Nothing is more important than a child."[113]

As resources became available in the early 1980s, all women were to have an ultrasound examination between their eighteenth and twenty-first weeks of pregnancy to check for congenital malformations.[114] By 1984, mass genetic screening through alpha fetoprotein analysis was being done on Cuban-designed ultra-micro ELISA (enzyme-linked immunosorbent assay) equipment called SUMA.[115] Ultrasound and alpha fetoprotein analyses for all fetuses far exceed medical norms even in the First World, where they are used primarily for those in high-risk categories. Because neither test may be medically necessary for every case, this practice demonstrates a misallocation of resources to gain symbolic capital through the commitment to provide prenatal care of First-World quality or better.

The content of these programs is very significant, but more impressive is the active commitment on the part of the Ministry of Public Health to seek out pregnant women, go to their homes if they do not attend appointments or educational lectures, actively follow up their progress, and insist on institutional childbirth. The first three tasks have been accomplished with the aid of the mass organizations and now are carried out by the family doctors. The fourth, the institutionalization of childbirth, is interesting because it demonstrates the government's willingness to finance what it proclaims to be important.

Hospital childbirth with physicians delivering infants requires a greater expenditure of resources than perhaps is necessary. It also goes against the current trend of dehospitalizing all medical procedures possible and of allowing nurse-midwives to deliver babies. In the developed countries with which Cuba likes to compare itself in the health sphere, the trend is toward birth clinics where paramedical personnel—nurse-midwives, obstetrical nurses, or midwives—deliver the babies. In the developing countries, because of the limited number of physicians and facilities available as well as the costs involved, the trend has been to train paramedics to perform these duties or to allow the traditional midwives to handle them. Hospitalization is not always necessary or even desirable. In fact, it has been suggested that the institutionalization or hospitalization of childbirth in Cuba has turned a perfectly natural process into a pathology.[116]

Why then is Cuba going against the current medical trend? Why does the government spend more on childbirth than seems necessary, judging by other countries' experiences? The initial incentive for hospital childbirth was to assure hygienic conditions and safe procedures, since home delivery was frequently detrimental to the health of both mother and child. In rural areas during the early years of the revolution, hospital delivery greatly decreased infant and maternal mortality because hygienic conditions were lacking in homes.

Because hygiene is still a problem in a great many remote areas, and particularly in mountainous areas, rural women living in less than adequate conditions are sent to a maternity home one to two weeks before their expected delivery date.[117] There they live in sanitary conditions under the auspices of the Ministry of Public Health and are taught hygiene, nutrition, proper child care, cooking, sewing, embroidery, knitting, and other domestic skills, as well as how to breast-feed. When their time comes to deliver, they are transferred to an adjoining or nearby hospital where they generally stay four to five days.[118]

Rural women in remote areas are not the only ones whose environment is inadequate for childbirth at home. Living conditions in urban areas are not always good either, because the housing shortage has forced many married couples to live with their parents or in very small quarters where basic plumbing is sometimes shared with other families. According to the 1979 demographic survey, 17.2 percent of the housing stock (386,382 units) were inhabited *bohíos* (thatch-roofed huts, often with dirt floors), 2.2 percent (49,976) of them in urban areas.

Another type of substandard housing, rooms in *cuarterías* (buildings that may have been intended for uses other than housing, or old apartment blocks subdivided into single rooms rather than apartments), provided lodging for individuals and families in both urban and rural areas. They total 5.4 percent of total housing (121,129 rooms), with 5.1 percent (114,229 rooms) in urban locales.[119] Moreover, data from the 1981 Housing Survey indicated that although some of the housing shortage was alleviated by a government decision to allow people to build and repair their own dwellings, many of the structures built between 1976 and 1981 by do-it-yourselfers contained very serious structural flaws.[120]

In addition to crowding, other hygiene problems exist. Water has long been rationed for several hours a day in some Havana neighborhoods.[121] As a result of the worsening economic situation caused by the virtual elimination of trade with the former Soviet Union and Eastern European countries, there have been many more electrical cuts than in the past. By 1992 there was a weekly schedule of blackouts affecting every Havana neighborhood. The water supply has decreased because of the loss of electricity for pumping and the lack of chlorine for water purification. Moreover, the trade crisis vastly increased shortages throughout the economy, including such basic consumer necessities as toilet paper, detergent, soap, toothpaste, and food. Thus a brief stay in the hospital can be like a vacation for many Cuban women, providing an escape from otherwise difficult conditions and uncomfortable and crowded surroundings.[122]

The second reason Cuba spends more than may seem necessary on childbirth is that the health of pregnant women and children is seen as a major determinant of the quality of life and the productive capacity of future generations. The investment made at this stage yields great returns in later stages of the child's life. These children experience less illness, require less curative medical care, and possess greater potential for development and educational achievement, which lead to greater work capacity and higher productivity. This investment in maternal and child health pays off in the long-term improvement of the social infrastructure required for greater societal development,[123] which is necessary for further accumulation of symbolic capital. Hence, human capital investment seems to justify this policy of institutionalization of childbirth.

Finally, the institutionalization of childbirth is partially explained by symbolic politics, because even if the trend in First World countries is away from institutionalized childbirth, most countries consider hospital-based medicine First World medicine. Cubans, on the other hand, might argue that hospitalization is necessary to reduce the infant mortality rate even further to ensure that not a single child is lost. Infant mortality is taken so seriously that each infant death is analyzed by the family doctor and polyclinic and/or hospital medical staff and by the municipal health director.[124] In Guantánamo province, there is a command post for infant mortality and the rate is checked daily.[125]

Cubans have invested heavily in neonatal intensive care units fully equipped with the latest Western technology available at the time of purchase and staffed by highly trained specialists. These units exist even in outlying municipalities like Baracoa, Guantánamo, historically one of the most socioeconomically backward and remote areas of Cuba.[126] Although the physical surroundings in which they exist may not compare with those of the developed countries, these units have the components necessary to accomplish their mission. Whatever the motive, the prestige Cuba gains by providing medical care in this specific field that approaches First-World standards is significant.

PROGRAM FOR THE INTEGRAL CARE
OF CHILDREN

Concern for the evolution of pregnancy and for childbirth does not end with the birth. The Cuban government places very high priority on the healthy development of children and thus devotes considerable effort to the prevention of disease. This effort begins with an evaluation of a newborn's living conditions and its mother's knowledge of proper childcare.

Two weeks after delivery, a nurse visits the mother and infant at home in order to check on their health, evaluate the sanitation of their living environment, determine whether the mother is breast-feeding, and make an appointment for the mother and child to see the physician in the polyclinic. This is only the beginning of a series of examinations that takes place periodically, but with decreasing frequency, over the next four years of the child's life. Where family doctors practice, medical surveillance is constant.

The program for the integral care of children provides preventive and curative care for all children under the age of fifteen, with the primary effort devoted to the first four years of life. This critical period of development is carefully monitored through programmed visits by the medical team to homes and the day-care centers or kindergartens, as well as through visits by the children to the polyclinic. The aims are to monitor the growth and development of children under the age of four, ensure that all children have the complete series of vaccinations, assess each child's agility and mental and physical development, and check for speech and hearing problems.[127]

Polyclinic norms require 7 examinations, the number considered ideal in the United States,[128] but in Cuba 3 of these occur in the home, so that the medical team can also assess hygiene and sanitation.[129] By 1984 the norms had apparently changed to 8 well-baby clinic visits during the first year of life, but the national average for 1983 was already 8.7 visits.[130] This statistic indicates that most polyclinics were surpassing the national norm.

In 1987 well-baby visits for children less than a year old were up to 9.7 nationally, with the highest number (13.1) being recorded in Guantánamo province as a result of the work of the family doctors in the mountainous zones. Most provinces registered over 9.0 visits that year, but two had less than 8.0 (7.2 in Sancti Spíritus and 7.8 in Isla de la Juventud).[131]

The figures for 1989 indicated an increase to 11.0 well-baby visits per year for the country as a whole, with the City of Havana in first place with 14.0 consultations and Guantánamo province second with 12.3, down 0.8 from 1987. The Isle of Youth brought the national average down with a rate of only 6.7 well-baby visits per year, a rather striking phenomenon compared with the rest of the country and somewhat surprising because this island has the second highest number of doctors per inhabitant.[132]

The well-baby norms for family doctors in Baracoa municipality require 24 visits for the first year, 12 in the home and 12 in the doctor's office. If a child under one has a medical problem, the child must be seen on a weekly basis.[133] In general, children between the ages of one and two are required to have 3 checkups per year, and those between two and four, 2 yearly checkups, with 1 in the home in both cases.[134] Again the family doctors' norms are stricter, requiring 4 yearly examinations either in the office or the home for healthy children between one and four. The norms always dictate greater attention for those with problems of physical or mental development.

Actual practice in 1989 revealed that doctors saw children aged one through four an average of 5.3 times that year, of which 1.7 visits were for well-baby care.[135] This number was exclusive of consultations in day-care centers. Children attending a day-care center or kindergarten are also seen in those institutions on a regular basis either by the resident nurse or resident family doctor or by local polyclinic doctors as their schedule permits.[136] These examinations occur in addition to all other regularly scheduled care. There were an average of 3.3 medical checks on children in day-care centers in 1987, 5.9 for children less than one year old, 5.3 for those between one and two, and 2.7 for those over two.[137] These numbers had dropped to 2.9 consultations in 1989, with 4.9 for children under one year of age, 4.4 for one-year-olds, and 2.4 for those two and over.[138] These numbers decline because formal visits become less necessary in neighborhoods where family doctors have more continuous contact with their patients.

There has been some variation in the degree to which norms are fulfilled even within the same municipality, as illustrated by the cases of two pediatricians who worked under the same municipal health director. In both cases they overfulfilled rather than underfulfilled the red book norms and presaged the practice of family doctors more than three years later. For example, at Punta Brava in 1981, the pediatrician said that children over the age of one but under the age of four should be seen four times a year. After the age of four there is less danger of accidents in the home and of problems resulting from poor hygiene because the children are at day-care centers or schools, where there are resident nurses, good hygiene, and careful supervision. The pediatrician also said that she spent four hours per week doing consultations at the day-care centers.[139]

According to a pediatrician working at the Elpídio Berovides polyclinic in the same municipality, there are twenty-four well-baby consultations during the first year of life rather than seven, as indicated in the 1977 norms, or eight, as indicated in *Granma* in 1984; four visits during the second year rather than the two prescribed by the red book; and two per year until the age of six instead of the age of four.[140] Twenty-four patient visits the first year of life is extraordinary and seems somewhat excessive. This practice appears to turn infancy as well as childbirth into a pathology.

Given the enormous concern for children's health shown by the highest level of government,[141] it is quite possible that these pediatricians or their polyclinic directors have increased the frequency of patient visits in an effort to reduce pediatric morbidity and mortality even further in their areas. Increases in the number of patient visits are considered to be accomplishments; they are reported as such and frequently cited by government officials, because these consultations do not necessarily imply ill-health but rather indicate an increase in preventive measures.[142]

Pediatric preventive health care includes an attempt to eradicate all vaccine-preventable diseases. Cuba's internationally recognized success in this endeavor is well documented.[143] Despite the stated goals and acclaimed success, in 1980 the percentage of children less than one year of age given the basic immunizations was not quite what one would expect: DTP (diphtheria-tetanus-whooping cough)—first dose, 78 percent; DTP—second dose, 67 percent; polio vaccine—first dose, 102 percent; polio vaccine—second dose, 103 percent; measles vaccine, 48 percent; and BCG (tuberculosis) vaccine, 99 percent.[144]

The most successful immunization campaign has been that against polio. The sugar-cube vaccine was administered by the CDRs under the supervision of the Ministry of Public Health. The CDRs conducted the campaign until 1991, when the vaccine was supplied by the Soviet Union in a vial and thus required administration by the family doctor after mobilization of the population by the CDRs.[145] The decentralization of vaccine administration to the block level and the seeking out of those in need of vaccination by the CDR block committee health liaisons assures that all children will be reached. These efforts probably also account for the claim that more than 100 percent of children received the polio vaccine. Overzealous CDRs either made bookkeeping errors, which raise suspicions about their efficacy, or administered more of the vaccine than necessary.

The tuberculosis vaccine is administered prior to the infant's departure from the hospital after childbirth, or if birth occurs at home, within twenty-four hours.[146] This practice results in near-universal coverage. The other immunizations are administered later in the first year of life, which may explain why some children have not received all of their vaccinations. Given the norms of attention to infancy, it is surprising that the immunization rates cited above were not higher. The family doctors have set out to improve them.

Measles vaccine was not given priority in the vaccination campaign because no one died from that disease. Only in 1971, when officials realized that the illness was a drain on resources did measles vaccination become part of the national immunization campaign. In one year Cuba increased its measles vaccination coverage from 50 percent to 71 percent. This increase resulted from a political commitment that translated immediately into resource allocation.[147]

Cuba has made steady improvement over the years in the rate of children immunized with all three doses of DPT. Among children less than one year of age, 99.5 percent got the complete series of DPT vaccinations in 1985, and in 1986 this went up to 100 percent.[148] Data for 1989 indicate that over 90 percent of all at-risk people were administered a whole range of vaccinations depending on their age group, with only one exception: DPT for those aged one through five reached only 87.9 percent of that population. Variations by province in 1989 were insignificant.[149] Beyond the vaccinations recommended by the World Health Organization, Cuba has administered over three million doses of its own meningitis B vaccine to the at-risk population.[150]

In Latin America, only Chile and Costa Rica had immunization rates slightly higher than Cuba's in 1979 and 1980, but no country surpassed Cuba by 1988.[151] Both Chile and Costa Rica have had a long-term active commitment to public health, unlike most nations of Latin America;[152] therefore their successes in immunization are not surprising. A comparison of Cuba's immunization rates to the Latin American average of over 60 percent in 1989 suggests that Cuba's immunization program deserves praise and emulation. Its success no doubt adds to Cuba's symbolic capital.[153]

The Cuban government has made a reality of its slogan, "There is nothing more important than a child." Not just in health, but also in education and recreation, there is a high-level government commitment to providing the greatest possible opportunity for the development of future generations. Actions of the Cuban government in the early 1990s in the face of economic collapse raise questions about Castro's vision of the future and whether it corresponds to that of the Cuban people. These, of course, are ideological questions that will be answered differently by those of different ideological persuasions. Nonetheless, a comparison with the United States is in order here because Castro has publicly stated that Cuba is competing with the United States in an effort to produce the best possible health indicators. Clearly, Cuba can compete in certain areas, but the United States has far more resources (human, fiscal, and physical) to bring to bear on any problem and will, therefore, always be in a better overall position than Cuba.

The Cuban commitment to children, however, contrasts with both the Reagan and Bush administrations' policies (rhetoric to the contrary aside) of budget cuts for various programs that directly or indirectly affect children's health. This fact is exemplified by Reagan's slashing of the public-health budget by 25 percent upon taking office in his first term and designating ketchup as a vegetable in school lunch programs, and by Bush's suggestion in June 1991 that the measles epidemic that had begun in 1990 be studied rather than that mass immunization be funded immediately for children under the age of two, as suggested in the measles white paper presented by an advisory committee to the National Vaccine Program six months earlier.[154] Both actions suggest an unwillingness to invest in prevention. In Cuba, on the other hand, human capital investment is considered to be profitable in the long run.

In the health sphere, the Cuban government has committed considerable resources to ensure the healthy development of all children, attempting to prevent disease rather than waiting to cure it. Although prevention is the primary focus of their program, pediatric curative facilities have been expanded as well. Infant and pediatric cardiovascular surgery are performed regularly, and research into in utero cardiovascular surgery is under way.[155] By 1984 there were twenty-nine pediatric intensive care units throughout the island and hemodialysis units in pediatric hospitals.[156] The intensive care units were built in response to the dengue epidemic in 1981 and may not represent the most useful allocation of resources, but they are symbolically significant and indicative of the philosophy that no cost should be spared when a child's life might be at risk.

PROGRAM FOR ADULTS: DISPENSARIZATION

One of the hallmarks of the Cuban health system has been the aggressive monitoring of patients with chronic diseases. Special attention through a program called dispensarization (as in the former Soviet system) is given to those who are disabled, over sixty-five, suffering from specific chronic or contagious diseases, or exposed to health risks on the job. These patients are actively sought out for observation and treatment.[157] Under the Family Doctor Program, there are no national norms for the number of patient visits, but because the doctors are responsible for their patients' health, they tend to see their patients much more frequently than they did under the previously established norms for the polyclinics.

Patients with nontransmittable chronic diseases, including ischemic heart disease, arterial hypertension, cerebrovascular disease, diabetes, bronchial asthma, and epilepsy, as well as patients with contagious diseases such as tuberculosis, leprosy, and syphilis, are examined in the polyclinic four times yearly and in their homes once a year, with the exception of the syphilitic patients who are checked in the polyclinic four times a year but not in the home. Statistics revealing morbidity and mortality from these diseases are also monitored closely, and the program itself is evaluated on a monthly basis by the medical staff, as are all polyclinic programs.[158]

The polyclinics and the family doctors keep either computerized records or a book or file of dispensarized patients listing all patients with these illnesses as well as those considered at high risk of contracting them. If these patients do not show up for their polyclinic appointments, the medical staff visits as many as possible at home. The aim is to visit all at home, but this is not always possible.[159] The Family Doctor Program provides even closer monitoring of dispensarized patients, because the physician and nurse team assigned to each city block and to rural areas is able to check on and, if necessary, examine these patients daily.

The Cuban health system has succeeded in reducing both mortality and morbidity through the efforts of the medical teams and family doctors in seeking out, educating, and treating those who are chronically ill, and through application of preventive measures wherever possible. Although there are still many flaws in the system and many instances in which norms are not carried out fully, compliance is adequate to produce very good health indicators and therefore symbolic capital. But the work of the medical practitioners alone is insufficient to assure good health. Popular participation and health education are key factors, particularly where prevention on a national scale is concerned.

Beyond Primary Care: High Technology Medicine

A distinguishing feature of the Cuban primary care network is the secondary- and tertiary-level support facilities that back it up. Throughout the island at the end of 1989, there were 263 hospitals of various types, 420 polyclinics, 163 dental clinics, 229 dispensaries, 3 medicinal spas, 148 maternity homes, 23 blood banks, 11 medical research institutes, 153 homes for the aged, of which 36 were senior citizen day-care centers, and 23 homes for the physically and mentally impaired. These facilities provided 6.0 medical assistance beds per 1,000 inhabitants and 1.3 social assistance beds per 1,000 people.[160] As of September 1991, the resources included the offices of the 15,141 family doctors who provided direct patient care.[161]

There were no geographic imbalances in Cuban medical facilities, except that those provinces designated as regional centers had slightly more beds per capita than did the other provinces and the City of Havana province had considerably more beds per capita because it is a national referral center. The most technologically sophisticated hospital in Havana, the Hermanos Ameijeiras, as a stated policy reserves 70 percent of its capacity for patients from other provinces, and the national medical research institutes also reserve inpatient space for national referrals.

Cuba has been improving the quality and increasing the quantity of its medical personnel in the secondary and tertiary health care facilities to further expand the provision of high-technology diagnostic imaging and medical care. Imaging is done with nuclear magnetic resonance (NMR), computerized axial tomography (CAT scanners), digital subtraction equipment (DIGIMAG), and ultrasound, as well as with other techniques. Medical procedures include heart transplants (since 1985), heart-lung transplants (1987), coronary bypasses, pacemaker implantation (1964), renal dialysis and transplants (1970), microsurgery to replace lost fingers and to perform ophthalmological procedures (1977), bone transplants, corneal transplants, pancreatic transplants, combined kidney and pancreatic transplants (1985), bone marrow and liver transplants (1985), partial splenectomy (1987), neural transplants to treat Parkinson's disease (1987), breast reconstruction by implantation of endoprostheses (1986), angioplasties, esophagus transplants (1991), implantation of Cuban-made artificial hearts (1991), extracorporeal lithotripsy, hyperbaric oxygen chamber therapy, and laser acupuncture, inter alia.[162]

In recent years Cuba has been successful in applying new medical procedures quickly. Only four months after the Yale Medical School's Hospital, Yale-New Haven, had performed its fifth heart transplant, Cuba's Hospital Hermanos Ameijeiras had performed its tenth. The first Cuban heart transplant was performed in December 1985, and by May 1987 twenty heart transplants had been performed.[163] Seventy heart transplants (ten in 1990 alone) and three heart-lung transplants had been performed by December 1990 with a survival rate of 88 percent.[164] On July 6, 1987, the state of Connecticut still did not have a single extracorporeal lithotripsy apparatus, despite what health officials claimed was a need for it, yet Cuba had been applying this noninvasive procedure for crushing and removing kidney stones since April 1986.[165]

Following the lead of a renowned Soviet ophthalmologist, Dr. Fiodorov, the Cuban government established the high-technology Center for Ophthalmological Surgery that allows the surgeon to operate on several patients simultaneously. From its inception in mid-1988 until November 1990, the center's ophthalmologists had performed over 24,500 operations, of which 12,039 were to correct myopia.[166] A Latin American doctor who himself underwent surgery there was truly impressed by the state-of-the-art facilities and quality of care he received.[167]

Techniques used by Cuban ophthalmologists are considered very sophisticated even by U.S. standards. Ocular ultrasound and computerized tonometry are advanced diagnostic tools. Vitrectomy is a very complicated procedure performed only by ophthalmological surgeons with very specific subspecialty training in vitreoretinal ophthalmology. Likewise, phacoemulsification, the implantation of intraocular lenses, and radial keratotomy are also indicative of very advanced techniques.[168] Cuban ophthalmological surgeon Dr. Orfilio Peláez developed a technique to halt, and in some cases reverse, retinitis pigmentosa, a disease that ultimately causes blindness. From November 1987 through January 1991, this surgical procedure had been performed on 1,917 patients, of whom 317 came from 20 different countries.[169]

Cuban neurosurgeons performed their first neural tissue transplant in 1987, and in the spring of 1988 the Cuban government established the Iberian–Latin American Center for Nervous Tissue Transplants and Regeneration at the National Neurotransplant Center. In its first twenty months of operation, the center's neurosurgeons treated over 150 people, including patients from abroad. Although it started as a very small facility with only 48 beds, the center has been expanded to 160 beds.[170]

World-class Cuban orthopedic surgical advances include revascularization of the spinal cord (1990), which in 1993 was still performed only on an experimental basis in the United States, and very advanced experimental microsurgery to graft nerve tissue to the spinal cord in cases where the spinal cord had been severed.[171] Rehabilitation services are highly advanced, particularly at the Frank País Orthopedic Hospital in Havana,[172] where many war casualties from Nicaragua, El Salvador, and the former Soviet Union have been treated. The external fixator (RALCA), developed by Dr. Rodrigo Alvarez Cambras, has been used to treat hip fractures in the elderly, allowing them to walk again within six days of application of the device.[173]

At the postoperative level, Cuba's intensive care units (ICUs) across the island are well equipped with high-technology monitoring devices and a large number of staff per patient.[174] Specialized intensive care burn units are very sophisticated, have one nurse per patient, maintain doctors on duty around the clock (rather than just on call), and treat patients with Cuban-developed epidermal growth factor (a biotechnology product), which closes wounds and speeds healing.[175]

The Hermanos Ameijeiras Hospital, which took close to two decades to complete, is a testimony to the allure of symbolism in the medical realm. Initially conceived as a new building for the National Bank of Cuba, the structure was finally finished as a much-needed 950-bed hospital in 1982 at a cost of 60 million pesos and an additional U.S. $62 million in hard currency for medical and nonmedical equipment.[176] The elegance of the building itself compares with that of the local five-star hotels, and the 24-floor structure affords patients breathtaking views of the sea and the city. Rehabilitation patients with whom I spoke were not eager to leave their luxurious (by Cuban standards) surroundings. But it is not the marble floors and walls of the lobby or the views for which this hospital is known.

The Ameijeiras was established as a world-class hospital that could provide the latest technology and procedures available in the most developed countries and that could serve as a site for training personnel to use these innovations. It is also a major research facility with computer and telex links to international research institutions. To achieve its goals, the government sends between 140 and 160 doctors, engineers, biologists, biochemists, and others to twenty-nine countries for training in how to introduce new technologies and techniques at the hospital. Because much of this technology has been extended to regional centers in the provinces, the Ameijeiras accepts only the most complicated cases, such as heart transplants and bone marrow transplants. Because of its sophistication, the Ameijeiras generally has about 35 residents from other countries in training.[177]

A 1988 assessment of the hospital by a ranking Pan American Health Organization official concluded that the staff "conduct research and use technology at the international cutting edge in the 38 medical specialties in which services are rendered."[178] The symbolic capital Cuba gained by this appraisal is very significant and has partially justified the enormous investment the country has made.

In sum, positive health outcomes have boosted Cuba's prestige, as has the health system that engendered them. As this chapter illustrates, the organization of the health system combines First World (doctors and high technology) and Third World or community-based (outreach) approaches. It provides the population with the security of knowing that they will be treated both in a health facility and at home and sought out if they miss their appointments. Moreover, Castro has made clear that where health is concerned, only the highest quality equipment should be used, particularly in the surgical specialties.[179]

The health system, in its organization and programs, provides the moral architecture that distinguishes Cuba from most other developing and developed countries. In important speeches Castro and other officials frequently refer to what they see as the moral superiority of their health system and to its real and symbolic successes.

Cuba's health ideology can be summed up by the idea that the health of the individual is a metaphor for the health of the "body politic," because the Cuban government judges its own efficacy on the basis of the health of the population. Low infant mortality rates, low general morbidity rates, and long life-expectancy at birth symbolize governmental success and add to Cuba's symbolic capital both domestically and internationally. These achievements enable Cuba to conduct medical diplomacy.

3

Health Education
and Popular Participation

Achieving the status of world medical power was a mythic feat for which many Cubans strived, not just those in the medical profession. Because the Cuban people identify strongly with the rest of the Third World and because their own economic development has been retarded by their colonial heritage,[1] the government has been able to rally them to contribute to this effort. Thus construction brigades and other nonhealth-sector personnel have taken it upon themselves to fight for a successful medical system that symbolizes socioeconomic development and scientific achievement. Health education provides the arsenal of weapons and popular participation provides the army to fight against disease and thus against the legacy of colonialism and underdevelopment.

Education, which has been an integral part of the Cuban approach to improving health since the beginning of the revolution, has become even more important because Cuba has long since solved health problems typical of developing countries. To achieve higher life expectancy at this stage of development, one of Cuba's goals in becoming a world medical power, necessitates a reduction in, and better management of, chronic degenerative diseases, which are also the main cause of death in the developed countries. A health-literate population is essential in order to realize this goal, and Cuba is well suited to this task because the government exercises central control over the media, educational curricula, and health services.

Popular participation in the implementation of health programs has been critical to the success of the Cuban health system, particularly in the early years. Mass vaccination campaigns, rural and urban hygiene and sanitation drives, mass screening of women for cervical cancer, early detection of pregnancy and provision of prenatal care, and blood and organ donations are some of the activities that have depended for their success on participation by the mass organizations' health liaisons.[2] Popular participation is also education in the broadest sense, because individuals and communities learn self-reliance and problem-solving techniques as well as factual information necessary for solving their problems.

This chapter explores health education in general as well as a few examples of recent health education campaigns to change lifestyles that increase risk of the two major causes of death in Cuba, heart disease and cancer. AIDS is discussed briefly as part of the epidemiological program but is included in the issue of health education. Popular participation is considered here both in the planning and implementation of programs, with the latter examined through the intersection of symbolic politics, health education, and popular participation in the campaign to eradicate dengue fever.

Health education and community participation are not just Cuban priorities but reflect the international consensus of the World Health Organization that such strategies will result in better health conditions. Both health education and popular participation have strengthened Cuba's ability to provide medical aid abroad, not just because of the symbolic capital garnered through the achievement of better health conditions at home and the extension of medical services but also because other nations have benefited by adapting aspects of these Cuban endeavors.

Health Education

Health education, on both the individual and the mass level, has been an integral part of the treatment of all patients, particularly adults. On the individual level, health education is supposed to be a part of each patient's consultation with the medical staff.[3]

This has occurred primarily in home visits where the medical team has more time than in the polyclinic to address educational issues.[4] The top priority of the Family Doctor Program, however, has been to promote health through education.

Family doctors have made health education a part of daily life because they tend to use both professional and social interactions with their patients for educational purposes. A family doctor who attends a party in the community, for example, invariably is asked health-related questions, and a doctor who meets patients at the grocery store often takes the opportunity to impart some type of health education.[5]

On the group level, health education takes place at lectures in various forums: the waiting rooms of polyclinics and family doctors' offices, the workplace, and meetings of mass organizations, most particularly the CDRs. Health education emphasizes the prevention of disease, its early detection and control, and the importance of using the health services. The specific themes addressed are the health hazards of smoking; proper nutrition; the benefits of exercise; personal and environmental hygiene; prevalent diseases in the community and their diagnosis and control; use of health services; and for those with health risks or chronic diseases, knowledge of their specific problem.[6]

The polyclinics offer health lectures, *audiencias sanitarias,* in special meetings of the CDRs. The frequency of lectures varies from once every two months at the Policlínico Comunitario Docente in Holguín to once every four months at the Policlínico Punta Brava in La Lisa.[7] This variation may result from the difference in types of polyclinic. In the early 1980s, Holguín was used to train medical students but Punta Brava was not used for this purpose.

Prior to the Family Doctor Program, health liaisons from the CDRs were trained to assist polyclinic workers in health promotion on their blocks in Popular Health Schools (*Escuelas Populares de Salud*) which met once a month.[8] These health liaisons have played a major role in the extension of health coverage by participating in immunization campaigns, helping the polyclinic staff locate and arrange new appointments for patients who fail to show up for their appointments,[9] conducting health surveys, and assisting in sanitation and hygiene work. The Popular Health Schools also educated the CDR health liaisons in general health issues to increase their level of knowledge so that, in turn, the liaisons could teach the other members of their CDR block committee.[10] Since the establishment of the Family Doctor Program, the health liaisons fulfill fewer functions and work in coordination with the family doctor from whom they also receive their training. Primarily they work on environmental hygiene and sanitation and on encouraging blood and organ donations. The other duties they previously carried out are now handled by the family doctors themselves, thereby reducing community participation in health matters. As one ministry official put it, "In a qualitatively superior era, the mass organizations do less."[11]

Members of the FMC who train as *brigadistas sanitarias* (health brigade members) participate in classes given by the polyclinics' nurses in first aid, giving injections, and general health information with an emphasis on women's health. *Brigadistas* assist the polyclinic staff by seeking out pregnant women and discussing with them the need for prenatal care, seeing that all women in their district have had their regularly scheduled Pap smears, going to the homes of women who miss their prenatal exams or other clinic appointments, educating the women in their area in various health issues, and performing other health functions.[12] The *brigadistas* also have had their role revised but to a lesser extent than the CDRs. Their main responsibility is to educate women about health issues affecting women in the most general sense (as women and mothers) and to mobilize people at the request of the family doctor whom they assist in specific health-related tasks and from whom they receive training. Although the number of tasks may have decreased, the number of *brigadistas* in 1991 (65,000 out of a population of 4 million women aged fifteen and over) has remained high.[13]

School children are also given health education classes, principally in first aid and, as a stimulus to career development, in the nature of the health professions. These classes are conducted by nurses and *brigadistas* as two- to three-week courses in first aid provided through the Red Cross to the children in health "interest clubs" (*círculos de interés*) or taught during extracurricular activity period at schools.[14] The Pioneers, a youth organization for those under the age of 14 similar to the Soviet Pioneers, also provides classes in first aid for its members. The Pioneers who take these classes actually help provide first aid by assisting the Red Cross staff on Saturdays or after school.[15] As a result, some Cuban children have a fair idea of what is involved in health care and also of how to treat minor traumas. This knowledge represents a contrast to recent reports of "health and hygiene illiteracy" among Soviet youth.[16]

Various types of special interest clubs are organized in part by family doctors to improve health, both mental and physical, and to provide health education. The children's health interest circle is one example, but there are also adolescents' clubs which, among other things, discuss sexuality and sex education; pregnant women's groups, where discussion tends toward prenatal and well-baby care; and grandparents' clubs, which promote exercise and social integration.[17]

Dental clinics also have *audiencias sanitarias* for the CDRs, in which dentists and dental nurses meet with various CDR block committees twice a year. The dental team also makes monthly visits to the work centers in their health area to give brief lectures during coffee breaks or lunch, if possible. Lectures on proper dental hygiene, tooth decay, and false teeth are given daily in the waiting rooms of dental clinics.[18]

Health education talks are also given in the waiting rooms of the polyclinics. These talks vary with the types of patients to be seen as well as with the circumstances. In a polyclinic in Holguín, for example, doctors and nurses were scheduled to give lectures in various waiting areas at 8 A.M. and 2 P.M. In pediatrics these lectures were on hygiene and feeding, the importance of vaccinations, the psychomotor development of children, and breast-feeding. In general medicine they were on obesity, the health hazards of smoking, the use and abuse of health services, the importance of vaccinations, venereal diseases (discussed privately with each individual), risk factors for chronic diseases, and the dispensarization program. In obstetrics and gynecology, the subjects were sex education, psychoprophylaxis,[19] and breast-feeding.[20] Lectures were scheduled daily so that there always would be some sort of educational activity in the waiting room.

Special health education meetings are held for patients in the dispensarization program. These meetings entail education through group dynamics. For instance, in a group dynamics session for hypertensives, the discussion leader, usually a social psychologist, nurse, or physician, asks an open question such as "What do you know about your illness?" The answer of one patient promotes a discussion by the others who either add to or contradict what the first patient said. In this way the level of the patients' knowledge about their disease becomes clear, and any gaps or misinformation can be dealt with by the discussion leader.[21] This method of group dynamics has proved successful in educating specific patient populations.

In addition to these lectures, there are health education booklets available on loan through the polyclinics and day-care centers. One such booklet, called *Popular Health Themes,* provides ninety-five pages of clear, simple explanations of various health issues and a glossary of terms. Discussions of diseases describe the diseases, their causes, and their prevention, and essays explain what constitutes good hygiene and nutrition.[22]

In addition, for over thirty years the National Directorate for Health Education has been reviewing primary- and secondary-school teaching materials in different fields to see when and how health education can be added. For example, in courses on geography the discussion of environmental pollution leads to discussion of adverse effects of pollution on health, and in chemistry classes the topic of proteins leads to discussion of proper nutrition. Teacher-training programs include a course on health education as well.[23]

Informal interviews with Cubans in various geographic settings and educational backgrounds during numerous field research trips indicate that some of the health education has been effective but that there are important exceptions. One of those exceptions, the program on AIDS, is discussed below. Cubans also seem more knowledgeable about hygiene, diseases, common ailments and their treatment, the nature and structure of the health services available to them, and health-career options than they are about nutrition and exercise. This finding confirms that there is a need for greater attention to health education but also indicates that efforts made thus far have not been in vain.

MEDIA COVERAGE OF HEALTH ISSUES

The Cuban media's prominent coverage of health topics indicates government commitment to improving the health of the population. Until late 1990, when the energy shortage led to decreased television broadcasting and the shortage of paper led to drastically reduced print media circulation, the mass media regularly provided various forms of health education. In the late 1970s and early 1980s, for example, a television series on health graphically presented the nature of the human body, its functions, and its potential illnesses. The programs dealing with the circulatory system and heart disease provided sound instruction and easily comprehensible information.[24] There were also television and radio programs on dental health that provide comprehensive information about what causes cavities.[25] Because the only two television channels offer little choice of programming, people tend to watch whatever is on. For this reason, it can be assumed that the health programs reached a considerable part of the population.

In the mid 1980s, a television series on nutrition that was aimed at youth mixed popular music performed by top stars with interviews with Dr. Manuel Peña Escobar, a medical professor who also holds a Ph.D. in nutrition. The show's rock video format was popular and Dr. Peña's careful explanations dispelled myths about nutrition.[26] Popular formats were also used in the late 1980s and early 1990s in a number of educational TV programs on AIDS. One of these programs, in addition to providing clear information about AIDS, presented interviews with people on the street in various parts of Havana to assess their knowledge of the disease and of how to avoid it.[27] Moreover, some programs included interviews with those who have tested positive for HIV. In one such interview, a youth mentioned having one hundred sex partners in a single year, the antithesis of the type of behavior the health officials are trying to promote. The message was clear and was followed with a statement of the ministry's position.[28] This type of programming has become common and has replaced socialist realism as the dominant media style.

Magazines published health columns regularly, but newspaper coverage was less regular until the early 1980s, when Castro's attempt to convert Cuba into a world medical power began. Most health news in both media has taken the form of reports on the many national and international medical conferences held in Cuba, reports on new medical devices or procedures such as a detailed description of brain surgery to treat Parkinson's disease, accounts of the experiences of Cuba's internationalist health workers in other Third World countries, and a regular health column, "What the Doctor Says," providing medical advice on specific health problems. Some magazine articles have taught the health consumer how to detect and manage a particular disease with a physician's help. Intentionally or otherwise, all of these articles symbolically underscore Cuba's medical prowess.

Along with the reports and columns on health that have appeared in the various newspapers and magazines, frequent full-page educational exhortations by the Ministry of Public Health have succinctly addressed one major health issue. For example, these exhortations appeared in what is perhaps the most widely read magazine, *Bohemia*, from February 1983 through January 1984: "Boil water for the whole family"; "Put yourself into motion . . . get into shape" [to promote jogging]; "Every month after your period, examine your breasts. Consult your physician if there is any change"; "Cleaning and hygiene for the elimination of the *Aedes aegypti* [mosquito]"; "A cytological exam—the early detection of uterine cancer—is a woman's right."[29]

Particularly noteworthy was the excellent news coverage of the 1981 dengue hemorrhagic fever epidemic. Dengue, often called breakbone fever, is a potentially fatal influenza-like illness reported to be the "most incapacitating fever known."[30] *Granma* ran daily articles and news items on the nature of the problem, its source, methods of eradicating the disease, and progress in stemming the epidemic and curing those already afflicted. Large scientific drawings of the vector, the *Aedes aegypti* mosquito, were even published on the front page of *Granma*. The government's ability to communicate rapidly and repeatedly with its citizens played a major role in eradicating dengue, and thereby in gaining symbolic capital.

The substantial increase in health coverage in the mid 1980s reflected Cuba's drive to become a world medical power. *Granma Weekly Review* ran 113 health and medical articles ranging from one paragraph to one page long, with most longer than one paragraph (the paper was 12 pages long), during 42 almost consecutive weeks from February 1 through December 13, 1987. Most issues contained at least two health articles; almost half had three or four; and a few had six or more.

Although these articles were informative, they also had the potential to stimulate patient demand for the health procedures and equipment described. The more informed the patient population, the more services it demands, potentially putting additional strain on the system to provide the latest equipment available. But the description of medical procedures and equipment increases public pride in the Cuban medical system and creates a feeling of greater security among the population, greater governmental legitimacy, and increased prestige (symbolic capital).

Governmental legitimacy flows from the satisfaction of the needs of the governed, with health being a particularly important need. Thus the more effectively the government satisfies the people's health needs, the more likely they are to see their government as legitimate. Obviously, health is only one of many factors contributing to legitimacy, and it may not be a very cost-effective one. Accordingly, it is quite telling that, of Cuba's priorities, the government uses health as an index of legitimacy.

THE CAMPAIGN AGAINST SEDENTARISM

Since the late 1970s, the highest priority for health education has been to alter traditional Cuban habits to reduce or prevent chronic degenerative diseases such as heart disease and cancer, the major causes of death both in Cuba and in developed countries. This priority results from the effectiveness and success of the revolution's early efforts to raise health levels to those of developed countries, a symbolically important achievement.

To combat sedentarism and foster physical fitness, the government promotes individual exercise such as jogging, group exercise, sports, and martial arts.[31] Beginning in the late 1980s, a fifteen-minute aerobics show aimed at youth aired on weeknights just before the evening television news.[32] Since 1980 the government has also promoted physical fitness among youth in conjunction with patriotic values and military preparedness through organizations called Patriotic-Military Societies, which teach martial arts among other skills.[33]

Sedentarism among the elderly came under attack in the late 1980s as well. Senior citizens were encouraged to join newly formed Senior Citizens' or Grandparents' Clubs (*círculos de abuelos*) that promote a number of activities including morning exercise programs conducted under the supervision of an exercise specialist from the Sports and Physical Education Institute (INDER) and the local family doctor. In one club the exercise leader was a one-hundred-year-old man.[34] By November 1988 there were 3,000 such clubs with 120,000 members, of whom about 80 percent were women.[35]

Although Cuba excels in competitive sports, as demonstrated by its numerous gold medals at international competitions, the general population is reluctant to exercise at all. Most Cubans would rather wait half an hour for a bus rather than walk a few blocks. Though the island has beautiful beaches, the people use them primarily for social gatherings rather than swimming.[36] If it were not for the economic crisis of the early 1990s, the campaign against sedentarism would be long and difficult. Perhaps one of the few benefits of that economic crisis is that the drastic reduction of petroleum supplies gave greater impetus to the antisedentarism campaign. Many car owners began to walk or ride bicycles because fuel was unavailable. Those who relied on buses had to turn to self-propulsion such as biking or walking.

With his usual skill at turning adversity into advantage, Castro himself said that the importation of hundreds of thousands of Chinese bicycles and the purchase of bicycle assembly plants would not only save petroleum but also decrease environmental pollution from the ubiquitous, heavily polluting, energy-inefficient Hungarian buses. Decreased pollution and increased physical fitness through biking and walking, he said, would thereby greatly improve the people's health. My personal observations in Havana in June 1991 corroborate Castro's view: sedentary, overweight people had become, in the fifteen months since my previous field research, thin or considerably thinner and appeared fit (because there were food shortages as well, people were deprived of the fatty foods they prefer); and the air was less polluted by diesel fumes because there was so little traffic. I made similar observations in July 1992, but since there was even less food available then, the appearance of fitness was probably deceptive.

Castro even asserted that those who lived within a ten-mile radius of their jobs would have to ride bikes or walk to work and that this would improve their health. He echoed statements made by environmentalists the world over that this is the age of the bicycle and that the bicycle is not just an inexpensive means of transportation for Third World countries such as China and India. He noted that it also serves countries such as the Netherlands and Sweden, which are among the most environment- and health-conscious. Castro can thus significantly draw upon these First World countries as models of biking societies to justify the switch from a more technologically advanced form of transport to a less advanced one.

NUTRITION CAMPAIGN

The major nutritional problem facing most developing nations is undernutrition or malnutrition because of inadequate food supplies, but in Cuba, until the summer of 1991, the problem was obesity. Although obesity has various causes, in Cuba, as elsewhere, it frequently results from simple overeating and from eating the wrong foods.[37] Accordingly, a campaign was launched to change dietary habits that lead to obesity.

The problem of obesity, however, has primarily been dealt with by encouraging exercise rather than by trying to change eating habits. A 1983 pamphlet produced by the Ministry of Public Health advised, "The easiest way to lose weight is through more physical activity," and, as the book *No Free Lunch* points out, "Eating less is only mentioned as a minor issue."[38]

Not until the 1987 food culture initiative did some government agencies and individuals actively promote proper nutrition. The exceptions were Dr. Manuel Pēna's television series on nutrition (mentioned above) and a nutrition campaign organized by the Cuban Institute for Research and Orientation of Internal Demand (ICIODI). This agency produced television and print media nutrition ads and distributed recipe pamphlets (minicookbooks) through its popular magazine, *Opina*.[39]

The Institute of Nutrition and Food Hygiene, in cooperation with UNICEF, produced a laminated paper "diet disc" that graphically provides a considerable amount of information on nutrition. One side contains pictures of three food groups: "Constructors and repairers (proteins), regulators (vitamins and minerals), energizers (carbohydrates and fats)," as well as three types of menus and the amounts of each food group necessary for a balanced diet. The menus are shown through a window as the top disc rotates over the bottom revealing breakfast, lunch, and dinner at three different caloric intake levels: 2,000 kilocalories for those whose physical activity is light, 2,500 for those who are moderately active, and 3,000 for those who are very active.

The other side of the disc has a table of exchange values for numerous foods by unit of measure, energy value, and protein, fat, and carbohydrate content. Finally, there is a table describing daily caloric needs by gender, age, weight, and physical activity. A companion pamphlet explains how to use the diet disc and lists the degree of physical activity required by various occupations. If used by consumers, this information could substantially alter the food culture and improve the health of the vast majority of Cubans.

Centuries-old habits and erroneous ideas as to what constitutes good nutrition, however, have been exceedingly difficult to alter. The government has been most successful in developing more adequate nutritional patterns among those born after the revolution rather than among those with well-entrenched conceptions of what should be eaten. The traditional Cuban diet, one that left people satisfied that they "had eaten," is a heaping plate of white rice with black beans or black bean soup, a large serving of roasted pork, a tuber such as *malanga,* followed by a very sweet dessert, such as candied fruit in syrup with white cheese, and espresso with a great deal of sugar.[40] This diet is high in total calories, starches, and saturated fats, and low in fiber.

It must be stressed that many Cubans, particularly in the rural areas and in the old urban slums, did not have the opportunity to eat all foods in this diet but ate only the rice and beans.[41] Unfortunately, they did not realize that they were better off nutritionally than the pork-eaters and so yearned for what they could not afford. Despite the attempt to change dietary practices through rationing, development of more nutritious agricultural products, heavily subsidized meals, and mass nutrition-education efforts, the Cuban diet through 1990, although compositionally different from what it was in the past, was still high in total calories, starches, and saturated fats, and low in fiber.[42]

Obstacles to a changed diet persist in Cubans' cultural views of the body. The idea that a fat baby is beautiful and healthy leads to pediatric obesity, setting a life pattern that is difficult to change.[43] Among adults, a little heftiness also is considered attractive. In fact, "How fat you are!" (*¡Que gordo estás!*) is a compliment.[44] This attitude is typical of those in developing countries and in situations of scarcity where people's status and wealth are often measured by their girth.

Nutrition education has been necessary in order to gain acceptance for foods such as eggs, yogurt, cheese, fish, and leafy green vegetables that were previously not consumed by much of the population. Other, more desirable foods eaten infrequently by many in the past, such as ice cream, milk, chicken, beef, pork, and citrus fruit, of course, required no health-education efforts.

Food that traditionally has not formed part of the Cuban diet has been introduced through heavily subsidized meals (fifty cents per meal) or free meals provided to workers and students in their cafeterias. Unfortunately, some of these foods, such as chickpeas and fish, were not prepared in a tasty way or were of low quality, thereby discouraging many people from eating them.[45] This situation is particularly problematic given the number of people affected by "social food provision." In 1991 a total of 692,000 people received three meals a day under this plan, and another 2.2 million received at least one subsidized or free meal outside their homes each day.[46] These numbers declined dramatically toward the end of 1991, and social provision of food ended in 1992 as the economic crisis worsened and food shortages became more severe.

Day-care centers also have introduced nontraditional foods into their menus, helping the children acquire a taste for foods that might not be served at home and thereby exerting pressure on their parents to provide them. The Ministry of Public Health has worked hard to educate both the employees of the day-care centers and the children's mothers to decrease the ingestion of sugar. The main problem is the addition of sugar to the children's milk. Family doctors try to persuade the mothers not to add sugar, because the children will not drink milk outside their home without it. If sugar is added at the day-care center but not in the home, then the health officials persuade the day-care center to gradually decrease the amount of sugar in the milk until there is none. This effort, carried out on a case-by-case basis and in coordination with the mother, demonstrates the lengths to which the health officials will go in an attempt to change eating habits early in a child's life.[47]

The provision of nontraditional foods has been accompanied by media efforts to convince the populace of the nutritional value of those foods. Despite these efforts survey data for 1979 indicated that "the typical Cuban erroneously believes that beef and chicken are more nutritious than eggs or fish,"[48] and that "only 13 percent of Cubans knew what foods contain carbohydrates and only 27 percent knew what foods are high in calories."[49] These figures suggest either the failure of Cuban nutrition education prior to 1979 or the tenacity of traditional ideas about food culture or both.

Nutrition education in Cuba has been constrained by the fact that food is a political issue on the international as well as the domestic level. Whereas it is internationally recognized that vegetable protein is both more economical and more nutritional than animal protein, Cuban vice president Carlos Rafael Rodríguez has stated that Cuba opposes the idea set forth frequently in international-development circles that vegetable protein is the solution to the developing countries' food-supply problems.[50] Vegetable protein appears to many in the Third World to be a second-class food compared to animal protein, which is associated with wealth and development. Ironically, many educated people in the First World, whom Third World peoples often seek to emulate, now prefer fish, vegetables, and grains to meat. In this case, the politics of symbolism works to the detriment of health in the Third World.

Because many food items are scarce in Cuba, rationing persists. Rationing increased, in fact, in 1990 and again in 1991 and 1992 because of vastly decreased Soviet trade, the elimination of Eastern European trade, and the curtailment of aid from both areas. Until the government can provide enough of each food item to satisfy consumer demand (now highly unlikely), it will not be able to alter the food preferences despite abundant scientific evidence to substantiate the superiority of vegetable protein to animal protein.

Once again, the economic crisis may have a somewhat salutary effect in that the government cannot afford to provide sufficient meat to satisfy popular demand (nor has it ever done so, for that matter). Consequently, people have no choice but to eat more vegetables, even though the government continues to seek less expensive ways of raising poultry and hogs by using feed made from the residue of sugar production processes and biotechnology. At the same time, the austerity-induced food program is replacing imports, both ingredients for other products such as wheat flour for bread and finished products such as canned ham, with domestic foods. For example, flour has been made on an experimental basis from tropical tubers. The food program, however, cannot supplant all of the staple foods previously imported.

The choice and allocation of foods is highly political in Cuba because control over the economy is centralized and because most basic foodstuffs are rationed. Government decisions, therefore, have real and symbolic significance, as they may call into question the very legitimacy of the regime. This fact is quite clear in the case of the milk ration.

After the revolution each child under the age of seven was promised a liter of milk per day. Despite repeated objections from nutritionists that half a liter is sufficient, the government persisted in providing a liter of milk to these children. This program was accomplished at considerable social cost, because all food items are heavily subsidized. Vice President Rodríguez explained the matter in 1980 to Medea Benjamin, an author of *No Free Lunch:*

Before we can tell people they don't need so much milk, there must be plenty of milk available for everyone. If we did it before that ... the people would say: "Here they come with technical arguments, when all they want to do is take away half a liter of milk from the kids." These are political problems ... and the people's feelings must be taken into account. We can't be 100 percent scientific because politics won't allow it.[51]

Rodríguez's point was clear: any nutrition program that entails a reduction in consumption, even though justified by international scientific literature and practice, will cause considerable political criticism. Such an action would decrease governmental legitimacy because of the government's perceived inability to meet the population's basic needs. Milk, in this case, is associated with children and is symbolic of development, and any decline in the ration would be seen as a step backward.

Other basic products and services have the same symbolic relevance. During the "special period in peace time" beginning in late 1990, milk was rationed and became largely unavailable to the general public as the government reserved supplies for children under the age of seven, for the elderly, and for the infirm. By mid 1992 even the latter two groups often were unable to get milk. The situation had to be explained as a "war economy" measure, as something extraordinary to meet the unique adverse circumstances Cuba faced, but this measure (among other similar ones) nonetheless has led some to question their government's ability to meet their basic needs and thus their government's very legitimacy.

ANTI-SMOKING CAMPAIGN

The political and symbolic problem of restricting a rationed good also arises with respect to the campaign against smoking. In 1981 more than three-quarters of the adult Cuban population smoked.[52] Since Cuba is a renowned producer of tobacco, attempting to convince the population of the adverse effects of smoking is a sensitive point for the government. Because the finest Cuban tobacco is exported to earn sorely needed hard currency, some Cubans might think that the antismoking campaign is merely the government's justification for decreasing domestic access to a commodity still rationed.

In 1971 the rationing of cigarettes and cigars was modified in order to discourage smoking. The ration was decreased and limited to people already over sixteen years of age. This move was supposed to provide an economic incentive not to smoke, because the non-ration price was five times higher than the ration price, and fewer people were then eligible for the ration.[53] Given the high percentage of adults who still smoke, it is clear that this economic disincentive has failed. Further, it is not at all clear that the 1971 ration change was made to improve the population's health rather than to increase tobacco exports at a time when Cuba failed to meet its goal of a 10-million-ton sugar harvest.

Data for 1976 indicate that Cubans then smoked 113 packs of cigarettes per year per capita, and by 1984 this had risen to 125 packs.[54] In 1985 more than 42 percent of the Cuban population over the age of seventeen smoked, making Cuba third in the world in number of smokers per capita. Cigarettes and alcohol consumed 25 percent of the family budget in 1986 despite a decrease in cigarette purchases.[55] One could argue that this figure may only reflect a lack of alternative goods to purchase, but other goods were not in short supply at that time, as both survey and health data corroborate.

A 1986 survey in one section of Havana indicated an alarming increase in the number of female smokers, particularly those in their childbearing years. More than a third of women over the age of fourteen smoked, of whom 55 percent were between the ages of twenty and twenty-nine.[56] Data for 1987 revealed that 35 percent of all women and 65 percent of all men smoked and that about 6.5 percent of the teenagers from thirteen to eighteen years of age and just over 15 percent of those nineteen to twenty-four smoked.[57] By 1990 this picture had improved: among the population over the age of thirteen, the prevalence of smoking was down to 35 percent, and only 24 percent of women and 47 percent of men smoked.[58]

Smoking-related illnesses, particularly respiratory and cardiovascular diseases, caused more than 30 percent of all deaths in Cuba in 1987. Lung cancer afflicted 25 percent of those who died of cancer, and cancer of the larynx afflicted 2 percent. Both diseases were then on the rise. Smoking caused 91 percent of the lung cancers in men and 66 percent of those in women.[59] Data for 1989 indicate that 44 percent of all deaths were caused by smoking-related diseases, a 14 percent increase over 1987.[60] For these reasons the Cuban government has been attempting to educate and cajole the population into refraining from smoking. Castro himself gave up smoking publicly in August 1985, announced that he had quit in 1986, and presented himself as a role model.

Cuba began to promote abstention from smoking in 1960 through prohibition of cigarette advertising, health warnings on cigarette packages, and education of health workers. In 1976 the Ministry of Public Health established a National Commission for Health Promotion that singled out smoking, sedentarism, and obesity as obstacles to better health. But the current antismoking campaign dates to the formation of a national working group in 1986, coordinated by the ICIODI, to direct the work of the many agencies involved.[61]

By the late 1980s, smoking was prohibited by law in all health facilities, classrooms, meeting and conference rooms, domestic flights, buses, certain workplaces, and sports areas.[62] Norms discouraging smoking were put into effect that prohibited officials from smoking publicly, and television and the press were forbidden from presenting positive images of people smoking. Smoking was also discouraged in restaurants and commercial and service facilities.[63] In 1990 the campaign against smoking was taken to primary schools, where it became part of every child's education beginning with the first grade.[64]

Since 1986 Cuban television has run a series of rather frightening but well-made public service announcements exhorting people not to smoke,[65] and the press has printed numerous articles on the dangers of smoking. The current antismoking campaign seeks to improve the health of smokers and of nonsmokers who passively inhale 20 to 30 percent of the smoke around them. Because smoking decreases not just life expectancy but also performance at work, at school, and in sports, special emphasis is placed on preventing youth from beginning the habit. Another priority target group, for obvious reasons, is pregnant and breast-feeding women.

During the first year of the antismoking campaign organized by ICIODI, there was a 6 percent decrease in smoking. A Cuban official has compared this favorably with the 40 percent decrease obtained by Norway over a ten-year period.[66] All Cuban provinces reported at least a 4 percent decrease, but one-third more than doubled that decrease. The two provinces indicating the lowest decrease were the least developed, Granma, and the most developed, Havana.[67] Between 1980 and 1990, the prevalence of smoking among those aged thirteen and above decreased by 14 percent.[68]

From 1985 to 1986, domestic cigar and cigarette sales decreased by 35 billion packs of cigarettes and 10 million cigars for a revenue loss to the state of 60 million pesos. The overall decrease in cigarette and cigar purchases from the time the campaign began until the spring of 1987 was 6.9 percent.[69] In late 1990 and early 1991, the availability of cigarettes declined because of the austerity program. Nery Suárez Lugo, who coordinates the antismoking campaign for ICIODI, contended that cigarette riots, as occurred in the Soviet Union, were avoided because of the previous work ICIODI had done to discourage smoking and provide programs to assist people to quit, and because cigarettes were still available albeit in reduced quantity.[70]

When asked about the contradiction between exporting tobacco and waging a war against smoking at home, officials tend to evade the question.[71] Just as in 1971, the Cuban government faced serious economic difficulties and a hard-currency crunch. Although the state loses domestic revenue with decreased cigarette sales, it gains in foreign exchange with more of the product to export. Moreover, long-term savings because of improved worker health and productivity make the war against smoking economically sound, whatever the motives. Increased life expectancy and reduced morbidity resulting from decreased smoking would enhance Cuba's prestige and thus add to its symbolic capital.

POPULAR PARTICIPATION IN ADMINISTRATION: PEOPLE'S HEALTH COMMISSIONS

Popular participation is a critical element in the PAHO strategy to achieve health for all by the year 2000. PAHO h as made clear that popular participation should not be conceived of merely as assistance in the implementation of programs but rather as communities' responsibility for their own health. This requires active involvement in the identification and resolution of community health problems.[72] Few countries have achieved notable popular participation even in program implementation. Some have incorporated community participation in theory only, and in other countries the principle has been applied on a local level in an uncoordinated fashion.[73] Cuba is the only PAHO country that has achieved popular participation in any form on a national level (although Colombia has the potential do so).[74]

Popular participation as education is a fundamental element of the People's Health Commissions. Participation by community representatives on the polyclinics' advisory boards creates greater social cohesion and allows nonadministrators and nonhealth workers a voice in polyclinic operations. The polyclinic director and department heads (executive committee) must meet on a monthly basis with community political and mass organization representatives in a people's health commission that analyzes, among other things, progress toward goals previously set; the executive committee's report on the health status of the population and any factors that might require community participation; specific health, hygiene, or sanitation issues raised by the mass organization representatives; and the evaluation of work on the basic-area health programs.[75]

With regard to decision making, the experts in the technical fields have prevailed, leaving only minor issues like the cleanliness of the facilities or hours of operation to the community representatives. The ultimate aim, however, is to have greater popular participation in decision making and planning.[76] Because the mass organizations' representatives on the People's Health Commissions lacked medical training and had less general education than their medical counterparts, their participation was minimal at best. The meetings served more of an educational than a participatory function.[77]

Greater administrative decentralization since the 1976 establishment of People's Power Assemblies (municipal, provincial, and national legislatures) has meant local control over the operation of municipal health facilities and increased ability of nonhealth workers to participate in decision making.[78] The polyclinic became accountable to the Ministry of Public Health on issues of norms, policies, and methodology and to the municipal People's Power Executive Committee in administrative and operational matters. Consequently, the municipal health director must report each month to the corresponding People's Power executive committee as well as to the municipal mass organization representatives.[79]

In theory, mass participation in the decision-making process has been transferred to the People's Power Assemblies, which operate local services. But since these services are under the normative and methodological control of the Ministry of Public Health, actual decision making and planning do not take place in the assemblies but rather in the ministry and at the local level of administration by ministry appointees.

POPULAR PARTICIPATION
AND THE EPIDEMIOLOGICAL PROGRAM

The Ministry of Public Health has been adept at containing and eradicating contagious diseases. Through the epidemiology program, it surveys the communities to detect, register, treat, and follow up persons with acute respiratory or diarrheal diseases, tuberculosis, venereal diseases, leprosy, malaria, and other communicable diseases. Diseases that can be prevented through vaccination are controlled in that manner.[80] Health education aims to teach the general population to recognize these diseases and their causes and to report them to the health officials when detected in their communities.[81] Family doctors now carry out this program in their areas, thereby assuring even better disease control. Sources of infection, be they an ill person or some other carrier of a disease, are sought out and treated; efforts to combat AIDS and dengue in this way are discussed below.

AIDS

Whereas Cuba, as an island nation with a very good public health system, has been able to eliminate or greatly decrease the prevalence of many contagious diseases, AIDS presented particular problems because for over three decades Cuba has provided development and military assistance to many Third World, particularly African, countries. As a result, hundreds of thousands of young Cubans have served abroad, in areas where the incidence of AIDS is high.

Contact with foreigners abroad and in Cuba has been the principal source of infection because Cuba has no intravenous drug problem, prostitution has been minimal and unorganized until the recent economic crisis, open homosexuality is uncommon and there are no public meeting facilities for gay people, and blood products have not been imported since 1986, when Cuba began screening its own blood supply. Once contracted, however, AIDS can easily spread within Cuba because of the high incidence of premarital and extramarital liaisons and the rapidity with which marriage and divorce occur.[82]

Demonstrating the capabilities of the Cuban medical system and its ability to enforce compliance with public health measures, the Ministry of Public Health announced in 1987 that by 1989 the entire population over the age of fifteen would be tested for HIV, the AIDS virus,[83] though only 6 people had died of AIDS in Cuba and only 21 confirmed cases had been reported. Of the almost 1.5 million people tested in 1987, 172 were identified as carriers.[84] By January 1989 it was claimed that "about 80 percent of the sexually active adult population" (3.5 million people) had been tested for HIV, of whom 268 tested positive. At the same time, only 84 AIDS carriers were detected among 300,000 Cubans returning from Africa, and all of them were tested and counseled before their return to Cuba.[85]

Data for the end of June 1990 indicate that 8 million tests had been carried out, detecting 449 positive cases of whom 325 were male and 124 female. Sixty-three persons had shown symptoms, and 32 of them had died. A year later there were 605 positive cases, of whom 433 were male and 172 female, with an average age of 24 for the whole group.[86] Because people at high risk of infection are tested repeatedly, it is difficult to assess exactly how many have been tested. Cuban data do suggest that a very large proportion of the population is being tested even if this does not include all of those who are sexually active.

To prevent an epidemic, all but four or five AIDS carriers have been quarantined initially whether or not they manifest symptoms, and those with symptoms, of course, have been hospitalized and treated. Quarantine is voluntary, according to a ministry official, but considerable pressure is brought to bear on those who resist. It is contended that most people decide to enter the sanitoriums because they desire treatment, fear infecting their family and friends, and fear rejection.[87] The complex of homes provided to those quarantined is luxurious by Cuban standards, the food abundant, and the treatment humane, but the conditions most likely do not compensate for the loss of freedom.[88]

Those living at these sanatoriums have unlimited but controlled contact with their families and friends, are allowed to go out for various social purposes, and get weekend passes to go home, but only under the watchful eye of a relative or a designated medical student. The ministry's policy has evolved since 1986 when the first

AIDS cases were discovered and confined, so that now, rather than quarantine, the ultimate goal is to educate and treat those affected to enable them to return to their communities, jobs, families, and friends. This policy had been stated in 1990 but had not yet been acted on. As the economy deteriorated, patients did not want to leave the sanatoriums because they would eat far less and live in much worse conditions outside.[89]

Whereas the at-risk groups and HIV carriers in the United States find the government, insurance companies, much of the medical profession, their employers, and landlords largely unsympathetic to their needs, Cubans find that although their government gives them no real choice but to undergo quarantine (despite rhetoric to the contrary), it is also making great efforts to provide them with considerate medical attention, drugs available on the international market, and experimental treatments devised locally. Moreover, patients confined to the sanatorium are paid their normal salary even though they can no longer work, and they do not have to pay for either residency or treatment. Where possible they work or study within the confines of the sanatorium, but many have no occupation other than recreational handicrafts. Many Cubans oppose quarantine simply because they resent what they perceive as the "good life" of those in the sanatoriums who are not yet symptomatic. They resent the material conditions of the sanatoriums, which are better than those available to most Cubans, and the fact that those quarantined do not have to work to get paid.[90]

Whereas U.S. observers argue that neither mass screening nor quarantine is necessary, some health officials from Latin America have expressed admiration for Cuba's ability to conduct mass screening. One official commented that only Cuba had the technical ability to do it.[91] Insofar as the Cuban people expect their government to safeguard their health, and given that the state espouses the protection of societal health over the rights of the individual, many Cubans, although not necessarily those adversely affected by mass HIV screening and quarantine, may agree with these practices.

In fact, this popular expectation of governmental protection from illness has a negative side. Many Cubans feel safe from AIDS precisely because their government has been so successful in the past in eradicating disease and because it has carried out mass screening and institutionalized all of those affected. They wrongly believe that all HIV carriers are in sanatoriums, and they do not seem to recognize that not all of the infection chains may have been discovered.[92]

This failure to recognize the danger of AIDS has occurred despite the production of considerable health promotion materials and regular newspaper articles, television shows, and radio programs that thoroughly discuss the causes, nature, prevention, and consequences of AIDS.[93] AIDS prevention pamphlets are simple and clearly written, emphasize safe sex, and explain that condoms are inexpensive, easily obtainable at pharmacies, and most important, do not interfere with sexual pleasure.[94]

Cuba's approach to AIDS and dengue are similar in that the government has made a tremendous effort to combat both diseases. Some observers look at the successful dengue campaign as a model for the AIDS endeavor, but because the natures and causes of the two diseases differ, these efforts differ greatly also. One, of course, can only be brought under control by a change in human behavior and the other only through the manipulation of the dengue vector's environment. What is common to both is the mass educational effort (successful in one case but only marginally so in the other) and institutionalization (hospitalization) of victims of the disease and in the case of AIDS, of carriers too. In both instances an all-out effort, right or wrong, has been made to reduce the incidence of disease, not without great cost in both hard currency and human resources. Quarantine is a human rights issue, and only time will tell if it can stem the tide of AIDS and thus possibly be justified. The Cuban medical system is able to limit the AIDS epidemic and thereby avoid the crushing burden on its hospitals and extended care facilities that the United States faces. That Cuba developed the equipment (SUMA) and reagents to perform mass screenings for AIDS symbolically places it among the developed countries, and Cuba's ability to launch a national screening program symbolizes its biomedical prowess. Furthermore, both developed and developing countries' health officials have asked for Cuban assistance in establishing AIDS sanitoriums.[95] Among the developing countries, only Cuba has and uses these capabilities, rightly or wrongly.

SYMBOLISM AND SUBSTANCE:
THE BATTLE AGAINST DENGUE FEVER

The campaign to eradicate hemorrhagic dengue fever, a potentially fatal disease that was introduced into Cuba in May 1981 and reached epidemic proportions by mid June 1981, affords an excellent example of the intersection of symbolic politics, health education, and the participation of mass organizations in health efforts. In his annual July 26 speech in 1981, Castro stated that there was no focal point in the world for the serotype of dengue found in Cuba at that time; therefore, he said, it must have been introduced into Cuba deliberately.[96] In 1984 he claimed that some "counterrevolutionaries confessed to having carried out biological operations against Cuba at that time."[97]

Castro did not directly accuse the United States of biological warfare in his 1981 speech but devoted almost half of it to that possibility and strongly suggested that this was the case. There is considerable documentation that the U.S. Army had been working on biological weapons for decades and that dengue was well suited to biological warfare.[98] Recognition of this fact led Castro to his allegation. The dengue campaign thus epitomizes the intersection of symbolic politics and health through the ensuing symbolic war between Cuba and the United States.[99]

The nation was put on war footing to do battle against dengue. The Ministry of Public Health organized a national campaign to eradicate the dengue vector, the *Aedes aegypti* mosquito. The news media carried daily stories on the nature of the disease, the vector that causes it, and a set of seven norms that the ministry had established for the detection and eradication of *A. aegypti*. There were graphic descriptions of the mosquito as well as of its favorite breeding places.

Since *A. aegypti* lays its eggs in bodies of standing water or in anything that will hold water—particularly old tires, buckets, flower pots, and pets' water dishes—the campaign included a general cleaning of the entire country to eliminate garbage, trash, and junk that might be a breeding place for the vector.[100] This general tidying up was like a ritual cleansing, symbolic of the decontamination of society and expulsion of the allegedly U.S.–perpetrated disease.

The entire population was mobilized to fight the *A. aegypti* through the mass organizations, the unions, and the Communist party. Members of the CDRs, called *cederistas,* were mobilized to seek out and eliminate breeding places in their neighborhoods, to fill and distribute bags of the larvicide Abate on their blocks, and to attend special health lectures (*audiencias sanitarias especiales*) on methods of eliminating the vector. Discussion of these ministry directives took place in 70,224 block committees and was scheduled to be repeated in all 81,000 block committees.[101]

Administrative groups were established in each CDR zone, presided over by a *cederista* campaign coordinator and composed of representatives of the FMC, the National Association of Small Farmers (ANAP), a health activist, and the Federation of Middle School Students (FEEM) or Federation of University Students (FEU).[102] Each group was responsible for helping direct the anti-dengue campaign at the neighborhood level, a campaign in which each person was to become a vigilante for health.[103]

The FMC was also mobilized to assist the CDRs, as well as to carry out general environmental cleaning and to help educate the population about the symptoms of dengue and the necessity for immediate medical attention. FMC workers insisted that those with symptoms be seen at the nearest health facility. FMC members helped the FMC health brigade and hospital personnel in whatever way and wherever possible.[104] They also helped women with hospitalized children attend their children at the hospitals.[105]

The union, the Confederation of Cuban Workers (CTC), also mobilized its members to carry out inspections of their workplaces and to apply larvicide to any actual or potential breeding places on the premises. Once the call was made to the unionists to mobilize, training sessions were set up immediately so that the program announced on July 15 would be carried out between July 20 and July 31. Certificates (moral incentives) were awarded to work centers that had eradicated the source of dengue.[106]

The ANAP asked its members and all small farmers and peasants to redouble their efforts to eliminate potential sources of the mosquito and to apply various larvicides to all possible breeding places. Further, the ANAP called for the establishment of committees for control and inspection to ensure that the health rules and measures would be followed in the rural areas.[107]

In addition to mass mobilization, the Ministry of Public Health also conducted a program of aerial spraying, covering more than 240,000 hectares by July 6. It reported in *Granma* the workplaces that failed to comply with ministry regulations, attempting to embarrass them into action. In these reports the ministry indicated that although it was the duty of the administration of each workplace to carry out these health directives, the union should rectify the situation itself if the administration failed to act. The ministry also announced in the newspaper those workplaces that would receive fines for failure to comply with these public health measures under decree-law 27.[108]

Finally, a "health army" (*ejército de la salud*) was established comprising 13,061 trained men and women rigorously selected by People's Power, the municipal health administrations, the FMC, and the Union of Young Communists, with the assistance of the party. The health army was charged with the continuous inspection and elimination of real and possible breeding places and equipped with backpack larvicide sprayers.[109] This group of trained volunteers would remain available to carry out vector elimination in the future. In 1988 health-army workers (now paid rather than volunteer) dressed in grey uniforms emblazoned with *Aedes aegypti* were still inspecting buildings every month.[110]

As a result of this massive effort by the Cuban people and by the health professionals who worked overtime daily, there were only 158 fatalities (101 children and 57 adults) out of the 344,203 cases of dengue reported. More than 116,000 dengue victims were hospitalized in improvised intensive-care units established in all hospitals, but there were only 9,128 severe and very severe cases among children and 1,097 among adults. The last case was reported on October 10, 1981, four months after the outbreak had reached epidemic proportions.[111]

The dengue vector was eradicated and the epidemic quelled, but at a cost to the Cuban government of 42,732,720 Cuban pesos (approximately U.S. $53,415,900 at the official exchange rate), half of which was spent in foreign exchange,[112] not to mention the loss of life, the debilitation of many people, and the enormous expenditure of human resources. No government in the Third World and few in the developed countries could have achieved as much as rapidly as the Cubans did, because most lack this national capacity to mobilize.[113]

In the final analysis, the dengue campaign had all the trappings of a war effort. Enthusiasm was whipped up through daily news articles and radio and television announcements. An emulation campaign or socialist competition was carried out in which work centers received certificates for liberating their workplaces from the dengue vector. A health army was created, complete with uniforms and assault equipment (larvicide sprayers). Everyone participated. This was an all-out assault against public enemy number one. The battle against the mosquito brought people together as only an external threat can.

In addition to enhancing communal bonds,[114] the dengue campaign had great symbolic importance. It was an opportunity for the collectivity to achieve a clear victory over an enemy and thereby rebuild communal self-esteem and honor. The latter was particularly important because the epidemic occurred only one year after the 1980 Mariel exodus in which 125,000 Cubans went into exile. Despite the popular images of hundreds of thousands of Cubans marching in the streets (*el pueblo combatiente*) in support of the regime and against the Mariel exodus—propaganda images produced both for export and internal consumption—Mariel was a wrenching experience that tore apart families and friends.[115] The collective effort against dengue helped recreate social cohesion.

The symbolic victory over the dengue vector was also important because of threats from the Reagan administration, particularly Secretary of State Alexander Haig's threats to "go to the source" of rebellion in Central America and to hold Cuba hostage for Afghanistan. The Cuban government responded with increased vigilance and the reestablishment of territorial militias. Military training for militia members became a common sight on weekends and in the evenings. That Cuba would not have an opportunity to win a military victory over the United States made it all the more important to win one over dengue, because the dengue "invasion" was a metaphor for a U.S invasion. Thus the victory over dengue represented victory over the United States. Once again, Cuba accumulated symbolic capital from a successful health campaign.

In sum, popular participation and health education are intertwined. Participation is education and education is necessary for social change. Social change occurs when increasingly larger numbers of people participate in "activities that direct attention away from the self and toward the collectivity, activities that wordlessly but dramatically teach the lessons of development and underdevelopment."[116]

Health efforts in which the community participates serve this function of promoting societal transformation. Participation and health education stimulate the people to take responsibility for their own health and that of their community. By creating a population literate in health matters and able to implement health programs, the Cuban government has extended the reach of its health care providers, reduced morbidity and mortality, and thereby increased its symbolic capital and legitimacy. This accumulation of symbolic capital lends credence to Cuba's claims that it is becoming a world medical power and concretely adds to the repertoire of experience Cuba is able to share with other developing nations through its medical diplomacy programs. And as the campaign against dengue illustrates, popular participation and health education can be used successfully for larger, symbolic political ends.

4

Domestic Factors Underpinning World Medical Eminence

A country that aspires to utilize medical diplomacy must first have achieved considerable success in developing its own health resources, and it must have attained health indicators worthy of emulation. Cuba has made very impressive gains in the health sphere that are important not only in and of themselves but also because the government uses them successfully for symbolic advantage. This explains why the government has been making such an extraordinary effort to decrease infant mortality, increase life expectancy, improve all other health indicators, and produce so many doctors.

By concentrating its resources in the health field both domestically and internationally, Cuba already has become a showcase for achievement in health. Its success has been highly acclaimed by Dr. Halfdan Mahler, the Director General of the World Health Organization until mid 1988, and Dr. Carlyle Guerra de Macedo, Director General of the Pan American Health Organization, as well as by a number of medical professionals from the United States and other capitalist countries who have gone to Cuba to observe its health system.[1] Both Dr. Mahler and Dr. Guerra de Macedo, in fact, have glorified the values embodied in the Cuban experience by making Cuba the site of numerous international health conferences over the years, particularly, but not only, conferences addressing primary health care.

Cuba's health accomplishments are striking enough to sway even the country's most bitter enemy. Despite the United States's hostility toward Cuba, a 1982 U.S. government document states that

the Cuban revolution has managed social achievements, especially in education and health care, that are highly respected in the Third World. . . . [These include] establishment of a national health care program that is superior in the Third World and rivals that of numerous developed countries.[2]

Although critics may argue that, for example, life expectancy has improved in all countries because of generalized medical advancements, Sergio Díaz-Briquets's exhaustive analysis of the mortality decline in Cuba concludes that the revolution's amelioration of the urban-rural gap and the Havana-interior gap and its provision of universal health care "appears to be the main causative factor behind Cuba's impressive gain in life expectancy."[3]

Cuba's success was built on a solid base. Prerevolutionary Cuba had relatively good health indices, but its statistics were neither complete nor reliable. Maldistribution of health resources was acute, with Havana siphoning off most personnel and monies. Although there was a good overall physician-to-population ratio, few physicians practiced outside of the cities and most were in Havana. Half of these doctors fled shortly after the triumph of the revolution. Malnutrition, parasites, and other diseases of poverty afflicted the majority of rural dwellers. Sanitation facilities and potable water were scarce everywhere, including in the capital.[4]

Thus Cuba's internationally acclaimed postrevolutionary success in the health sphere spurred Castro to announce in January 1985 that Cuba had stopped comparing its health statistics with those of other developing countries and had officially begun comparing them to those of the United States.[5] Furthermore, Castro claimed that Cuba was competing with all capitalist countries and expected to surpass their health indicators by the year 2000 in its drive to become a world medical power.[6] By 1991 geopolitics has made this goal merely a pipe dream.

Table 3: Selected Health Statistics for Cuba, the United States, the Soviet Union, and Latin American Averages, Developed Countries Averages, and Developing Countries Averages (LDCs), 1986

Item	Cuba	U.S.	USSR	L.A.Avg.[a]	Developed Countries Averages	LDC Avg.
Public health expenditures per capita (US$)	84	783	270	31	521	11
Population per physician	455	482	235	947	376	1,946
Population per hospital bed	190	190	80	360	100	590
Life expectancy at birth	73	75	69	66	73	61
Infant mortality (per 1,000 births)	15	56	24	56[b]	14	79
Percent population with safe water[c]	82	100	100	71	97	54

[a] Latin American averages include Cuba.
[b] Data for most developing countries, except Cuba, understate infant mortality because of the inadequacy of registration systems.
[c] Data are for any year available from around 1986.

SOURCE: Ruth Leger Sivard, *World Military and Social Expenditures 1989* (Washington, D.C.: World Priorities, 1989), 50–51.

Cuba's Success:
Comparative Health Indicators

A comparison of Cuban health statistics with those of both developing and developed nations demonstrates that the Cubans have had good reason to compare themselves with the United States and to consider themselves a competitor because, as table 3 shows, their health indicators are closer to those of the developed nations than to those of the developing nations. Cuba's success in achieving these health indices is illustrated by the infant mortality rate and life expectancy at birth, two indicators that are very difficult to alter once a level of health comparable to Cuba's is attained. Although caution must be exercised in making international comparisons of social data because of the inadequacy of many statistical systems and because of varying data quality and methodologies, among other factors, it is useful to look at comparisons for trends, however conditional they may be. The following data are therefore suggestive but not definitive.

Already in 1982 Cuba's infant mortality rate was only 1 point higher than the average rate for all of the developed countries and 73 points lower than the average rate for all of the developing nations. It was also lower than all of the then Warsaw Pact countries' rates, except for East Germany and Czechoslovakia, and was the lowest rate in Latin America.[7] The same comparisons made for 1986 reveal that Cuba's infant mortality rate was still 1 point above the developed countries' average, 5 points above the U.S.'s rate, 54 points below the developing countries' average, 7 points below the Warsaw Pact's average, 41 points below Latin America's average, and, of course, still the lowest rate in Latin America. Among the Warsaw Pact countries, only the German Democratic Republic had a lower infant mortality rate than Cuba in 1986.[8]

In 1984 Cuba's infant mortality rate was 15 per 1,000 live births, only 4.2 points higher than the U.S.'s rate and one of the fifteen lowest in the world.[9] Data for 1985 indicated a slight increase in Cuba's infant mortality rate to 16.5 per 1,000 live births.[10] Cuban authorities vowed to redouble their efforts to again lower the rate to below 15 per 1,000 live births for 1986.[11] Given the importance the Cuban government has placed on reducing infant mortality as part of the strategy to become a world medical power and given its competition with the United States, it is not surprising that this rate decreased beyond what was predicted to 13.6 per 1,000 live births in 1986, 13.3 in 1987, 11.9 in 1988, 11.1 in 1989, 10.7 in 1990, and rose to only 10.7 in 1991 despite the economic crisis.[12] (See table 4 for provincial differences over time.)

The latest data for the United States indicated an infant mortality rate of 10.6 per 1,000 live births in 1985; 10.4 in 1986, 10.1 for 1987, 10.0 for 1988, and a preliminary rate of 9.7 for 1989. In all U.S. cases, the rates for African-Americans were double those for whites and almost double the national rate.[13] These data suggest that Cuba has substantially narrowed the gap between its infant mortality rate and that of the United States and thereby has accumulated considerable symbolic capital.

Once the infant mortality rate has decreased to the level achieved by both Cuba and the United States, medical intervention and genetic

Table 4: Infant Mortality Rates (Deaths per 1000 Live Births) by Age
Group and Province, 1979, 1989, and 1990

	Less Than 1 Year			Less Than 7 Days	
Province	*1979*	*1989*	*1990*	*1979*	*1989*
Pinar del Río	20.4	11.2	8.3	12.9	5.4
La Habana	19.0	9.7	9.8	10.8	5.1
Cd. de La Habana	16.2	10.4	10.0	9.5	5.0
Matanzas	14.9	10.7	12.1	9.1	5.2
Villa Clara	15.6	9.2	7.6	9.7	3.8
Cienfuegos	17.3	8.2	9.9	12.0	3.7
Sancti Spíritus	20.5	12.6	7.7	12.1	6.6
Ciego de Avila	20.2	12.6	11.5	12.4	5.7
Camagüey	18.3	10.6	11.4	10.5	5.5
Las Tunas	26.1	13.2	12.9	17.1	7.4
Holguín	18.5	11.6	12.0	9.1	5.9
Granma	23.9	11.9	13.5	12.7	5.5
Santiago de Cuba	19.5	11.8	11.4	11.5	5.4
Guantánamo	24.1	12.0	10.9	12.7	5.8
Isla de la Juventud	14.7	10.9	10.4	8.8	5.8
Average	19.4	11.1	10.7	11.3	5.4

SOURCES: Ministerio de Salud Pública, Dirección Nacional de Estadísticas, *Informe anual
1979* (La Habana: MINSAP, 1980), xvi–xvii; *Informe anual 1989* (La Habana:
MINSAP, 1990), 34; and *Granma Weekly Review,* January 20, 1991, 4.

screening become much more important. Neonatal mortality (early
mortality is less than seven days, and late mortality is seven to twenty-
seven days), the primary component of infant mortality in the more
socioeconomically advanced countries (including Cuba), is directly
related to biological factors and to the quality and sophistication of
hospital care. It is by far the most difficult and costly rate to reduce
because heavy investments must be made in high-technology hospital
infrastructure and services to do so.[14] Consequently, had it not been
for the economic devastation of change in the former socialist world,
Cuba's infant mortality rate probably would have continued to decrease as further efforts in that direction continued. These efforts
included installation of perinatal intensive care units in all maternity
hospitals in 1987, increased genetic screening for congenital abnormalities, and the intensified efforts of the family doctors.[15]

Table 5: Life Expectancy at Birth by Province, 1977–78, 1982–83 and 1985–90

Province	1977–78	1982–83	1985–90
Pinar del Río	72.87	74.91	75.51
La Habana	74.27	75.25	76.01
Cd. de La Habana	72.01	73.42	74.21
Matanzas	73.53	74.75	75.51
Villa Clara	73.87	75.66	76.01
Cienfuegos	74.30	75.16	76.01
Sancti Spíritus	73.83	75.29	76.01
Ciego de Avila	72.87	74.96	75.51
Camagüey	72.09	74.49	74.21
Las Tunas	73.21	75.31	76.01
Holguín	72.83	75.36	76.01
Granma	72.70	74.97	75.51
Santiago de Cuba	72.34	74.17	74.21
Guantánamo	72.15	74.97	75.51
Isla de la Juventud	73.01	74.77	75.51
Cuba	72.72	74.22	75.22

SOURCE: Reproduced from Ministerio de Salud Pública, Dirección Nacional de Estadísticas, *Informe anual 1987* (La Habana: MINSAP, 1988), 9, and *Informe anual 1989* (La Habana: 1990), 23.

Cuba has also achieved status comparable to that of the United States in life expectancy. In 1982 life expectancy at birth in Cuba was surpassed only by Japan, Sweden, Switzerland, Denmark, Iceland, the Netherlands, and Norway, and was equaled by the United States, Canada, Australia, Belgium, and France.[16] Life expectancy at birth in Cuba was 74.2 years in 1985, whereas in the United States it was 74.7 years.[17] The 1985–1990 life expectancy projection for Cuba was 75.2 years, the 1990–1995 estimate was 75.7 years, and the preliminary figure for the United States for 1988 was 74.9 years, with a projection for 1990 of 75.6 years.[18] Since at this level of health, increases in life expectancy are minimal and difficult to achieve, it is unlikely that either Cuban or U.S. life-expectancy data will significantly outstrip the other country's in the next few years now that they have achieved parity, a symbolically significant achievement for Cuba. (See table 5 for provincial differences over time.)

The five major causes of death both for the general population and for infants were the same in 1982 for Cuba and the United States.[19] In 1987–1988 the major causes of death were the same for the general population, and four out of five were the same for infants.[20] Only in medical expenditures per capita did Cuba lag far behind the United States,[21] suggesting that "expenditure on health services more often reflects the health of the health services than the health of the people."[22] Cuba's lower per capita expenditure to achieve health indices similar to those of the developed countries suggests that health care is not as expensive as one might imagine and that health care alone will not improve the population's well-being, but that meeting the entire population's basic human needs, including medical services, through resource redistribution will.

Money is necessary but not sufficient to improve a people's health. Government intervention is essential to guarantee access to health care and to guarantee, therefore, greater effectiveness of the medical system. Comparisons of Canada, the United States, and Britain "suggest that among these three countries health is inversely related to health-care costs, but directly related to the degree of governmental intervention in health care delivery."[23] The government of Cuba is the sole provider of health care,[24] and gives high priority to allocating resources—fiscal, physical, and human—to achieve its health goals.

THE CREDIBILITY OF CUBA'S HEALTH CLAIMS

The credibility of Cuba's claims depends in part on the reliability and consistency of its demographic statistics. There is little debate about the statistics; most experts have concluded that the data are "of very high quality".[25] Since 1972 Cuban health statistics have been considered very reliable by the statistical office of PAHO.[26] Recent research evaluating Cuban data over time has confirmed the experts' view that the statistics are complete and trustworthy.[27]

That the Cubans do not hide negative trends in their health statistics as the Soviets did from 1971 until 1989 indicates their honesty in reporting their population's health status whatever it may be.[28] Moreover, Cuba's data are carefully scrutinized from a variety of perspectives and have been upheld.[29] The reliability of these data substantiates Cuba's success in dramatically lowering the infant mortality rate and in raising life expectancy to levels characteristic of developed nations. Since in Cuba health indicators are measures of government efficacy, the government's claims that in the near future Cuba would achieve health indicators that would surpass those of the United States very well might have been credible had the world around Cuba not changed so rapidly.

In fact, studies in the United States before 1982 indicated that the infant mortality rate in the United States would increase for the post-1982 period as the effects of decreased federal spending for welfare and other social services for the poor were felt and as the effects of unemployment, lack of health insurance, and hunger became more pronounced.[30] Although the overall infant mortality rate did not increase, the rate of decrease slowed considerably from 1982 on, and the neonatal death rate increased in 1985. The actual number of both early and late neonatal deaths and post-neonatal deaths (between twenty-eight days and eleven months) increased, the former in 1983 and the latter in 1985.[31]

The Children's Defense Fund cited a 3 percent increase in post-neonatal infant mortality nationwide, the first such increase in eighteen years. The fund claimed that this increase resulted from low birth weight and from a delay in or absence of neonatal care, and that its cause could ultimately be found in the Reagan administration's cuts in medicaid, maternal and child health programs and supplemental food programs, and in the increased poverty in America. The fund's report indicates that twenty-six out of thirty-three states reporting prenatal care data for 1982 showed an increase compared to previous years in the percentage of women receiving late or no prenatal care.[32]

U.S. Census Bureau data corroborate the Children's Defense Fund findings. Between 1985 and 1987, there was an increase in the percentage of women who either began prenatal care in their third trimester of pregnancy or who had no prenatal care at all, and this increase roughly corresponded to the percentage of women who gave birth to infants of low birth weight (6.9 percent). Only 74.4 percent of women who gave birth in 1987 had prenatal care in the first trimester.[33]

Comparable data for Cuba are not available, but data in table 6 indicate that in the areas where family doctors worked in 1988 over 90 percent of the pregnant women in all but two provinces began prenatal care in their first trimester. There has been a steady increase in the number of prenatal consultations per childbirth since 1970

Table 6: Pregnancies Detected by Family Doctors by Province, First Six
Months of 1988

| | Trimester of Gestation | | | | | |
| | (1) | | (2) | | (3) | |
Province	N	%	N	%	N	%	Total
Pinar del Río	996	90.7	90	8.2	12	1.1	1098
La Habana	761	91.0	65	7.8	10	1.2	836
Cd. de La Habana	8179	94.4	457	5.3	33	0.4	8669
Matanzas	960	95.1	46	4.5	3	0.3	1009
Villa Clara	1626	94.4	90	5.2	7	0.4	1723
Cienfuegos	635	91.6	56	8.1	2	0.3	693
Sancti Spíritus	389	89.2	46	10.6	1	0.2	436
Ciego de Avila	326	94.8	15	4.4	3	0.9	344
Camagüey	1093	92.3	87	7.4	4	0.3	1184
Las Tunas	375	87.0	51	11.8	5	1.2	431
Holguín	1224	92.6	94	7.1	4	0.3	1322
Granma	1877	92.9	123	6.1	21	1.0	2021
Santiago de Cuba	3730	92.8	267	6.6	22	0.6	4019
Guantánamo	1804	84.9	276	13.0	45	2.1	2125
Isla de la Juventud	436	95.2	20	4.4	2	0.4	458

SOURCE: Reproduced from Ministerio de Salud Pública, *Médico de la familia: Información estadística* (La Habana: MINSAP, September 1988), 19.

when the number was 7.0. Consultations rose to 11.4 in 1980 and
15.1 in 1989.[34] By 1970 over 90 percent of births took place in
hospitals, and by 1973 98 percent occurred there.[35] The overall percentage of infants born with low birth weight in 1989 was 7.3 percent, only 0.4 percent above the U.S. figure.[36]

According to the 1985 Harvard Physician Task Force on Hunger
in America, the epidemic of hunger affecting approximately twenty
million people in the United States resulted from the Reagan administration's budget cuts of $12.2 billion from the food stamp and child
nutrition programs. Therefore, "Clinics in poor areas report cases of
Kwashiorkor and marasmus, two 'Third World diseases of advanced
malnutrition,' as well as vitamin deficiencies, diabetes, lethargy,
'stunting,' 'wasting,' and other health problems traceable to inadequate food."[37]

This situation contrasted with that in Cuba, which had "eliminated
almost all malnutrition, particularly among children."[38] Measuring
weight for height (to detect acute malnutrition) in preschoolers

according to the World Health Organization's methodology, the Cubans found that only 0.9 percent of the children were malnourished in 1987.[39] This was an improvement over 1980, when almost 5 percent of the total population suffered from malnutrition.[40] Even according to a 1972 study of childhood growth and development, there were no cases of second- or third-degree malnutrition, and only 3 percent of the 56,000 children examined suffered from milder first-degree malnutrition.[41] These findings compare very favorably with rates for the member countries of PAHO, where the average rate of malnutrition in 1980 was 52 percent, with 14.7 percent classified as moderate or severe.[42] By the end of the 1980s PAHO indicated that in its region "the prevalence of [total] malnutrition ranged from 2.1% to 38.0%," but that in Cuba, "There are few apparent cases of malnutrition, and in general they are secondary or associated with specific social and familial problems."[43]

Cuba's death rate from avitaminoses and nutritional deficiencies for children under the age of five in 1980 was 3.8 per 100,000 population, a rate surpassed in this hemisphere only by the United States, Canada, Puerto Rico, and Martinique. For the sake of comparison, the high end of the spectrum was 121.2 per 100,000 population in Guyana.[44] Actual deaths due to nutritional deficiencies for the same age group in 1988 numbered only 2 in Cuba but 33 in 1987 in the United States (latest U.S. data).[45]

Until the economic crisis of 1990, food in Cuba was available on the free market, but the basic foods necessary for an adequate diet were rationed to insure universal distribution. Food had become scarce by late 1990, and the number of items rationed increased to assure that the deleterious effects of the crisis would not redound to any one sector of society but would be shared by all. An emergency food program was begun in an effort to substitute local produce for Eastern European and Soviet imports no longer available, but domestic conditions do not allow the cultivation of certain crops such as wheat. Although the variety, quality, quantity, and availability of rationed foods leave much to be desired, no one had gone hungry prior to June 1991. The chances that this will occur, however, seem greater than before.[46]

During the 1980s, while the U.S. government decreased provision of prenatal care, maternal- and child-health programs, and supplemental feeding programs with its severe budget cuts, Cuba strengthened its provision of these health programs and continued its longstanding policy of providing supplemental food for pregnant and breast-feeding women and for children under the age of seven.[47] Moreover, Cuban polyclinic personnel and mass organization liaisons have sought out those women who fail to attend prenatal appointments, educational lectures, and well-baby and pediatric appointments, and have urged them to continue their prenatal care. Family doctors have done likewise. In fact, in 1986 the Family Doctor Program already had greatly decreased the infant mortality rate in areas in which they worked, particularly in the remote mountain areas where the rate decreased to less than 10 per 1,000 live births (less than the overall U.S. rate).[48] This rate was down to 6 per 1,000 live births in one remote mountainous area in 1990 and below 8 per 1,000 that year for the entire provinces of Villa Clara and Sancti Spíritus, both of which are largely rural.[49]

In a concerted effort to further decrease infant mortality, Castro ordered the construction of perinatal intensive care units in all maternal-infant hospitals.[50] In situations in which infant mortality rates are low, deaths result from genetic defects and other internal factors that require sophisticated medical treatment, particularly in the perinatal period.[51] Infant cardiovascular surgery has been performed regularly to save lives, and research is under way to perform *in utero* cardiovascular surgery.[52] Since the majority of infant deaths occur in this period, Castro's strategy, though rather costly, should be effective.

The continued expansion of genetic screening to detect congenital abnormalities, with therapeutic abortions for those whose infants would not be viable, has also lowered the infant mortality rate, not to mention the costs of care for a seriously malformed infant with little potential to be a productive member of society. Alpha fetoprotein studies conducted in 1987 on over 80 percent of pregnant women detected 505 cases of neural tube defects that led to 495 abortions and 22 cases of sickle-cell anemia that resulted in 17 abortions. Amniocentesis tests for Down syndrome were fewer because of the need to weigh the costs and risks of testing against the benefits. Down syndrome was detected in 39 of the pregnant women who underwent amniocentesis and 32 aborted.

Although a little over one-third of the infant mortality rate (between 3.0 and 3.2 per 1,000 live births) is the result of genetic diseases, genetic disease diagnosis can reduce the rate by only about one point according to Dr. Luis Heredero, provincial director of genetics for the City of Havana. Heredero stressed that the purpose of genetic screening was not just to decrease mortality. Some pathologies could be treated in utero or through pediatric surgery later, and if forewarned both the woman and the child would receive special attention at birth.[53] For those women who choose not to abort, there are special homes and schools for the physically and mentally impaired that, like all other educational and medical services, are free and well equipped.[54]

The Cubans assert that women (the ultimate decision-makers in this case) are not pressured to abort.[55] However, given the intense effort to decrease infant mortality, it is possible that, the free-choice abortion policy aside, many doctors may strongly advise and even pressure for abortion. Certainly the statistics mentioned above suggest that this might be the case. Reducing infant mortality is not the sole justification for abortion; the main justification is, rather, the desire to provide the family with a better quality of life and to prevent the suffering of the unborn child. There are no internationally accepted standards on this matter since the potential quality of life of both the unborn child and the parents must be carefully considered. Whether or not one considers abortion an ethical option, this procedure certainly has given Cuba an advantage over other countries in the race to decrease the infant mortality rate.

Cuba's universal free-education and health-care coverage, medical outreach programs, food rationing, general amelioration of socioeconomic conditions, and high priority on reducing infant mortality apparently irrespective of cost, have contributed significantly to Cuba's success in lowering its infant mortality rate to almost the same rate as that in the United States. These factors have made it more likely that Cuba would have further decreased its infant mortality rate relative to the U.S. rate rather than the reverse had the economic crisis of the early 1990s brought on by the disintegration of the socialist bloc and the Soviet Union not occurred. In so doing Cuba would have accumulated considerable symbolic capital by achieving one of its objectives in attempting to become a world medical power.

Given the current circumstances, the government is trying to maintain the health indices it has thus far achieved and still asserts that health, particularly that of infants and children, is the number one priority. By contrast to other Latin American governments, whose austerity plans have disproportionately affected the poorest segments of society, Cuba's austerity measures are designed not just to weather the economic storm, but to minimize social dislocation for all and to develop economically. In spite of a likely setback from this crisis, Cuba has accumulated substantial symbolic capital for its notable accomplishments thus far.

The Availability of Human Resources

Unlike health care systems in other developing countries, China, and the Soviet Union, Cuba has established a health-care system that, even in rural areas, is physician-based rather than paramedic-based. By the end of 1986, Cuba had 25,567 physicians, or one doctor for every 399 inhabitants, and in 1990, 38,690 doctors, or one doctor for every 274 people.[56] Projecting the general population and the physician-to-population ratio for the year 2000, Cuba would have had approximately one physician for every 196 inhabitants had the socialist world not crumbled, a ratio that far exceeds not only the island's own medical needs but also the physician-to-population ratios of the most developed countries.[57] Projections for the year 2000 for the United States indicate that there will be one physician for every 405 inhabitants.[58] Cuba's ratio would have given the country a considerable lead in the physician-to-population ratio.

Why would Cuba have had so many doctors by the year 2000? Castro believes that there are never too many doctors. If Cuba doesn't need them, then other countries do. Castro envisions not only "a doctor on every fishing boat, on every merchant ship, in every school, in every factory, on every block,"[59] but also a massive increase in biotechnology research, continuing education for physicians, and an increase in the provision of international medical aid. In 1984 Castro announced plans to train another 50,000 doctors by the year 2000 for a total of 75,000 M.D.'s, of whom 10,000 would provide international aid; 20,000 would provide primary care in the Family Doctor Program; 35,000 would staff the primary, secondary, and tertiary health-care facilities and research institutes; and 10,000 would provide a reserve so that all physicians could take a sabbatical once every seven years to update their medical knowledge and skills apart from their routine continuing education.[60] In 1986, however, the plan was reduced to 65,000 physicians by the year 2000 with the same distribution of personnel except that the 10,000 M.D. reserve for sabbaticals would be temporarily suspended, and 5,000 of the 35,000 who would staff the health facilities would instead be family doctors assigned to factories and schools.[61]

According to 1988 calculations of medical school promotions and graduations, the Ministry of Public Health expected to have all urban and rural areas fully covered by family doctors by 1995 at the latest, rather than by the year 2000. Barring unforeseen changes in the medical school dropout rate and the percentage of graduates incorporated into the Family Doctor Program, this goal should have been accomplished easily according to my calculations had the economic crisis not occurred.[62] Projections for the year 2000 called for the same total number of doctors, but those available for international duty had been reduced because of changing geopolitics and combined with sabbatical relief and reserves available for short-term replacement duty (vacation, illness, promotion, and leave). These categories would add up to a total of 10,000.[63] A PAHO report written in 1990 suggested that the residual category was for internationalists and those doing basic research or producing medical technology.[64]

Although paid sabbaticals for physicians are not unusual in communist countries, they are remarkable even for noncommunist developed countries and extraordinary for a small developing nation.[65] Whether or not this plan is implemented immediately, the mere fact that it was considered seriously and that it may eventually have been implemented is surprising for a developing nation with serious economic difficulties. The plan is indicative of Cuba's commitment to quality health care.

At the same time that Cuba was greatly increasing its pool of physicians, it was also producing a large number of other health personnel compared to other countries in the region. Conversely, the trend in most developing nations has been toward a shortage both of doctors and nursing personnel, as well as toward a shortage of nurses relative to the number of physicians. In those developing countries in which there is a good nurse-to-physician ratio, it is generally a result of the low number of physicians rather than of an adequate physician-support system, whereas in developed countries it may reflect adequate coverage for hospital-based and long-term care.

The nurse-to-physician ratio is important because it promotes efficiency in health-care delivery and extends scarce resources by allowing the doctor to delegate routine work to the nurse. The 1980 goal for the PAHO region was 237 nursing personnel for every 100 medical doctors. This goal, of course, was based on the assumption that most countries would have insufficient numbers of doctors and that this ratio would be efficient. Although Cuba did not meet the 1980 goal because it produces both many physicians and many nurses, it did reach the goal by 1987 by vastly increasing the number of nurses in training. In 1989 it had just under 2 nurses for every doctor, but only 1.7 for every doctor in 1990.[66]

In 1984 Cuba's ratio of physicians to 10,000 population was almost double that of Latin America's, and Cuba's ratio of nurses to 10,000 population was almost seven times that of Latin America's.[67] Since these data are no longer published by PAHO, a current comparison cannot be made. Suffice it to say that Cuba has continued to produce very large numbers of both doctors and nurses but has sought parity in numbers for the Family Doctor Program. In 1990 Cuba had 36.5 doctors per 10,000 population and in 1989, 60.9 nurses and 47.4 middle-level health technicians per 10,000 inhabitants.[68]

From 1959 through 1989, the Cuban government had trained 157,064 nurses and other intermediate-level health technicians, 2,465 university-trained nurses, 6,642 dentists, and 36,807 doctors.[69] Medical school enrollments for the 1989–1990 academic year totaled 27,924, of whom 53.9 percent were female. So many women have become doctors that the official policy for some years has been to try to achieve parity between men and women in enrollments so as not to make medicine strictly a feminine profession. In addition, at the university level there were 3,037 dental students, 6,293 graduate nursing students, and 51 graduate health technologists, and at the vocational high school level there were 21,712 students, of whom 15,620 were studying nursing.[70] For the 1990–1991 academic year, there were 26,888 medical students, 2,980 stomatology students, and 7,970 graduate nursing students.[71]

Medical-education policy has changed to reflect changing needs rather than to respond to any crisis resulting from the "special period." The Cubans finally realized that they did not need to continue training so many doctors because they will have more than enough to fill all of the projected posts before the year 2000 and because the dropout rate had stabilized at about 10 percent for the first year and between 5 and 10 percent for the second year. After the second year, there generally are few if any dropouts.[72] First-year medical school enrollments were at 5,500 until 1988 but decreased to 4,500 in 1989, 3,500 in 1990 and 1991, and are projected to decrease somewhat in 1992, although there was no decision as to how much.[73] The emphasis now is on increasing specialty training, which would consist of the obligatory Comprehensive General Medicine residency and second residencies in other medical fields.[74] There were already 17,291 medical specialists and 12,479 residents in 1990, which means that 45 percent of all Cuban doctors are specialists and 77 percent are either specialists or in training as specialists.[75]

The nature and numbers of nurses being trained has also changed. Since 1987 the goal has been to require university-level training for nurses. The last class of nurses to be trained as middle-level technicians entered school in the 1990–1991 academic year. Henceforth, the quality of nursing is expected to improve and the numbers to increase in proportion to the decrease in the number of medical students. These changes ensure that there will be no wasted infrastructure in the medical schools and that total enrollments will remain steady because doctors, stomatologists, and nurses train in the same school. There will be no change in the numbers of stomatologists trained because there is still need for more.[76]

The Cuban government views health policy partially but not entirely as a reaction to the ever-increasing needs, demands, and desires of the populace. This view has been expressed by former Minister of Public Health Dr. José A. Gutiérrez Muñiz, who stated that the health services' "objectives are not only . . . to satisfy the community's demands, but fundamentally to cover needs, often not [yet] felt by the population."[77] Cuban health education, particularly through media coverage of new techniques and technologies, has created the demand for continuous expansion and improvement of health-care delivery and services.

Yet the realization that physicians are a good export commodity, politically and economically, also helps explain Cuba's past human resource policy.[78] Altruism, the lure of hard-currency earnings, and other political aspirations such as the accumulation of symbolic capital also motivated Cuba's greatly increased production of physicians. Whether or not one agrees that Cuba's massive production of doctors is warranted in strictly medical terms, this policy appears justified in light of these and other long-range objectives such as placing a doctor on every block.

DISTRIBUTION OF MEDICAL PERSONNEL

More important than sheer numbers is the actual distribution of medical personnel across the country. Because the Cuban government has controlled entry into medical school, the type of training received, and employment upon graduation, it has been able to produce the quantity and variety of physicians needed according to its long-range plans. Problems such as understaffing of physicians in hospitals in the eastern provinces have been remedied with specialists from Havana filling the gaps on five-year assignments until enough local people could be trained. And family doctors have been dispatched from Havana to provide primary care to dispersed rural populations. Less-developed specialties also have been given priority in medical education.[79] Nonetheless, distributional differences persist, as can be seen in table 7, but can be explained in large part by the imperatives of a regionalized, hierarchically organized national health system.

The most pronounced distributional difference is that between City of Havana province and the rest of the country. Approximately 20 percent of the total population lives in the province, yet in 1989 41.3 percent of the physicians worked there, down from about 63 percent prior to the revolution. The disparity between the percentage of total population and the percentage of doctors per province is generally 1 to 2 percent except in Granma and Holguín provinces, where it is 3.5 and 4.0 percent respectively. There is exact parity in only two provinces, Santiago de Cuba and Isla de la Juventud.[80] Why do these distributional differences persist despite revolutionary policy to ameliorate the rural-urban gap and the Havana-interior gap?

First, the capital houses the major research institutes, tertiary care and specialty hospitals, many of the pharmaceutical and medical products industries, more medical schools than the other provinces (each has at least one medical school except La Habana), and the Ministry of Public Health. Regionalization of the unified national health system requires a geographic hierarchical ordering of services with referral from one level of care to the next. For efficiency and cost-effectiveness, it is reasonable for these entities to be in close proximity and in the area of highest population density, Havana. As mentioned earlier, the Hermanos Ameijeiras Hospital's policy is to

Table 7: Distribution of Medical Facilities and Staff by Province, 1989

Province	Population 1989 (1,000s)	N Hospitals (1,000s)	Hospital beds per 1,000 population	Population per M.D. and D.D.S.	
Pinar del Río	687.2	18	5.1	414	2,027
La Habana	638.7	8	2.1	454	1,398
Cd. de La Habana[a]	2,088.8	47	11.4	146	1,016
Matanzas	604.8	10	4.6	342	1,575
Villa Clara	803.6	17	4.1	333	2,040
Cienfuegos	360.0	6	4.1	393	1,800
Sancti Spíritus	425.7	21	5.2	449	2,087
Ciego de Avila	360.8	9	4.0	497	1,860
Camagüey	735.8	23	6.3	392	1,931
Las Tunas	489.4	12	4.6	559	2,472
Holguín	984.4	24	4.2	523	2,395
Granma	783.3	23	4.4	569	2,543
Santiago de Cuba	982.3	27	6.1	302	1,554
Guantánamo	489.4	16	4.6	460	1,793
Isla de la Juventud	72.7	2	7.7	288	1,398
Totals	10,506.9	263			
Averages			6.0	302	1,621

[a]Figures for Ciudad de La Habana include tertiary care facilities and specialized hospitals and medical personnel that receive islandwide referrals and treat foreigners.

SOURCES: República de Cuba, Ministerio de Salud Pública, *Informe anual 1989* (La Habana: MINSAP, 1990), 19, 90, 94–96.

reserve 70 percent of its beds for referrals from other provinces. Other major cities house secondary- and some tertiary-care facilities based on the geographic and demographic imperatives of regionalization, but Havana remains the major referral center.

Second, physicians on internationalist missions or working in administrative positions are included in the totals for the provinces whence they come. In assessing the 1985 distribution of personnel, the Director of National Development for the ministry wrote that 29.9 percent of all physicians provided medical care in City of Havana province and 7.0 percent in Santiago de Cuba province at a time when 20 percent of the population lived in Havana and 3.6 in Santiago, and when according to aggregate figures, 42.1 percent of the physicians practiced in Havana and 8.1 percent in Santiago.[81] The director included a residual category of 16.5 percent who did not provide patient care but could be assumed to be in administration, teaching, or research positions, or employed by other ministries or by the party. These data also indicate that 10.5 percent were on internationalist missions and were not included in the provincial totals.[82] Thus the apparent 1986 maldistribution (and because of the similarity in numbers, the 1989 one by implication) seems to be a fiction.

Third, in 1986 City of Havana province had the lowest life expectancy in Cuba and a higher incidence of some diseases than other provinces; therefore the Habaneros may have needed more medical care than other Cubans.[83] The higher incidence of certain ailments may be a result of better reporting because of the greater number of doctors, but the lower life expectancy indicates that the problem is real. Certainly there is greater crowding in Havana, greater environmental pollution, and thus a less salubrious life. The infant mortality rate was the second lowest on the island, suggesting that it is better to be born in Havana than to live there.[84] (See tables 4 and 5 above.) This was no longer the case in 1989 when both Cienfuegos and Villa Clara provinces registered lower infant mortality rates than Havana. In that year the latter was tied with two other provinces for the lowest life-expectancy.[85]

Fourth, the rather high ratio of doctors to population on the Isla de la Juventud is the result of the large number of secondary boarding schools for both Cuban and foreign youth. This proportion of doctors to population is an expression of governmental concern for the development and well-being of youth. Fifth, those provinces that are predominantly rural, such as Granma and Las Tunas, have fewer physicians because, as in most countries, fewer are willing to live in rural areas, and because the population is so dispersed that a considerable increase in the number of physicians, perhaps beyond what would seem reasonable, would be required. For this reason the government established medical schools in all the provinces to train local people who would stay in their home provinces upon graduation. Also, the Family Doctor Program has been sending physicians from Havana and other cities to live in the more remote rural areas to seek out (often on horseback) and treat dispersed populations. Although the Cuban government has considerably narrowed the distributional gap, it still is working toward greater equity in health resources, though its efforts have been hampered by the collapse of socialism elsewhere.

By contrast the U.S. government is unable to rectify distributional imbalances in either specialty or geography without a radical change in policy (such as the creation of a national health service or a community service requirement for all graduates). U.S. physicians cannot be sent to underserved areas unless they are paying back educational loans or working for the U.S. Public Health Service. Even then, if conditions are not satisfactory they can leave. Further, federally employed physicians comprised only 4 percent of all U.S. physicians in both 1983 and 1987, indicating the limits of government control over their distribution.[86]

The following example of the United States's difficulty in ameliorating the maldistribution of physicians is quite revealing. According to Dr. Jo Ivey Boufford, president of New York City's Health and Hospitals Corporation, a 1986 program of financial incentives to encourage doctors to serve in poor areas attracted only 111 applicants, of whom half were not qualified. "Others dropped out because they would not be on the staff of a city hospital or because they could not expect to get rich." Thus the doctors' homesteading program added only 5 new doctors to serve the poor.[87] Despite some distributional differences, all Cuban provinces fare considerably better than the Latin American average in physicians and nurses per 10,000 population.[88] Compared to other countries, both developed and developing, in which rural areas and urban ghettos are underserved if served at all, Cuba has a rather equitable distribution of medical personnel.

By the year 2000, Cuba would probably have had slightly more than twice the number of physicians per inhabitant than would the United States if current projections remained valid. From a U.S. perspective, Cuba's very high doctor-to-inhabitant ratio might seem unwarranted. Despite projections of a much lower ratio, the U.S. Graduate Medical Education National Advisory Council (GMENAC) report warns of an increase in the existing surplus of physicians in the United States by the turn of the century. The GMENAC report calls for "rapid and decisive action if a gross oversupply is to be averted."[89] In a fee-for-service environment, the problem of oversupply is critical to the health of the physicians' finances, because through the American Medical Association they control entry into the profession and attempt to keep the supply insufficient to meet the demand.

This notion of a surplus of doctors in the United States is largely a function of maldistribution. Distributional problems on a scale experienced in the United States, as noted before, are not permitted to arise in Cuba. It could be argued that the cost for Cuba of training so many physicians is very high, but this is not the case because the medical school infrastructure is already in place so that it costs the state little more to have, for example, forty students in a class than it does to have twenty.

Other means of improving health, such as improved sewerage, potable water supply, and housing, are even more costly than training and deploying doctors.[90] Nonetheless, these infrastructural improvements were being carried out in the 1980s in a frenzy of both public and private construction, but the economic crisis of the early 1990s led to a moratorium on the construction of almost all new social projects.

Some setbacks have occurred as well. Progress made in the provision of potable water, for example, was offset by the inability of the state to import chlorine beginning in mid 1990 because of the financial crisis. Sixty-five percent of the total population and 82 percent of the urban dwellers were connected to water supply systems by 1988, and over 90 percent of the water had been chlorinated until mid 1990. In addition, there was still considerable insufficiency in sewerage systems in 1988, although some new systems were under construction at that time.[91] Once again, after completion of projects underway, no new ones would be executed for the short term.

Because Cuba has a large pool of educated and skilled laborers and the infrastructure to produce more without recourse to hard-currency expenditures, it is cheaper to make changes that require human capital rather than fiscal capital. It is, therefore, more cost-effective for Cuba to train more health workers of any sort or to provide health education to the population than to use scarce hard currency to buy chlorine to treat the water. An educated populace such as Cuba's can simply be instructed to boil water before using it. Moreover, doctors are more visible and more versatile than chlorinated water. This is one of the host of reasons Cuba has produced so many physicians.

DISTRIBUTIONAL ISSUES AND HEALTH STATUS

Distributional disparities in health status arise in all countries, even the most developed. The factors that lead to these differences in any country are myriad, but chief among them are "poverty, illiteracy, rurality, density of professional services."[92] In Cuba the Family Doctor Program has increased the density of professional services precisely in those areas of poverty, less education, and rurality. An important question is whether the deployment of physicians on a fairly equitable basis has in fact made a difference in the people's health. After all, as even the Cuban leadership pointed out in the early days of the revolution, medicine alone would not cure the people's ills.

Although this question cannot be definitively answered because of the lack of consensus about acceptable measures and because of the complexity of the problem, it is possible to assess equality or inequality in health resources, outcomes, and processes (see tables 8 and 9). This may provide some suggestive evidence about the health system's effectiveness across provinces. Caution is in order here because the socioeconomic conditions of each province differ and may have a greater effect on health outcomes irrespective of medical action than does the medical system itself. Perhaps what the following data show is only whether the revolutionary government's commitment to ameliorate the Havana-interior gap can be demonstrated by the relative equality of health conditions. This equality is symbolically significant because few countries have achieved it across regions.

Differences in the infant mortality rates among Cuban provinces persist but have declined markedly since the revolution. This decline is demonstrated by the sharp decrease in the difference between the highest and lowest rates from 1979 to 1989, which can be seen in table 4 above. As would be expected, three provinces that have been historically less developed registered the highest infant mortality rates in 1979: Las Tunas, Guantánamo, and Granma. But by 1989 only Las Tunas still had one of the highest rates; its rate was, in fact, the highest. Guantánamo and Granma had both benefited from large infusions of family doctors as well as from socioeconomic development projects. More important, the variance among these rates was insignificant in 1989.

Table 8: Outcome Indicators by Province, 1989

Province	Infant Mortality Rate (per 1,000 live births)	Low Birth Weight (percent)	Life Expectancy at Birth
Pinar del Río	11.2	7.0	75.51
La Habana	9.7	4.5	76.01
Cd. de La Habana	10.4	6.8	74.21
Matanzas	10.7	7.1	75.51
Villa Clara	9.2	6.3	76.01
Cienfuegos	8.2	7.5	76.01
Sancti Spíritus	12.6	6.3	76.01
Ciego de Avila	12.6	7.2	75.51
Camagüey	10.6	7.2	74.21
Las Tunas	13.2	7.5	76.01
Holguín	11.6	7.7	76.01
Granma	11.9	8.5	75.51
Santiago de Cuba	11.8	8.2	74.21
Guantánamo	12.0	8.7	75.51
Isla de la Juventud	10.9	6.1	75.51
Cuba	11.1	7.3	75.22

SOURCE: Ministerio de Salud Pública, *Informe anual 1989* (La Habana: MINSAP, 1990),

The three provinces with the worst ratio of doctors to inhabitants in 1989—Granma (the worst, with one doctor for every 569 inhabitants), Las Tunas, and Holguín—as would be expected had relatively low rates of visits to the doctor, but interestingly not lower rates of well-baby visits. Both Holguín and Granma were among the three provinces with the lowest budgets for health, but this did not necessarily translate into poorer outcomes.[93] Life expectancy in Las Tunas and Holguín was among the highest in the country, and in Granma province it was in the midrange for the country as a whole. Only Las Tunas registered a significantly higher infant mortality rate (13.2 per 1,000 live births) than the national average and one of lowest number of prenatal visits per pregnancy (12.6), but neither that nor the ratio of doctors to population necessarily explain why infant mortality was higher there than elsewhere in Cuba. One thing should be made clear: Las Tunas's ratio of doctors to population, its infant mortality rate, and its number of prenatal care visits were ex-

Table 9: Process Indicators by Province, 1989

Province	Number of Visits with Doctors per Inhabitant				
	Gen. Med.	Ob.	Gyn.	Pedi. < 1 Yr.	Well Baby < 1 Yr.[a]
Pinar del Río	2.0	13.4	0.4	19.7	10.9
La Habana	2.6	17.7	0.4	20.2	9.8
Cd. de La Habana[b]	3.8	18.7	0.5	27.9	14.0
Matanzas	2.4	12.5	0.5	20.1	10.2
Villa Clara	2.7	16.7	0.4	22.8	10.8
Cienfuegos	2.7	15.0	0.4	22.3	10.2
Sancti Spíritus	2.2	18.6	0.5	19.3	9.5
Ciego de Avila	2.0	13.2	0.5	17.2	9.6
Camagüey	1.9	12.1	0.5	16.4	10.2
Las Tunas	1.3	12.6	0.5	15.3	10.1
Holguín	1.7	13.4	0.5	14.1	10.1
Granma	1.7	13.4	0.4	18.2	10.2
Santiago de Cuba	2.4	15.7	0.5	18.4	10.7
Guantánamo	1.6	12.9	0.4	18.0	12.3
Isla de la Juventud	3.1	14.5	0.7	16.3	6.7
Cuba	2.4	15.1	0.5 ·	19.9	11.0

[a]The well-baby figures are also included in the data for pediatric visits but are shown separately to assess preventive medicine.
[b]The data for the Cd. de La Habana include referrals from other provinces, so do not represent greater attention for Habaneros.

SOURCE: Ministerio de Salud Pública, *Informe anual 1989* (La Habana: MINSAP, 1990), 110–113 passim.

cellent by comparision with the rest of Latin America and also compare favorably with those of the developed countries.

Las Tunas also had the highest rate of early neonatal mortality (less than seven days), so it is conceivable that either doctors did not detect abnormalities that would lead to early death or the medical care provided in the hospitals was inadequate because the facilities or staff or the socio-economic conditions in which the mother lived were not up to par. Without information as to the cause of death, it is impossible to tell from the statistics what the problem was. More important, the early neonatal mortality rate for Cuba's worst case, Las Tunas, was only 8.5 per 1,000 live births compared with the overall U.S. rate for 1986 (latest available data) of 31.0 per 1,000 live births.[94] This comparison certainly creates significant symbolic capital for Cuba.

Granma province had one of the highest percentages of low birth weight babies (8.5 percent). This is not surprising because birth weight is primarily a result of the socioeconomic conditions in which the mother lived but can be largely rectified with early prenatal care and supplemental feeding. The national figure was 7.3 percent and the U.S. figure for 1987 (latest available data) was 6.9; therefore despite its relative poverty, Granma province does not lag much behind the United States.[95] That one of the poorest Cuban provinces can produce a birth weight figure that is so low and so close to that of the United States signifies noteworthy success for Cuban social programs in general and medicine in particular.

The range of differences among provinces for selected indicators of processes, outcomes, and facilities varies by indicator, as tables 8 and 9 demonstrate. For the purpose of this analysis, City of Havana was not included because most data for it incorporate national referrals and thus skew the numbers in Havana's favor. The least variation among provinces occurs with the number of gynecological visits per woman (0.3 between the highest and lowest number) and life expectancy at birth (1.80 years difference). The variation among provinces for life expectancy has declined steadily from 1977 to 1990. There was considerable variation between the highest and lowest infant mortality rates (5.0), percentages of infants with low birth weights (4.2), and population per doctor (281). As with life expectancy, there has been a continuous decline since 1979 in the variation among provinces for infant mortality rates.

The greatest variation among provinces was in process indicators: the number of visits to pediatricians varied by 8.7 between the highest and lowest within that category, the number of well-baby visits differed by 5.6 from high to low, and visits to obstetricians varied by 6.5. The actual number of visits at the lowest end of the range, however, is quite good by any standards, as are the infant mortality rate and percentage of infants of low birth-weight. The distribution of hospital beds by province is relatively even except for those areas designated as regional or national centers, which is to be expected in a regionalized system. In 1990 new hospitals were completed in some of the provinces that until then had not performed as well as others on health indicators: Las Tunas (which got two new hospitals), Holguín, Granma, and Villa Clara.[96]

The allocation of health expenditures per inhabitant in 1987 (average of 89.7 pesos) also varied in the pattern that would be expected for a regionalized health system, as table 10 shows. When superimposed on a map of Cuba, it becomes very clear how carefully selected the locations for greater expenditures were. The City of Havana, as the national referral center, was the province with the highest expenditure (151.5 pesos per person), followed by the Isle of Youth (122.4 pesos), which gets special medical attention because of the many boarding schools located there. The other provinces with greater expenditures than the rest are regional centers. If both the City of Havana and the Isle of Youth are excluded from the calculation of variation, then the disparity between the province with the highest expenditure and that with the lowest is 21.4 pesos per person.[97] These variations should not be interpreted as a sign of poor health conditions, poor facilities, or poor health. They do point to areas in which the Cubans should work to further ameliorate the conditions of life in the less-developed provinces, yet they suggest to the rest of the world an ability to resolve centuries-old imbalances.

The distributional problems Cuba faces in the health field are gradually disappearing as resources are channeled to those areas in greatest need. That Cuba has been successful in decreasing these regional variations over time clearly indicates the central government's commitment to improving rural life in particular and life in the provinces in general. Because medical services are delivered as part of a multisectoral development program, it is difficult to separate out exactly what percentage of the decrease in mortality rates and the increase in life expectancy is attributable to purely medical or public health interventions. Nevertheless, because today medical and health services are highly correlated with decreases in mortality, it must be assumed that they have played a large role in the amelioration of urban-rural and Havana-interior differences. This, of course, is highly significant in the further accumulation of symbolic capital.

Medical Education

Cuban medical education has been decentralized since early in the revolution, and now almost all medical personnel at all levels are trained locally in the province from which they come. Curricular innovations have further decentralized medical education

Table 10: Current Expenditures per capita for Public Health, Rank, and
Percent of Budget for Salaries by Province, 1987

Province	Rank[a]	Per Capita Expenditures (in pesos)	Percent of Budget for Salaries
Pinar del Río	8	75.1	58.8
La Habana	12	66.2	63.5
Cd. de La Habana	1	151.5	54.6
Matanzas	3	84.0	61.4
Villa Clara	10	69.6	57.2
Cienfuegos	6	78.6	56.1
Sancti Spíritus	5	81.8	57.5
Ciego de Avila	11	67.5	57.7
Camagüey	3	84.0	57.7
Las Tunas	9	73.2	54.6
Holguín	14	62.6	55.0
Granma	13	65.5	58.4
Santiago de Cuba	4	82.0	57.7
Guantánamo	7	77.5	57.1
Isla de la Juventud	2	122.4	52.9
Averages		89.7	56.8

[a]Ranked with regard to per capita health expenditures. One is the highest expenditure.

SOURCE: Ministerio de Salud Pública, Centro Nacional de Información de Ciencias Médicas, *Algunos indicadores de salud en Cuba* (La Habana: MINSAP, n.d. [typescript]), p. 5 in "Informe viaje a Cuba," PAHO internal document HSI/84/2.1 (53/90), May 2, 1990, anexo, 5.

to the community level. Teaching polyclinics instituted in the 1970s have further extended their educative role with the introduction of the Family Doctor Program. Now they are the primary sites of training for the Comprehensive General Medicine residency and continuing medical education for family doctors and nurses.

In 1981 Castro established a commission to reevaluate the type of physician Cuba needed and the medical education necessary to create such a professional. It was imperative, he said, to improve medical training if Cuba was to become a world medical power.[98] During the four years prior to the initial family doctor experiment in 1984, numerous health and education officials analyzed Cuba's medical goals as enunciated by Castro, actual medical needs both domestic and international, and the nature of the existing health care and medical education systems.[99] The result was not only the Family Doctor Program and the three-year residency in Comprehensive General Medicine but also an entirely new medical school curriculum based on a thorough assessment of the best foreign medical schools' curricula.

A panel of experts identified 286 health problems that the new graduate, a basic general doctor (MGB), should be able to treat both on the individual (preventive, curative, and rehabilitative) and community (epidemiological and environmental) levels. The experts then determined 760 skills the students would have to master to deal with these problems, and these were combined with the basic knowledge, both theoretical and clinical, one should acquire in order to perform the stated tasks well.[100] From there the new curriculum was created in response to the stated goal of training the highest caliber primary-care specialist possible.

The new curriculum presents information in integrated modules organized from a biological-systems rather than a disciplinary standpoint. For example, the module called "regulation in the human body" includes the nervous system, the endocrine system, the reproductive system, and the metabolic system. Another module deals with "functions of distribution, nutrition, and excretion" and includes the circulatory and respiratory systems, the urinary and digestive systems, and nutrition and energy. More importantly, medical education begins with a module on "society and health" that includes epidemiology, hygiene, health organization and administration, social psychology, biostatistics, and demography. Because of the importance of social medicine, both the first and last semesters include modules in public health as well as in biomedical subjects.[101]

The curriculum exemplifies an "integrated teaching, assistance, and research approach" to community-based medical education. From the very beginning, students are involved in theoretical, practical, and investigative work, although at a very elementary level. Cuba is not the only country in which this type of medical education exists, but it is one of the only ones in which community-based medical education is universal throughout the medical school system. The Netherlands, Canada, Brazil, Egypt, the Philippines and other countries all have one or more medical schools in which community-based medical education is the norm.[102]

The Cubans are convinced that their new medical school curriculum is worthy of emulation by others, and so they designed a step-by-step guide that explains how to analyze, plan, and change medical school education from one based on a purely biological perspective to one based on an integrated sociomedical approach. This guide is presented in the form of a paper delivered in 1988 by Vice Minister of Health Dr. Fidel Ilizastigui Dupuy at an international primary-care conference held in Cuba and sponsored by the World Health and Pan American Health Organizations and the Network of Community-Oriented Educational Institutions for Health Sciences (the Netherlands). In this paper Ilizastigui reiterates Cuba's position on the primacy of doctors in the health-care system when he asserts that the World Health Organization's goal of "Health for All by the Year 2000" implies high-quality health care. The Cuban view is that this can only be provided by physicians, although they believe that in countries that do not have the resources to employ physicians any type of health practitioner would do.[103]

A Canadian medical professor from McMaster Medical School who has known ranking Cuban health officials for more than two decades suggested that the new Cuban curriculum and the Family Doctor Program were modeled after the McMaster paradigm but that at Castro's behest the Cubans went even further in their use of family doctors by putting them on every block. He suggested that the use of the McMaster model came about because the driving force behind this curricular change and the primacy of primary health care, Dr. Cosme Ordóñez Carceller, had been a frequent visitor at McMaster since the 1960s.[104]

What is important here is not whether the new curriculum is original, but the fact that Cuba trains all doctors in response to the perceived needs of the population to be served rather than according to the dictates and models of medical imperialism: fee-for-service, hospital-based, high-technology curative medicine that is the basis of medical school curricula in the developed countries and that is therefore copied by almost all developing countries whether suitable to local conditions and needs or not. Moreover, this model was promoted and funded by nongovernmental organizations such as the Rockefeller Foundation. That Cuba has broken away from the established and, one might add, neocolonial or medical imperialistic model and finally created a medical school curriculum in accordance with domestic needs and conditions affords Cuba enormous prestige and influence (symbolic capital) that is quite appealing to potential Third World beneficiaries of Cuba's medical diplomacy.

The Symbolic Significance of Cuban
Health Achievements

It is symbolically important that the guidelines contained in the World Health Organization's resolution, "Health For All By The Year 2000," are strongly reminiscent of those of the Cuban health system, with the notable exception that the resolution recommends the use of paramedical personnel rather than relying solely on physicians in primary care.[105] Not surprisingly, international health officials have often compared Cuba very favorably with the "Health For All" model; Cuba already had achieved its goals in the early 1980s. This success, of course, further enhanced Cuba's ability to provide international medical assistance.

The dispensing of medical aid abroad is intertwined with the government's plan to become a world medical power. Becoming a world medical power symbolizes scientific achievement or, at a minimum, achievement in a highly sophisticated technological field. Although eliminating the diseases of poverty is primarily related to improving the standard of living (which results from public health measures and simple medical procedures) going beyond this point requires the use of high technology to diagnose, treat, and abate or even cure the diseases of development. Since Cuba has eradicated the diseases of poverty, it now focuses on maladies afflicting the developed world, the prevention of which requires changes in lifestyle, and the diagnosis and treatment of which often depend on high-technology medical intervention.[106]

Lifestyle changes are important aims of the Family Doctor Program; however, the real and symbolic importance of being able to diagnose, treat, and abate the chronic degenerative diseases cannot be emphasized enough. Many developing nations have neither the equipment nor the personnel to accomplish these goals, and those that do suffer from a shortage as well as a maldistribution of resources and from the inability of the majority of the population to pay for such services. This fact makes the free provision of both high-technology medical services and primary care to the entire Cuban population a remarkable achievement.

Cuba's ability to conduct medical diplomacy is a logical outcome of having developed a health-care system capable of accumulating symbolic capital by garnering international accolades for its out-comes, processes, infrastructure, human resources, and equality of access. Without this domestic medical success, any gesture of provid-ing medical aid to other countries would be neither credible nor much appreciated.

5

Biotechnology, Biomedical Research, and Medical-Pharmaceutical Exports

Science and Development

Cuban scientific endeavors are part of an overall socioeconomic development strategy that from the earliest days of the revolution sought the incorporation of science as a means of rational and planned societal transformation. The production and exportation of biotechnology, medical, and pharmaceutical products was a natural outgrowth of this scientific process that was employed first and foremost to remedy domestic problems but was capitalized on later to convert acquired knowledge into export earnings. The abilities to conduct biotechnology and biomedical research and to produce exportable products signify Cuba's accomplishments in a complex scientific arena and thereby increase Cuba's symbolic capital and the power of its medical diplomacy.

The appeal of science as a major tool of development has been particularly common in developing nations with socialist ideologies because of socialism's "scientific" analysis of the movement of history and because science itself provides rational means by which to achieve development goals that then legitimate the regime.[1] It is therefore not surprising that Fidel Castro has repeatedly stated since 1961 that Cuba's future must be one of scientists and that Cuba must not only take advantage of the scientific-technical revolution but also participate in it. This precept has been applied to all aspects of socio-economic development in Cuba.

In the biomedical field, Cuba's Minister of Education, José Fernández Alvarez, contended that "we think the next century is the century of biology. Microbiology and biochemistry will be used to solve problems, achieve higher production, feed humans, and improve health."[2] To speed up the process of funding projects and establishing new laboratories, the Biological Front, a high-level policy-making body, was formed in 1981 to circumvent the ever-present bureaucratic red tape.[3] By 1990 Castro had claimed that biotechnology was "one of the most promising industries in the medical field," and designated it as one of three top priority sectors (with food and tourism) that would receive continued investment in a time of severe economic crisis and fiscal retrenchment.[4] With this high-level impetus, Cuba, unlike most developing nations, has made strides in the development, testing, and distribution of biotechnology and genetic engineering products.[5]

It is indeed rather astounding that Cuba should make biotechnology such a high priority in its development plans. No other country has done so, with the possible exception of Japan, which has the necessary industrial, scientific, and technological infrastructure and the capital to finance long-term projects that may or may not be fruitful.[6] Why then has Cuba made the decision to invest so heavily in biotechnology, and will it be profitable?

Although great importance has been placed on the use of biotechnology to improve food production, particularly to produce disease-resistant seeds inexpensively, I examine only Cuba's biotechnology development strategy in medicine. This strategy entailed finding a model product to develop (interferon), training personnel to conduct research, and producing concrete results (exportable products) to justify the investment. These issues are examined, along with various expert assessments of the quality of Cuban biotechnology, to evaluate the Cuban program, its potential and, most important, its symbolic significance.

The Interferon Model

Where does a developing country begin a biotechnology enterprise? Lacking a scientific infrastructure or highly developed molecular biology faculties at its universities, Cuban biotechnology and genetic engineering began as a further specialization in clinical medicine. In the early 1980s interferon, a protein that inhibits virus development in a cell, was thought to be a potential wonder drug, particularly as a cancer treatment. It was therefore chosen as a model for developing genetic engineering and biotechnology techniques. This decision to study interferon and invest in biotechnology was made by Fidel Castro himself after he learned about experimental work with interferons for the treatment of cancer in a meeting in 1980 with Dr. R. Lee Clark, the president of M. D. Anderson Hospital of Houston, Texas. Castro dispatched two medical doctors to Dr. Clark's cancer hospital for advanced training. There they learned that the best laboratory in which to study interferon was in Finland.[7] Thus in January 1982, after a group of Cuban scientists were trained at the Helsinki laboratory of Dr. Kari Cantell, the inventor of the technique for isolating interferon from leukocytes, Cuba established a similar laboratory with Dr. Cantell's advice and began purifying interferon.[8] In the same year, the Center for the Breeding of Laboratory Animals (CENPALAB) was conceived to meet the demands of biotechnology and increased biomedical research. CENPALAB opened in 1986, but construction was not completed until 1991, by which time there was considerable production of germ-free and specific pathogen–free (SPF) animals, as well as diagnostic kits and immunochemistry reagents.[9]

By the mid-1980s the Center for Biological Research (CIB) scientists' second-generation interferon, recombinant alpha-2b interferon cloned in yeast, was being used in clinical studies. According to researcher Patrick Gray of California-based Genentech, "The Cuban 'production system is pretty much like that of other groups using yeast alpha factor,' but 'what is different is that they're using it to produce interferon for clinical purposes.'"[10]

Cuban scientists have used interferon experimentally for the treatment of various viral diseases and tumors and have claimed some success in the treatment of plantar warts, laryngeal papilloma, hepatitis B, dengue fever, inoperable lung cancer, herpes zoster, and leukemia.[11] Their 1990 marketing information indicates that they have obtained positive results using interferon for the treatment of two dozen afflictions.[12] This success probably results from their application of interferon to a wide range of diseases in clinical trials to see whether serendipitous results might occur, irrespective of whether the scientific literature points to its potential use.

Cuban scientists can perform clinical tests very rapidly after the initial development of a product, because unlike U.S. scientists they do not face Food and Drug Administration (FDA) regulations that greatly delay clinical trials. Moreover, Cuban researchers automatically have at their disposal the entire population as clinical trial subjects, if they so desire, because of the link between research and the provision of medical care through the national health service. This does not mean that Cuban clinical trials are immoral, unethical, or unsafe, but simply that they are quicker.[13] They may, however, not always conform to international standards primarily because the Cuban doctors are morally opposed to placebo trials; they do not believe in withholding treatment. Otherwise, they claim to follow the World Health Organization (WHO) and FDA protocols.

Although the Cubans can be criticized for such heavy emphasis on interferon, which in the mid 1980s was no longer considered the wonder drug many once thought it to be, they regard it as "a 'model' to develop the infrastructure for cloning and protein harvesting."[14] Cuban scientists Manuel Limonta and Luis Herrera have stated that they

view it [interferon] as a model in two ways. One, for acquiring the necessary skills to do advanced molecular biology—DNA splicing, vector construction, sequencing and synthesizing genes and proteins, etc.—and also as a model for the purification, scale-up, clinical testing and eventual general use of biotechnology products.[15]

This, however, may be simply an ex post facto rationalization rather than a premeditated plan.

Harvey Bialy, the research editor of *Bio/Technology*, suggests that the Cubans have been successful in using the interferon model for the purposes described above as evidenced by the types of research papers and findings they have presented at international meetings, the new projects they have undertaken, and the rapid diversification of their research and development interests. Although Cuban scientists have gone beyond simply working with interferons, these proteins are still an important part of their research.[16]

Because interferons are immune system regulators, there is continuing and, in the early 1990s, renewed interest in alpha, beta, and gamma interferon and interleukin-2, all of which are being tested in many countries as "immuno-modulators, anti-virals and anti-cancer drugs."[17] In fact, one analyst suggested that "alpha interferon almost serves as a paradigm for all of these biological response modifiers [interferons, interleukins, and colony stimulating factors]" that are at the forefront of biotechnology research.[18] Cuba works with all three.

Already in 1986 Cuba was "the second-largest producer of natural human leukocyte interferon, after Finland," and had been able to capitalize on this status by signing a marketing agreement with a major Austrian drug exporter, Chemie Linz, to sell interferon products under the trademark of Leuferon in Europe, Latin America, Asia, and Africa.[19] By 1988 the agreement was no longer in effect because, as a Cuban official said, Leuferon was not commercially viable even before Chemie Linz was acquired by Austria Tabac. Although one might assume a likely reason for Chemie Linz's cancellation of the agreement would be political pressure from the Reagan administration as it tightened its economic embargo against Cuba, that was not the case. In the mid 1980s interferon simply was not considered to be as useful as was once thought.[20] The point, however, is that the Cubans were successful enough to make such a deal.

In the 1990s, the worldwide market for interferons began to expand as clinical results indicated their increasing utility. According to a U.S. pharmaceutical industry securities analyst, "Alpha interferon is at the springboard of several anti-viral and anti-cancer indications that make it look like it could be a $1 billion drug."[21] Worldwide sales were already over $300 million annually, according to 1990 estimates, and they are expected to triple by 1994, partly because there are an estimated 225,000 hepatitis patients in the United States who are potential inteferon users, along with an estimated 20 percent of the populations of developing countries.[22]

Why then is Cuba not in a good position to capitalize on recent breakthroughs in interferon treatments despite being one of the largest producers of interferon? First, the international market is mostly divided between two pharmaceutical giants, Schering Plough and Hoffman LaRoche, and two other producers: the Ares-Serono Group of Italy and Sumitomo Pharmaceuticals of Japan.[23] Second, Cuba cannot compete with the multinationals and gain a share of the world market primarily because Cuba copies patented products without license and markets them, and therefore cannot sell to countries that recognize U.S., European, and Japanese patents. Cuban interferons could be sold only for research use rather than medical use in those markets because all interferons are already patented there.[24] Third, without the slick marketing techniques, distribution networks, follow-up, and service of these established producers, it is highly unlikely that Cuba could gain a foothold in the market unless it were to find another major company (perhaps in a joint venture) to distribute its products now that Chemie Linz is not marketing them. Finding such a company would be highly unlikely except in the research market because an arrangement such as this would violate intellectual property rights. Fourth, the entire Cuban economy is geared to uncompetitive (subsidized and protected) production, and considerable time will elapse before substantive change can be made. Fifth, even if Cuba could compete with the transnationals, it could not, of course, supply the U.S. market because of a three-decade-old trade embargo against Cuban products and even against products with Cuban components.

Cuba may circumvent these difficulties by concentrating on the Third World market and that of the former Soviet republics until these nations agree to recognize patents, and by agreeing to barter, countertrade, or clearing accounts rather than require hard currency payable in cash. Developing countries, however, will be unable to afford interferon for most patients because the course of treatment for hepatitis B costs $3,640 per patient at current prices ($6.50 per one million unit dose), and hepatitis C $1,404 per patient.[25] Even if Cuba were to sell interferon considerably below the world market price and continue to accept barter rather than hard currency, there are other, more pressing, health priorities in developing nations that require their health ministries' scarce resources.

On the other hand, Cuba sold interferons to the Soviets in exchange for oil, among other things, as a component of the 1990 trade agreement between the two countries that included "300 million rubles in medicine, vaccines, products of biotechnology and high-tech medical items."[26] This increased initially to U.S. $800 million for the 1991 trade agreement (the first year in which all trade was calculated in dollars) but was later reduced to U.S. $730 million, probably because of negotiations over the items to be traded, the terms of trade, and rates of exchange.[27] Whether these amounts are calculated in rubles or dollars, the fact that Cuba sold such a large quantity of biotechnology and medical products to the Soviets is significant and demonstrates Cuba's relative success in one of the few markets that were open to it. It does not, on the other hand, suggest competitive ability on the world market.

Disintegration of the Soviet Union, internal strife within key exporting republics, and economic crisis in both the Soviet Union and Cuba, however, cast serious doubt on whether either side would be in a position to fulfill these trade agreements irrespective of their intentions.[28] The economist Miguel Figueras suggested that possibly only half of that contract might be realized.[29] In fact, by the end of 1991 no deliveries of Cuban biotechnology or medical products appeared in Soviet trade data. In April 1992 the economist José Luis Rodríguez said that only a small part of the 1991 contracts was fulfilled because of decreased imports from the Soviet Union (no Soviet ships, no trade).[30]

One of Boris Yeltsin's economic advisers, Igor Nit, suggested in late 1991 that the Russian Republic would be interested in Cuban medical and biotechnology products but that trade would have to be mutually beneficial and, of course, arranged with numerous Russian firms rather than through any central ministry.[31] Adapting to changing circumstances, the Cubans have made contracts in 1992 with Russia, Ukraine, Belarus, and Estonia that include biotechnology and medical products, but no specific details were available.[32] The new agreement notwithstanding, difficult logistics, high transportation costs, and, more important, the absence of political will on the part of the Russians to support the Cuban regime diminish the possibility of renewed trade on a large scale.

Human Resources Development

Cuba's science programs, of course, would fail without the requisite personnel to perform sophisticated research. Long-term government policy, therefore, has been to channel students into high-priority scientific fields. The capacity of the government to determine educational patterns according to development goals has resulted in an exponential increase in the number of scientists, engineers, and science technicians available by the mid 1980s to engage in research and develop new products either for import substitution or export as Cuba's baby boom generation comes of age.

Created in 1965 with only 12 scientists, Cuba's National Center for Scientific Research (CNIC) had a staff of 1,000 by 1983, of whom 350 were professionals; 100 to 150 were students carrying out advanced research; and 50 to 60 were researchers from other institutes participating in CNIC projects.[33] By 1983 there were 33,506 people working in all fields of science and technology in Cuba (one for every 295.5 inhabitants), of whom 11,174 were at the professional level. In the Ministry of Public Health alone, there were 5,552 scientific workers. Comparable data for 1989 indicate that there were 41,784 science workers in all fields (one for every 251.3 inhabitants), of whom 19,985 were professionals. There were 6,948 people working in scientific research at various levels of the Ministry of Public Health's institutes then, a decrease of 336 from 1987 levels (probably because nonphysician scientists such as biologists were then doing biomedical research).[34]

Many of the CNIC and CIB scientists have been trained in western Europe, primarily in France, Belgium, and Scandinavia. Others have been trained in Canada, the Soviet Union, and East Germany; some briefly trained at laboratories in the United States;[35] and others studied in Great Britain and Mexico.[36] Advisors to CNIC have included Czechoslovak and Polish microbiologists and the members of the North American–Cuban Scientific Exchange (NACSEX) who advise scientists at many other biomedical and biotechnology institutions as well.[37]

The year 1986 produced a qualitative and quantitative leap in Cuban research with the opening of a much larger and superbly equipped facility for the CIB's scientists, the Center for Genetic Engineering and Biotechnology (CIGB). The CIB has become a division of the CIGB. The opening of the CIGB was accompanied by an increase in the number of scientists, so as to take advantage of biotechnology to produce both human and animal vaccines and conduct more genetic research on plants.[38] Thus the biology faculty of the University of Havana graduated 749 students in the five-year period ending in 1990 and by 1991 had an annual enrollment of 850 in its three areas of specialization: biology, biochemistry, and microbiology.[39]

The human resources needed for increasing Cuba's biotechnology research capability are partially included in Cuba's plans for expanding the number of doctors by the year 2000, but many of these researchers are scientists rather than M.D.'s. In order to prepare students for biotechnology and other cutting-edge scientific research, the Cuban government established in 1981 a new type of high school (preuniversity) dedicated to scientific excellence. In the 1984–1985 academic year, only 200 out of 6,000 applicants were accepted after entrance exams in physics, chemistry or biology, and mathematics.

Unlike those at other Cuban preuniversity schools, the professors at this scientific preuniversity have also been selected on the basis of examination, and some are doctoral candidates in the European sense. In addition to the regular faculty, researchers and professors from the universities, the Academy of Sciences, and the National Center for Scientific Research regularly teach specialized courses at this school. The educational standards are considerably more stringent than at other schools, the student-teacher ratio is low, and there are well-equipped laboratories capable of providing direct experimental opportunities for all.[40]

The selection and recruitment processes for the various scientific research institutes are quite rigorous and vary from formal analytical examinations and various sets of interviews in English, to what amounts to an internship and independent research project for a small number of promising students. CIGB, as the premier institution, has a doctoral program and gets the best students, the latest technology, and the most resources, all of which cause resentment among the less well-endowed research institutes and university faculties, particularly because resources in general are scarce.[41]

Scarcity of resources in the "special period in peace time" has accentuated the government's desire for scientists to solve all of the problems of development, an effort that, in turn, will further stratify society according to scientific ability and ultimately according to the ability to produce something exportable or for import substitution. As a result, increased competition among research centers may be inevitable unless research efforts are consolidated and interrelated rather than separated. There is some indication that, in fact, consolidation of efforts has begun, as the university faculties have become involved in projects with research institutions and as scientists affiliated with those institutions have participated in the teaching and training of university students.[42] The biggest impediment to coordinated research among these institutions has been the lack of resources and research experience in biotechnology at the universities and other institutions as compared with the resources and experience available at CIGB.[43] In the "special period," transportation diffi-culties have meant that even those outside researchers allowed to use certain CIGB facilities have difficulty getting to CIGB regularly because it is so far from the center of town.

The Quality of Cuban Biotechnology

Are Cuban scientists competent to produce sound re-sults and good products? Cuban biogenetic engineering scientists' knowledge and the quality of their equipment were considered to meet U.S. standards as early as 1985.[44] In an assessment of his Cuban counterparts at the CIB that year, Harvard microbiology and molec-ular genetics professor Jon Beckwith asserted that they were "amaz-ingly *au courant,* sophisticated and creative in the field of genetic engineering."[45] The types of DNA and gene manipulation and cloning he witnessed at CIGB was similar to those he had seen in U.S. labo-ratories. Cuban scientists also asked questions similar to those asked by U.S. scientists and developed computer programs to analyze pro-tein sequences and DNA. It was clear to Beckwith that the Cuban government had made a substantial commitment to biotechnology by purchasing very expensive equipment and supplies, such as the latest high-pressure liquid chromatography equipment.[46]

Costly equipment at CIGB includes primarily Japanese products: a JEOL JMS-HX110 mass spectrometer, a JEOL JMS-T330 electronic scanning microscope that magnifies images by 200,000 times, a JEOL JEM2000EX transmission microscope that magnifies images 1 million times, and a Hitachi spectrophotometer. This equipment is housed in a central core area accessible from the laboratories that line both sides of the building on a given floor so that it can be shared. Less costly equipment is housed in the individual laboratories. Because in biotechnology only state-of-the-art equipment has been purchased, it comes only from capitalist countries. The former socialist countries have developed little biotechnology capability and were therefore not potential suppliers.[47] In fact, Cuba could now supply these countries with a number of items.

The international biotechnology expert Daniel Goldstein suggests that "all of Latin America together cannot reach the ankle of the Cuban endeavor" in biotechnology. He contends that Cuba is in an exceptional position in this field and is the only country in Latin America capable of copying biotechnology. However, no Latin American country, including Cuba, can now develop original products and processes, because these countries focus on off-the-shelf technology rather than basic science. Goldstein asserts that the leading Cuban scientists have been technicians who can clone sequences, but not one group has done original research basic to the development of new technology.[48]

Harvey Bialy concurs that the Cubans do high-quality focused technological work and says that "because of the extreme pressures they work under they have little time to pursue basic biological questions."[49] Cuban sources do not deny that their whole project is geared toward producing immediate, usable results rather than delving into questions of basic science. Their aim always has been one of harnessing science for socioeconomic development. More importantly, Bialy asserts that by continuing this cutting-edge biotechnology enterprise, the Cubans will be in a position to capitalize on future developments in the field. The real breakthroughs in biotechnology are yet to come, and without the CIGB Cuba would never be able to catch up with the developed world's biotechnology enterprises.[50]

Both Bialy and Goldstein insist that their criticisms be taken constructively in the context of their overall praise for Cuban biotechnology and the dearth of such scientific endeavors elsewhere in Latin America. Although Argentina, Brazil, and Mexico do conduct research, its breadth, scale, and sophistication are not comparable to the Cuban effort. Moreover, a 1989 PAHO evaluation stated that CIGB researchers had excellent training, used advanced methods, and were, therefore, highly qualified scientists working in a high-level research institute.[51]

These positive and negative comments have been corroborated by members of NACSEX, experts in various fields who have evaluated the Cubans' programs and facilities and advised them since the outset of their biotechnology endeavors.[52] In discussing the CIGB, Issar Smith of NACSEX called it a "state of the art" center with "ultramodern scientific equipment" and "modern techniques like DNA sequencing, oligonucleotide [small fragments of DNA] and oligopeptide synthesis and NMR [nuclear magnetic resonance] spectroscopy."[53] He also reiterated Goldstein's criticism of the lack of basic research at Cuban scientific institutions but mentioned that the Cuban scientists with whom he spoke, particularly at CIGB, recognized this shortcoming and were keen on rectifying it as soon as circumstances (read economics) would allow.[54] Economic necessity dictates science policy.

Robert Ubell, writing in *Nature,* stated that Cuban research centers have "unusually well-equipped laboratories." He was surprised by how up-to-date and expensive the equipment was and that virtually none of it came from the Soviet Union.[55] Ubell noted, however, that the U.S. trade embargo has been very costly to Cuba's scientific efforts. Procurement in Japan or Europe has increased the costs and time involved in obtaining equipment. As a result, Cuban scientists have had to learn to produce their own restriction enzymes, make tissue cultures, and establish virus collections.[56] Economic considerations have also led Cuban industry to manufacture equipment, such as that for electrophoresis and gas chromatography.[57]

The U.S. trade embargo has also affected the supply of current international literature available; thus some Cuban libraries have up-to-date literature while others do not. This problem was remedied in large part by the establishment in 1986 of the Central Library for Science and Technology. The library is stocked with 10,000 books and 7,000 journals in areas of research emphasized in Cuba.[58] As is common in the medical libraries, copies or summaries of materials circulate throughout the island. A wire service was established at the same time to disseminate the latest international public health and biotechnology news to all provinces.[59] Moreover, through the science and technology library researchers have access to foreign on-line data bases.[60] Remote on-line access to data is made possible through the network of scientific and technical information sites, including the National Library which had 2.2 million volumes by 1987.[61] Improved access to information was already evident in the citations used in articles in 1987 and early 1988 issues of Cuban biotechnology, public health, and medical journals. Shortages of paper in 1990 and 1991 probably will affect the dissemination of information in this field, but since it is a high-priority sector it may be affected less than others.

Biotechnology research is a privileged field with up-to-the-minute documentation available at the CIGB. In mid-June 1991 the CIGB library had major U.S. scientific journals for that month, some of which were also available on diskette. On-line data bases such as *Science Citation Index, Medline, Life Sciences, Current Contents,* and *Lilacs,* among others, were available and current. Recent publications from the U.S. National Academy of Sciences and from prominent European institutions were in evidence as well. The automation team at the library was setting up a local area network (LAN) to provide easier access to data.[62] Like many Cuban research institutions, CIGB has been connected to international electronic mail networks since 1992. All these resources should improve research capabilities.

Research, Product Development, and Trade

Will Cuban miracle drugs lead to economic and political miracles? That is the hope of the Cuban leadership. Domestic need has led to the import-substitution production of medical, pharmaceutical, and biotechnology products at considerable savings but not yet to economic miracles. The Cuban economist Miguel Figueras, however, predicted a threefold increase in biotechnology exports alone in 1991 to approximately $500 million. This volume would place this sector among Cuba's three largest export sectors.[63] Moreover, Fidel Castro has claimed that the sale of biomedical products makes investment in that field quite good: in 1990 Cuba earned 819 million pesos on investments of 130 million and the export sale of medicines alone that year equaled the export sale of tobacco (1990 data were not available, but 1989 tobacco sales were 83.6 million pesos and pharmaceuticals were 109.7 million pesos, whereas 1990 biomedical deliveries totaled U.S. $140 million). He contended that these products "have a guaranteed market, whether in competition with others or as something new."[64] Castro made no mention of what market was guaranteed, but it is unlikely that any is now that the CMEA is defunct. The Cubans, however, have been doing market research in various capitalist countries with an eye to exporting a variety of medical, pharmaceutical, and biotechnology products.[65] Castro himself has suggested that biotechnology exports will soon subsidize other areas of the economy. If these predictions are borne out, a highly unlikely event, then economic miracles may indeed occur.

Most biomedical and biotechnology research done in Cuba is destined for immediate application because science is viewed as a means of fostering development. For example, scientists at CNIC have been using genetic engineering techniques since the early 1970s and already at the beginning of the 1980s had been using monoclonal antibodies on alpha fetoprotein, among other research.[66] In July 1981 when Castro had asked to be apprised of developments in medical technology, he was informed about alpha fetoprotein analyses, a safe means of mass genetic screening to detect congenital malformations which would lead to a further decrease in the infant mortality rate and replace the more risky and invasive procedure of amniocentesis.[67] Castro quickly approved and funded projects to develop the technology to analyze genetic material and test women nationwide.

Work began immediately on the development of test kits and equipment that were less expensive than the universally standard ELISA (enzyme-linked immunosorbent assay). The result was SUMA (ultramicro analytic system), which used only a tenth of the reagents needed for a standard ELISA (the most expensive part of testing). SUMA was therefore suitable for cost-effective mass screening of blood supplies for HIV and hepatitis B as well as for individual screening for alpha fetoprotein, hyperthyroidism, allergies, HIV, and hepatitis B. SUMA equipment was first installed in pediatric hospitals and laboratories by 1984 and was soon in use nationwide.[68] In 1988 Cuba began to market SUMA which, according to an international expert, "does show an impressive array of performance characteristics."[69] Third generation SUMA-321s were available in 1990 and fourth generation SUMA-421s in 1992, which suggests that a new generation machine has been produced every two years since its initial development.[70]

Performance and cost aside, the Cubans have neither the marketing skills nor the networks to profit fully from their product development. For example, the Brazilian biotechnology firm Vallee Diagnosticos, which produces diagnostic kits for AIDS, hepatitis, and syphilis, purchased its technology from a U.S. firm for more than twice what it would have had to pay Cuba for the same technology only because it was unaware of the Cuban products at that time.[71] As the Cubans learn marketing techniques and as Cuban products and capabilities become better known in Latin America through scientific meetings and trade fairs, cooperative agreements with scientific institutions in various countries, and regional collaborative arrangements orchestrated by PAHO and the United Nations Development Program (UNDP), it is less likely that Cuba will be excluded from the market.

By 1990 the Cubans had sold seven SUMAs to Brazil, donated six to the Soviet Union after the Chernobyl nuclear accident and the

Armenian earthquake, and donated one to Pope John Paul II. The Soviet Union then agreed to purchase fifty SUMAs as part of their 1990 trade agreement with Cuba. Interestingly, however, Cuba has generally not sold SUMAs, but only the diagnostic kits such as those for HIV and hepatitis B. The hardware required to use the kits is supplied by the Immunoassay Center only for the duration of the agreement, and is installed by Cuban technicians.[72] Only in 1991 did Cuba agree to sell the SUMA hardware to the former Soviet Union.[73] The pre-1991 posture tends to corroborate the Brazilian health minister's claim that Cuba was unwilling to transfer technology in this field, although the "borrowed" equipment could still be copied.[74] Because Cuba has copied the products of others and does not recognize patents, it would be difficult for Cuba to legitimately complain about anyone who did the same thing.

Cuba has also provided SUMAs, reagents, and HIV diagnostic kits to Argentina and Ecuador as part of PAHO's regional program of Technical Cooperation Among Developing Countries (CTPD/CTP).[75] One would expect this effort to lead to future sales of these items either through bilateral agreements or CTPD/CTP–orchestrated arrangements.

The continuing economic crisis has led to the rapid commercialization of products, often before they have been extensively tested. Foreign critics are not the only ones who believe that Cuba has rushed biotechnology and medical products to the market. In reference to interferon, Dr. Alejandro Silva, head of the microbiology laboratory at the CIB, was quoted in 1986 as saying that "it's only been tested in animals so far. We need more results before commercializing this interferon."[76] Suppporting this view was Dr. Silvio Barcelona Hernández, a director of CIB, who stated that "for MediCuba to advertise the recombinant interferon is an error."[77]

The same criticism has been lodged against Cuba by foreign experts assessing the meningitis B vaccine. A 1989 World Health Organization document indicated great interest in the vaccine because it was the only one of its type in production.[78] But a 1989 PAHO document said, "To the best of our knowledge there is not a formal publication in any journal, and certainly not in an international journal, having a peer review system, of these data [results of clinical trials]."[79] This failure to make available the scientific data may have stemmed from Cuban officials' fear of closing their postdevelopment window of opportunity to market the vaccine if they were to make public the details of its characteristics and effectiveness.

Although the meningitis B vaccine had been available for sale since 1987, it was only undergoing the fourth of the six WHO-required trials in 1990. Thus the Brazilians were simultaneously using and evaluating the Cuban vaccine.[80] Uruguay reportedly agreed in February 1991 to exchange food for Cuban meningitis B vaccine, hepatitis B vaccine, and some reagents, but three months later was reported to be inquiring in relevant international scientific circles about the quality and effectiveness of the Cuban vaccines.[81] Mexico has not purchased the Cuban meningitis B vaccine precisely because the vaccine has not yet been subjected to all of the necessary clinical trials.[82]

A December 1990 PAHO document stated, however, that "22 million doses had been applied in Brazil and Cuba and that tests were begun in Viña del Mar (Chile), Antioquía (Colombia), and Buenos Aires [Argentina]."[83] It further mentioned that clinical testing had been conducted using the U.S. Food and Drug Administration norms (which does not imply FDA approval) in the first three phases of testing and that in late 1990 the vaccine was in phase 4 and had been registered for a patent but had not yet received one.[84] By August 1991 the vaccine still had not been approved by WHO but had shown evidence of effectiveness against meningitis B subtype B:4:P1.15. A WHO expert committee that studied the Cuban documentation that year recommended that field trials be conducted indefinitely.[85]

Cuba has sold Brazil a considerable amount of meningitis B vaccine since 1989, but conflicting figures exist as to the actual monetary value of the sales—either U.S. $230 million, U.S. $217 million, or U.S. $182.5 million through June 1991. The details of the sales are important in attempting to assess exactly how successful Cuba has been in marketing the vaccine. Moreover, they indicate how difficult it is to get good financial data from Cuba. Some sources suggest that 18 million doses were sold in 1989 for 1990 at a cost of U.S. $130 million or $7.22 per dose, and that 15 million doses were sold in 1990 for 1991 at U.S. $100 million or $6.67 per dose. Another source contends that the first sale (1989 for 1990) was for 10 million doses at $8.00 per dose and that this amount later increased to 15 million doses. This source says, however, that 1 million doses were not paid for, which reduced the price to $7.47 per dose for a total sale of U.S.

$112 million. The next sale (1991) was for 15 million doses at $7.00 per dose for a contract total of U.S. $105 million. Later sources indicate sales of U.S. $100 million at $10 per dose in 1989 for 1990 and U.S. $82 million or U.S. $82.5 million at $5.50 or $5.47 per dose in 1990 for 1991.[86] In 1987 the Cuban press cited the manufacturing cost per dose of meningitis B vaccine at $4.50, but this amount was based on pilot production rather than large scale commercial production.[87] Complaints about the cost by Brazilian Minister of Health Alceni Guerra led to the decrease in price between the two contract periods but not immediately to the technology transfer that the Brazilians wanted. Guerra subsequently accused Cuba of imperialistic practices.[88]

Conflicting reports of a technology transfer agreement under which Cuba and Brazil would jointly manufacture the meningitis B vaccine in Brazil and share the profits have appeared in both the Brazilian and Cuban press since April 1990. In that month a Cuban publication cited the Brazilian Minister of Health as saying that the project was under study but also that production would begin in 1992.[89] Yet no firm agreement existed at that time. A May 1991 Brazilian newspaper article indicated that the deal was on, but another report on June 30, 1991, this time in a Cuban newspaper but quoting a Brazilian health official, suggested that the two countries were still "analyzing the possibility." If and when it is implemented, the joint venture's annual production of vaccines against meningitis A, B, and C for the Brazilian market would reach between 50 and 100 million doses. Vaccine costs would plummet to about one-fifth of what Cuba charged for the meningitis B vaccine under the 1991 contract, then stated as U.S. $82.5 million.[90] An agreement was signed in January 1992 to begin the joint venture, but by spring it had been suspended because of the inefficacy of the Cuban vaccine in Brazil. Whether any joint production can be salvaged from the deal remains to be seen.

In an interesting bit of political posturing, Alceni Guerra claimed on June 20, 1991, that Brazil would purchase 15 million doses of meningitis B vaccine if Cuba would transfer the technology to manufacture it. This proposal occurred less than two weeks after the health department of the state of São Paulo suspended use of the vaccine because it was less than 50 percent effective. During a debate about the vaccine purchase in the Brazilian Chamber of Deputies, it was suggested that the competence of Cuban scientists was not in question but that insufficient documentation had been provided to properly assess the effect of the vaccine. Representatives of Brazil's own research institutes that were working on a similar vaccine complained about the lack of funding for their projects and suggested that the money spent on purchasing the Cuban vaccine would have allowed them to develop their own.[91]

The Brazilians bought the Cuban vaccine because about 50 percent of the cases in their latest epidemic were subtype B:4:P1.15, the type for which the Cuban vaccine had been developed and for which the vaccine was supposed to be over 80 percent effective.[92] It was inexplicable to the Brazilians why the vaccine was so ineffective if, in fact, the Cubans' tests were valid. For this reason, further tests were run.

The Cuban vaccine for meningitis subtype B:4:P1.15 and C may be 85 percent effective in Cuba but only about 54 percent effective in Brazil because of the prevalence of different subtypes of meningitis B there. The B portion of the vaccine is an outer membrane protein (OMP) vaccine that has great specificity, and that therefore is effective only against the precise subtype of meningitis from which it is made. The C portion is a polysaccharide vaccine that is effective against the entire serogroup, which explains why the Cuban vaccine is more effective against meningitis C in Brazil than against the strains of meningitis B prevalent in the areas tested. Because there is no truly effective vaccine against meningitis B, WHO is conducting field trials in Iceland on the various types of vaccine currently available, including the Cuban vaccine. Results should be available in mid 1993.[93]

Recent Brazilian test results on the effectiveness of the meningitis C portion of the vaccine indicate very good protection for children under the age of two, something that existing meningitis C vaccines do not afford. Oddly, this vaccine is not being explored by the Cubans even though it is very promising. Perhaps this is because several companies already make meningitis C vaccine but no one makes an effective meningitis B vaccine. The latter would be a scientific coup for Cuba if it were proven successful for the entire serogroup B. For this reason Cuban scientists are working on a recombinant meningitis B vaccine for which they have already expressed the protein. They are using this protein to produce an experimental vaccine, but no scientific data have been released yet.[94]

The Cuban meningitis B vaccine, however, became controversial in Brazil not for medical but for political reasons: the state of São Paulo bought it but distributed it to private practitioners instead of

to public health facilities.[95] More importantly, it has been argued that
no real meningitis epidemic existed but that a false epidemic was
being used to mobilize people as part of preelection campaigning,
exploiting their reaction to a real but unacknowledged epidemic under the previous military regime.[96] Thus, it was alleged, Brazilian acquisition of the meningitis B vaccine was more a political ploy than
a medical necessity. Moreover, it was supposedly purchased without
the full consent of the relevant technical experts.[97] It can be argued
that Brazilians suffer more pressing health problems than meningitis,
such as hunger and malnutrition, but those problems require an economic solution that may also mean a political change. Purchasing
meningitis B vaccine allows the government to appear to face a public health problem head on and is, therefore, symbolically important.

The vaccine was purchased, in part, to even out the trade deficit
Cuba held with Brazil. Of the 1991 sale, part of the money would go
toward Cuba's U.S. $38 million debt acquired through the purchase
of various food items, and part of it would finance the construction
of the vaccine factory in Brazil.[98] One knowledgeable observer contended that the health officials did not find the vaccine to be as
effective as claimed but that the foreign ministry wanted the deal to
go through for economic reasons; another claimed that the reasons
were also geopolitical in that the Brazilian government had decided
on a regional foreign policy that would not follow the U.S. trade
embargo against Cuba.[99] If the nonmedical factors were the determinants, it may prove difficult for Cuba to sell the vaccine widely without further testing and without provision of adequate scientific
documentation.

Despite some problems with the initial vaccine deal, particularly
with the delivery of one batch of poor quality, delays in the delivery
schedule, and the lack of timely scientific documentation, the city of
Rio de Janeiro agreed in January 1990 to buy other Cuban products:
sixteen thousand bottles of the vitiligo medication Melagenina and
other pharmaceuticals.[100] In 1991 the city of Niteroi (near Rio de
Janeiro) followed suit; it is opening a vitiligo treatment center with
the aid of Cuban specialists and the importation of Cuban Melagenina.[101] Although the initial problems with the meningitis vaccine
were quickly solved, they raised doubts about whether Cuba could
consistently manufacture high-quality vaccines and other medicinal
products in the requisite quantities. These doubts did not reduce

sales to Brazil, but they did give the Brazilians a bargaining chip for price reductions.

The Cubans seem to be rushing their hepatitis B vaccine to market as well. A PAHO report indicates that the CIGB has expressed the antigen in yeast "in an environment of scientific rigor," yet suggests that although the studies have been satisfactory thus far, they are incomplete. The report adds that "the remaining studies must be carried out in order to have a vaccine of proven safety and efficacy in accordance with WHO international standards."[102] In mid 1991 the Cubans were finishing the third phase of the WHO clinical trials, but an international health official who had seen the data did not know how the Cubans had reached the results they had.[103]

Reading between the lines, the PAHO report expressed concern that the hepatitis B vaccine would be marketed without proper clinical trials, particularly since only six of the twenty-three elements to the WHO protocols for the development of hepatitis B vaccine using recombinant DNA had been completed. The report noted, however, that good progress had been made toward another three, that the methodology for another had been established, and that prelimary studies toward still another had been carried out. The rest remained pending as of May 31, 1989.[104] The PAHO concern was well-founded, as Cuba announced later that year that it would sell the hepatitis B vaccine at below the market rate.[105] Only one month prior to this announcement, the CIGB had submitted a request to PAHO to fund field trials with the long-term objective of achieving WHO standards.[106]

Scientific data available in July 1992 indicate that the Cuban recombinant hepatitis B vaccine has produced good results. It was undergoing the certification procedure of the WHO/PAHO at that time, and if certified, which seems likely, it can be purchased by international organizations, particularly UNICEF which buys vaccines for the WHO regional offices' Expanded Immunization Programs (EPI). If this occurs and Cuba's price is right, the country stands to make considerable earnings because the EPIs are recommending the inclusion of the hepatitis B vaccine in their program of childhood vaccination.[107]

CIGB director Manuel Limonta has claimed that his institute is self-financing through the products it sells, although initially it was not clear whether he was referring to operating expenses or capital investment.[108] Later he suggested that capital expenses were amortized over time rather than covered by initial sales but that the CIGB was self-financing for operating costs.[109] Fidel Castro went further and asserted in late 1990 that "biology, biotechnology and the pharmaceutical industry are self-financing in convertible currency."[110] Sales figures suggest that the CIGB's current operating expenses and the initial capital investment (cited in *The Financial Times* of London as U.S. $110 million) have been covered by the sale of reagents, epidermal growth factor, HIV diagnostic kits, hepatitis B vaccine, and meningitis B vaccine.[111] Although initially developed by CIGB and the National Biopreparations Center, the meningitis B vaccine, a big hard-currency earner, has been produced and marketed since 1990 by another center developed specifically for that purpose, the Instituto Carlos Finlay (formerly the National Anti-Meningococcic Vaccine Center). Moreover, the actual capital investment made in CIGB is unclear because part of the expenditure was in hard currency (about U.S. $25 million) and part in Cuban pesos,[112] and because the Cubans generally do not include such information as the cost of land or surrounding infrastructure in their accounting. Sales to date have been primarily in the form of barter or countertrade, so that no actual hard currency has been realized, although hard currency was saved by not having to purchase other goods with it. In this sense it appears that Castro's statement may be correct.

Epidermal growth factor, produced by CIGB and marketed under the name Facedermin and now Hebermim, has been sold in Latin America, western and eastern Europe, and the former Soviet Union,[113] but no sales figures are available. As early as 1988, the Soviets were interested in large quantities of SUMA equipment and the accompanying reagents. The Cubans, however, did not have the production capacity at that time to supply them because most of their biotechnology and cutting-edge technology products are made in small pilot plants or laboratories until a potential market exists, at which time a research-production center is constructed. The Soviets needed supplies for approximately twelve thousand laboratories, but the Cubans were trying to meet domestic needs first and only then begin to expand production for export.[114]

The 1991 Soviet-Cuban trade agreement called for an increase over 1990 in Cuba's provision of eight types of high-technology medical equipment (including SUMA) and of pharmaceutical and biotechnology products such as interferon, Melagenina, epidermal growth factor, and vaccines against hepatitis B and meningitis B,[115] but the agreement collapsed with the disintegration of the Soviet Union as a unified market and political entity. Cuba and China signed a five-year trade agreement for 1991–1995 valued at U.S. $500 million that also included unspecified biotechnology, pharmaceutical, and medical equipment products.[116]

Domestic need for the enzymes used to cut large DNA molecules at specific points (the most basic step in recombinant DNA technology) led to their mass production for both domestic use and export. The Cuban medical products export firm MediCuba was already marketing six restriction endonucleases under the name of Enzibiot in 1986.[117] Four years later a new Cuban marketing firm, Heber Biotec, the sales agency for CIGB's products, listed in their sales catalog forty restriction endonucleases, nine modification enzymes, three industrial enzymes, two diagnostic kits (HIV- and IgG-based), three software programs, twenty-six monoclonal antibodies, three DNA molecular weight markers, a range of nucleic acid reagents for doing genetic engineering (three primers, forty-one nonphosphorylated linkers, seven adaptors, three plasmid-based vectors), various pharmaceutical products such as alpha, beta, and gamma interferons, human transfer factor, recombinant streptokinase, human recombinant epidermal growth factor, and hepatitis B surface antigen vaccine. Apart from these products, Heber Biotec also offered a service: oligonucleotide custom synthesis using high-performance liquid chromatography and gel electrophoresis.[118] This is an impressive array of products for a developing country that only recently joined the biotechnology enterprise.

Cuba produces good-quality reagents at well below the world market price; thus their products should be quite marketable. Reagents for the AIDS test generally cost between U.S. $2.30 and $2.70 on the world market. In São Paulo, Brazil, they cost $1.09 for each AIDS determination, and in Mato Grosso, Brazil, $5.00. Cuba could supply them for about $.50,[119] but in fact sells them for about 30 percent below the U.S. price.[120] Cuba is the only Latin American country to export restriction enzymes, and its reagents are used in many laboratories in Europe, not out of political sympathy for the revolution but because they are inexpensive and of good quality.[121]

According to Castro himself, one of the hottest items on the research agenda is a cholesterol-reduction drug the Cubans call Ateromixol or PPG, which purports to improve one's sex life as well. It is still in the research phase and is not being developed for the latter property, which is considered to be merely a beneficial side effect.[122] If this drug proves effective for either purpose, it will have considerable market potential.

Cuba is also producing more medical researchers for its eleven specialized medical research institutes, where applied and experimental research has led to the development and application of new medical procedures, equipment, and cures. Some of these medical developments are destined for export as well as for domestic use. Their international acceptance depends on quality, marketing, service, follow-up, utility, affordability, terms of trade, delivery schedules, and geopolitics. Some Cuban medical products have been marketed abroad for years, either by Cuban firms or by private companies from capitalist countries. For example, the RALCA external fixator is sold by Cuban agents in Central and South America, France, Japan, Mexico, and Libya.[123] This type of fixator and its successful experimental use in the United States was featured on a health segment of the CBS morning news program in the United States on January 14, 1991, after more than a decade of generalized use in Cuba.

MediCuba, which handles both imports and exports of medical products, has been exporting Cuban medical goods since 1978.[124] The Union de Empresas Productoras de Equipos Médicos (UEPEM), one of two consortiums of producers of medical equipment in Cuba, produces 143 items, some of which have been exported to Nicaragua, various African countries, East Germany, Czechoslovakia, and Vietnam, for a total of about one million Cuban pesos.[125] Cuba imports base chemicals to produce pharmaceuticals to supply over 80 percent of the domestic market and for export to capitalist countries, particularly those in Latin America, most of which are already Cuba's customers. In 1987 Cuba spent U.S. $34.6 million on imported base chemicals and in 1989 exported approximately U.S. $75 million in finished products, of which over two-thirds was destined for market economies.[126]

The Industria Cubana de Equipos Médicos (ICEM) produces a thirty-three page catalog of medical instruments, medical electronic equipment, and medical furniture and rehabilitation equipment, and the Fábrica de Equipos Médicos de Santiago de Cuba (RETOMED) publishes a sixty-three page catalog of laboratory equipment, dental equipment, lamps, optical products, medical electronics, and physical therapy equipment. Although the products available may be of good quality, some of the catalogs were rudimentary by international standards, exhibiting many spelling and grammatical mistakes in the English translation, and often offering insufficient product information. MediCuba catalogs for 1991 were much improved on all counts, and those available from Heber Biotec for 1992 approached international norms.

Because marketing is so important in capitalist trade relations, it is doubtful that these products will be successfully sold in large quantities except on favorable terms to the buyer or through barter arrangements with Third World countries, unless adequate service and follow-up can be guaranteed. As one international health official said, "Marketing is everything." If this is so, how can Cuba compete with the transnational pharmaceutical companies and medical equipment producers?[127] Barter and international cooperation agreements may be the answer.

Barter (as well as countertrade and clearing accounts) is still at the heart of Cuba's recent trade and cooperation agreements with various African, Latin American, and Middle Eastern countries, as well as with China, the former Soviet Union, and now the republics. These agreements have included an increase in cooperation (read aid and trade, particularly barter) in the health sphere whereby Cuba provides medical, pharmaceutical, and biotechnology products, and the other party furnishes whatever it can (agricultural or industrial goods) that Cuba either needs or can trade elsewhere (triangulate) for something more useful.

Because Cuba can provide medicines at well below world-market prices, the Venezuelan government has shown considerable interest in importing generic drugs from Cuba.[128] In these fiscally difficult times, many governments may find that importing medicines from Cuba is the only way they can meet domestic public-health demands.

It is unclear whether Cuba will be able to import sufficient quantities of the materials needed for the production of its high-technology medical products. A 1989 study indicated that at least 98 percent of the inputs into three such products, Cardiocid-M, Medicid-3M, and Neurocid-M, were purchased with hard currency.[129] These three items were part of Cuba's 1991 export package of medical technology to the former Soviet Union and probably make up part of the 1992 trade agreement with various republics. Therefore unless Cuba is able to get the inputs it will have difficulty meeting its contract obligations. Comments made by European vendors of laboratory equipment in July 1992 about sales to Cuba since 1989 indicate that hard currency is available for the biotechnology and medical-pharmaceutical research centers and industries, and it would seem reasonable to assume that inputs into production are attainable as well.[130]

The difference in price between products available in capitalist countries and comparable products produced in Cuba suggest that Cuba saves considerable hard currency by import substitution and that it could make a handsome profit by producing this equipment domestically and exporting it at any price above cost. For example, comparing the prices in 1987 contracts for medical equipment from capitalist countries that was comparable to Cuban-made products, a Cuban researcher, using an exchange rate of one U.S. dollar per Cuban peso, found that Cardiovit electrocardiogram equipment analogous to Cuba's Cardiocid-M was sold for $14,363.22. However it cost Cuba only $3,351.84 to make, so that as a result of domestic production Cuba saved approximately $11,000 per unit.[131] It must be noted that the dollar fluctuates and is actually worth fifty pesos (March 1993) on the black market and that this exchange rate is closer to its true value, so that the savings for Cuba might be greater than the researcher suggested. Likewise, the Spectrum 32 electroencephalogram equipment sold for $30,000, whereas the Cuban version, Medicid-3M, cost Cuba $16,074.85 to produce, for savings of about $14,000 per item. Finally, the Neuropack electromyographic analysis system was priced at $40,000, but the Cuban model, Neurocid-M, cost Cuba only $3,659.13 to make, for a savings of about $36,300 per unit.[132]

Although these costs are probably variable in that they do not include research and development costs and equipment depreciation (the Cubans do not know how to do true cost accounting yet), it is still quite likely that domestic production of this equipment is very profitable in spite of the high percentage of imported components. In 1986, for example, Cuba imported 81.1 million pesos worth of medical products, half of all products consumed domestically.[133] Had these been produced domestically, the savings would have been substantial. The costs of research and development in a command economy are very different from and incomparably lower than those in a capitalist economy. Moreover, the initial impetus to produce the equipment was import substitution undertaken to meet the needs of the ever-expanding domestic health-care system. With the infrastructure in place, the potential profits Cuba can make on these export items should substantiate the wisdom of the government's policy of making the export of medical products one of the highest priorities.

Although Cuba met only 31 percent of its domestic medical equipment needs in 1989 (while projecting it would meet 40 percent) and estimated that 45 percent would be met in 1990, the country began exporting this type of product in 1984, though not at the expense of meeting domestic demand. Some products the Cubans need have not been produced domestically because of the lack of inputs and technology, inadequate demand to warrant domestic production, or high cost of domestic production compared to the cost of importation. Between 1984 and 1989, total exports were calculated at 2.2 billion pesos, of which 33.8 percent was sold to the former socialist countries that began receiving Cuban medical equipment in 1987.[134]

By 1989 Cuba had already exported seventeen medical equipment products to Albania, Angola, Bulgaria, Bolivia, Ethiopia, Spain, Guyana, Hungary, Iraq, Kuwait, Mexico, Mongolia, Nicaragua, Uganda, and Vietnam. Projections by a Cuban researcher made in 1989, before the fall of the Berlin Wall, for trade with the CMEA countries between 1991 and 1995 included about 27.5 billion pesos of Cuban medical equipment exports.[135] High-level Cuban economists justifiably doubt this figure.[136] If one considers that the 1991 trade agreement between Cuba and the Soviet Union called for U.S. $730 million in sales of Cuban medical and biotechnology products, and if the Soviets had continued to purchase these products at the same rate, then over a five-year period Cuban gross earnings would be U.S. $3.65 billion.

Even adding possible sales to the other former members of CMEA, all of whom have smaller markets than the former Soviet Union, it becomes quite clear that the trade projection was more wishful thinking than reality. Moreover, trade with the former CMEA countries has virtually vanished since then, and it seems unlikely in the current political and economic climate that they will find barter or clearing accounts with Cuba the least expensive way to acquire certain medical, pharmaceutical, and biotechnology products. Some of the republics of the former Soviet Union are finding that trading with Cuba still makes sense, but the magnitude does not compare with that of past trade with the Soviet Union.

A Cuban student of international relations suggested that, given the economic difficulties of Third World countries, Cuba "intensify medical assistance in the immediate future, linking it to the provision of medicines and specialized instruments [produced in Cuba] for hospitals that the receiving country necessarily acquires abroad."[137] She maintained that Cuba should offer complete hospital complexes, or parts thereof, and build, equip, and supply them with material as well as human resources. She mentioned joint ventures as a means of meeting both Cuba's and other developing countries' needs, but these would require prior market analyses. Finally, she called for the strengthening of links between Cuba and international organizations such as WHO, PAHO, and UNICEF to allow Cuba to participate in future projects from the outset and to play a role in the design of the project and the construction and/or supply of facilities, equipment, and personnel.[138] The Cuban government has successfully applied all of these tactics in one case or another in its past efforts to increase medical exports, but much work remains to be done to expand these exports.

Miguel Figueras, economic advisor to the president of the State Committee for Economic Collaboration (CECE), said that there is a fine line between providing medical aid in a disinterested manner and indirectly "selling" Cuban medicines. He asserted that Cuba does not use its doctors for the sales promotion of Cuban medical products. If anything, he insisted, Cuban medical aid opens markets for the transnational pharmaceutical companies because the Cubans create a demand for medical products and the transnationals dominate the global market.[139]

As for projects with developed countries, Cuba has joint ventures with the Japanese firms Sakura Finitechnical (since 1982) and Meiji Seika to produce medical equipment for the Cuban domestic market and for export now that most of the domestic need has been met. The Japanese companies supply parts, components, know-how, and licensing, and the Cubans make and sell the final product. The tabletop sterilization equipment, Autoclave ASH-260, made with Sakura, cost U.S. $850 to produce in 1989, but the world market price was U.S. $2500. Total production for 1989 was only 2,058 units, and the estimate for 1990 was 2,501 units. When the initial 100 autoclaves were produced in 1982, all of the components were imported, but by 1989 only 34 percent came from Japan.[140]

Cuba has exported very few of these sterilization apparatuses because the first priority has been to furnish them to the family doctors. In 1987 only 90 were exported, at 1553.49 Cuban pesos each, for a total of 139,814 pesos. Among Cuba's clients were Hungary (which bought 2), Vietnam (25), Nicaragua (10), and Uganda (50). None were exported in 1988, and in 1989 only 20 were sold to Nicaragua at 2,500 pesos each, which is the world market price if one uses a conversion rate of one peso to the dollar.[141] Both 1988 and 1989 were years of major expansion for the Family Doctor Program, which probably accounts for diminished exports during those years. Export capacity was projected to increase when the family doctor network was completed in 1995, but export potential remains dependent on a number of factors, not the least of which is Cuban marketing abilities in a politically and economically hostile environment.

In agricultural biotechnology Cuba has saved millions of dollars a year through import substitution and increased productivity. For example, genetic engineering laboratories produce disease-resistant seeds for more than five basic crops.[142] The biochemistry group at CNIC has produced dry cells for poultry feed by extracting lysine from yeast.[143] CIB researchers have innovatively isolated a toxin that causes a hemorrhagic bovine disease and have been using it to develop a vaccine.[144] Biotechnology is also being used to improve the industrial efficiency of sugar mills through the addition of enzymes at various points in the refining process.[145] The hard-currency savings from these biotechnology interventions are sufficient to make the second CIGB (devoted to agriculture) self-financing as well.[146]

Whether or not Cuba is immediately successful in exporting its biotechnology, medical, and pharmaceutical products is critical for Cuba's economic, and thus political, survival, but the mere ability to export these products is symbolically important. If this accumulated symbolic capital can be converted quickly into material capital, then Cuban pharmaceuticals, biotechnology, and medical products will have done wonders for the economy and thereby helped sustain the political regime.

Biotechnology and Symbolic Capital

Through the development of biotechnology, the Cuban government has garnered a measure of domestic and international legitimacy. Cuba was in the competition in the early 1980s to house the United Nations Industrial Development Organization (UNIDO)–

sponsored International Center for Genetic Engineering and Biotechnology (ICGEB). Because of divisive politics and delays in the decision-making process, Castro went ahead with the construction of a similar center following the UNIDO plan but without UNIDO's financial support. Construction began in 1984 and took a little over two years to complete. The Center for Genetic Engineering and Biotechnology (CIGB) opened in July 1986 and was at that time one of the largest laboratories in the world, surpassed only by Monsanto.[147] Building this center brought Cuba enormous symbolic capital among researchers, government officials, intellectuals, and international organizations officials, all of whom have marveled at the facility and its capabilities.

The Cuban view of the problems with UNIDO decision making was substantiated by international reports. In 1983, Belgium, Cuba, India, Italy, Pakistan, and Thailand were still in the running to house the UNIDO center, but India seemed likely to prevail because of Sweden's support.[148] Both Sweden and Canada had withdrawn from the competition because of a "dominance of politics in the scientific debates."[149]

After many delays the decision was made in February 1984 to have two sites, one in Trieste and the other in New Delhi, each concentrating on a different area of research. The Delhi center was commissioned to deal with Third World problems.[150] After years of organization and debate, the ICGEB in New Delhi was supposed to begin operating in 1989,[151] but neither that facility nor the one in Trieste was operational in late 1990. In fact, according to a North American knowledgeable in this field, these centers are considered the white elephants of biotechnology, partially because there is no consensus on what research to do or how to do it, nor is there agreement on how to coordinate efforts. Further, much of the research in which these centers might engage is already carried out in the private sector or in universities and other research institutes.[152]

Writing in various publications about the privatization of biotechnology research and development, Daniel Goldstein levels a different sort of criticism at the international centers and their lack of utility even when they are operational. Goldstein is highly critical of their negative impact on scientific endeavors in general, particularly those in the Third World. He also condemns the nexus between transnational corporations and universities that leads to rapid patenting of research results and the failure, for obvious commercial reasons, to disseminate those results.

Moreover, Goldstein suggests that although the international organizations that promote biotechnology research in the Third World do so with good intentions, the results of their endeavors redound to the benefit of transnational corporations rather than to the peoples of the Third World. Clearly, he contends, the problems of the Third World studied by the scientists at these international centers may produce good results that will be in the public domain and that therefore will be easily patented by a transnational corporation and expensive for the developing countries to acquire. This process goes beyond just the continued loss by the Third World of their reservoir of germ plasm that has for some time been exploited by First World companies; it is also a type of brain drain but without physical migration and a deepening of the dependency of developing countries on those already developed.[153]

This privatization and commodification of biotechnology research is also decried by the New York–based joint Council on International and Public Affairs-International Center for Law in Development (CIPA-ICLD) Biotechnology Research Group for much the same reasons as are proposed by Goldstein. But for reasons similar to those in the developed countries, David Dembo, Clarence Dias, and Ward Morehouse of CIPA-ICLD also suggest the probable extension of this trend among those developing countries that have biotechnology capabilities.[154] Rather than engage in what is known in international organizations and development circles as TCDC or technical cooperation among developing countries, these Third World countries' "national self-interest may well tend to override Third World solidarity" because of the extreme competitiveness of the biotechnology race, in which dominance is equated with national security.[155]

Although the Cuban CIGB addresses Third World problems, makes results available to developing countries, and was intended to provide training for and collaboration with scientists from other Third World countries, the hard-currency crisis in which Cuba finds itself dictates that it too consider national self-interest (economic and hence political survival) over solidarity. Consequently, the Cubans have thus far refused to transfer possibly lucrative technology in this field to other countries; it is clear that if they do so, they will lose their potential market share just as others may have when Cuba copied their patented products.[156] In this sense, CIGB may be no different than Genentech or any other U.S. biotechnology or pharmaceutical company.

Although Cuba has made considerable gains, the country has neither the resources nor the experience to be at the forefront of biotechnology research. Cuban scientists have taken bold steps in certain areas but primarily have acquainted themselves with the literature and techniques that they have quickly mastered and successfully applied. Cuban scientists are good copiers of techniques developed elsewhere, but without doing basic research they are unable to create the real profit-making products. Because much of what they produce is patented elsewhere, trade with countries honoring patent laws will be extremely difficult.[157] Moreover, "Changes in instrumentation from one year to the next are so great that even American universities have trouble keeping up"; how, then, can a resource-poor developing country do so?[158]

Cuba does not have the scientific infrastructure to be at the forefront of medical research, but Cuban medical scientists have pioneered some techniques, treatments, and instruments. Whether these will gain acceptability outside Third World or socialist settings is debatable. Cuba's best prospects are for joint ventures with companies in the developed world in which their partner provides capital, marketing skills and distribution networks, and some know-how. In fact, the president of Heber Biotec said that he would accept any deal that allowed the company to control its own activities and be profitable, and that he was interested in a joint venture with anyone as long as it did not impede the development of Heber Biotec, CIGB, and Cuba.[159] This view was reiterated in July 1992 by Dr. Manuel Limonta Vidal, the director of the CIGB, who said that he would listen to any offer.[160] Joint ventures and mergers and acquisitions are common in the biotechnology field, where start-up companies begin small but are bought out by transnational pharmaceuticals if and when they demonstrate potential profitability.

The innovative biomedical products that Cuba has marketed have not been created through genetic engineering. The meningitis B vaccine is a traditional (outer membrane protein or OMP) vaccine, and SUMA is a very cost-effective refinement of the standard ELISA test equipment. The biotechnology products Cuba has marketed are those such as interferon, epidermal growth factor (EGF), and recombinant hepatitis B vaccine, all of which Cuban scientists have copied from elsewhere. Recombinant streptokinase may be an innovation, but natural streptokinase is very inexpensive and easy to produce;[161] this innovation has no great merit unless it can be shown to be substantially more effective or cheaper to produce than the natural product. Products such as nerve growth factor (NGF) are still in the research phase and are already produced elsewhere. Cuban reagents do have markets, but the global demand for them is tiny (perhaps about one hundred laboratories want one thousand bottles per year), and there is considerable competition.[162]

It is possible that Cuban work on epidermal growth factor, human transfer factor, nerve growth factor, and other products is somehow different from work by other scientists in either its expression or its effectiveness. But because the Cubans are less than forthcoming in providing documentation and because they remain obtuse on matters of intellectual property, it is not clear whether they have made innovations. Nonetheless, if Cuba can sell its biotechnology products to the former Soviet republics even though those products are not original, then those sales alone would justify the enormous expenditure made to develop the CIGB. But if the republics begin to recognize patents, as is likely as they integrate into the world capitalist system, then Cuba's biotechnology enterprise will have increasing difficulty in remaining self-financing.

As the Cubans have become more adept in the biotechnology and biomedical field and as their potential markets have changed, they have begun to seek patents for certain products like the meningitis B vaccine, recombinant alpha interferon, recombinant streptokinase, and the uses of various monoclonal antibodies. The marketing manager of the Center for Molecular Immunology (CIMAB), Dr. Juan Félix Amador Pérez, said that CIMAB staff were studying patents and patent law to see where they could get patents for their monoclonal antibodies and that it was more important not to violate other people's patents than to get their own.[163] This is a new twist for the Cubans, who now must sell in an unprotected (nonsocialist) market.

Patents present one of the most difficult problems for Cuban biotechnology exports. Patent law in this field is quite complex and what one can patent varies considerably across countries. Biotechnology patents are issued either for processes, methods of cloning and expression, or products. Changes in arriving at a recombinant substance must be substantial to warrant a new patent for the process or to claim that the product does not violate existing patents. If a different expression system only tinkers with an amino acid or two and does not affect the biological activity of the recombinant product, then the change is not sufficient to make the product or process new.[164]

Naturally occurring substances such as antibodies cannot be patented, but a use for them can. A patent may be requested for all uses of a monoclonal antibody to treat a specific disease, but either the patent office or the courts generally limit the scope of the patent to a narrow area. There is considerable litigation in the biotechnology field over who "owns" what processes and products. Loopholes exist in U.S. patent law allowing a company to produce a biotechnology product offshore that is already patented by another company in the United States and to import it into the United States without infringing on patent rights. Unfortunately for Cuba, the trade embargo precludes Cuba's entry into the U.S. market by this or any other means.[165]

On the other hand, Cuban biotechnology has benefited from UNDP funding of U.S. $2.2 million over a five-year period beginning in 1986. Cuba participates in the UNDP regional biotechnology program and "co-ordinates a project with Mexico and Colombia for the commercial production of penicillin amidase and 6-APA."[166] Moreover, Cuba plays an important role in the UNDP–Pan American Health Organization–Latin American Economic System (SELA) joint project of technical cooperation among Latin American and Caribbean countries in scientific development and health technology. The estimated regional market for health technology products in 1990 was approximately U.S. $1.5 billion, of which about U.S. $500 million was covered by intraregional production.[167] If Cuba can increase its share of this regional market and continue to receive funding from international organizations, then its biotechnology and medical export endeavors may well continue to be self-financing and become important sources of hard-currency earnings even if only on barter terms. Unfortunately, this endeavor along with the tourism program will not be sufficient to keep the economy afloat.

Criticisms of Cuba's biotechnology efforts are warranted but must be taken in the context of Cuba's accomplishments, which are noteworthy, and not just in the context of the Third World. No country in the Third World is doing the type of work the Cubans are, none does it on a scale that approaches theirs, and none does research in as many areas. Whether the CIGB is a high-technology white elephant or a gold mine is as yet uncertain. Irrespective of judgments about its true worth, the CIGB is perhaps as important for the symbolic capital it accumulates for Cuba in the eyes of scientists, policymakers, and international organizations officials who are awed by it, as for any actual biotechnology achievements. This symbolic capital has been an essential factor in Cuba's ability to conduct medical diplomacy.

What is notable here is the Cuban government's political use of the CIGB in both the domestic and international arenas as a symbol of the government's achievements, abilities, foresight, and determination to succeed against all odds. Because the fruits of biotechnology have not yet been harvested anywhere, Cuba is in a good position to take advantage of biotechnological breakthroughs from which other developing nations will be largely excluded. The new international division of labor will be between those who can manipulate sophisticated scientific and technological processes and those who supply raw materials and assembled goods. Castro wants Cuba to be among the former. Moreover, the conversion of symbolic capital into financial capital through trade and aid has suggested the wisdom of this seemingly farfetched project.[168]

Whether Cuba can continue to maintain a highly privileged scientific sector in a country that in other areas is rapidly returning to the preindustrial era is questionable. Tensions are bound to arise between this sector and the nonprivileged sectors of society, particularly among employees in those sectors who become marginally employed or unemployed because of the energy shortages and have to work in agriculture. Moreover, the enormous burden of saving the revolution is placed on those in the scientific sector who must search for ways to develop marketable products quickly. This haste to solve the problems of underdevelopment allows little time for basic research and thereby makes most work derivative rather than innovative. Nonetheless, Cuba's biotechnology capabilities have created considerable symbolic capital among scientists and politicians from both developed and developing countries, as well as among officials of international organizations. What is needed now are more markets, and these may come only through international organizations' technical cooperation programs and through countertrade or barter. Thus the overall policy of capitalizing on the development of biotechnology and medical exports is sound, but the current economic circumstances make long-term success unlikely.

6

Cuban Medical Diplomacy

Medical diplomacy has been overlooked in analyses of Cuban foreign policy, yet it has been an integral part of almost all the cooperation and aid agreements that Cuba has used historically to strengthen diplomatic ties with other Third World countries. Dozens of countries have received long-term Cuban medical assistance, and many others have received short-term aid in response to specific emergencies. Cuban medical aid affects millions of Third World people annually through the direct provision of medical care, and thousands annually through medical education and training programs both in Cuba and abroad. The positive impact of this aid on the health of Third World populations has vastly improved Cuba's relations with other countries and has increased Cuba's symbolic capital among governments, international organizations, and intellectuals who, in the Third World, often play an important role in the formation of public opinion and public policy.

Cuba has been particularly adept at using medical diplomacy to further its political and economic objectives and accumulate symbolic capital. Medical diplomacy or "collaboration between countries on health matters for the purposes of improving relations with one another . . . [produces] humanitarian benefit while simultaneously developing improved relations."[1] Because all peoples consider health necessary for personal as well as societal development, medical aid may be a more effective foreign policy instrument than other, more traditional, ones.

Domestic success in the medical field led the Cuban leadership to capitalize on accumulated symbolic capital and to make health an important part of its foreign policy. Since 1963 Cuba has provided civilian assistance to many Third World countries, despite its own economic difficulties. This assistance has taken the form of direct medical care and medical education both in the host country and in Cuba; donation of equipment, medicines, and supplies; disaster relief; epidemic control and epidemiological monitoring; facility construction; organizational, administrative, and planning advice; scientific research and exchanges; vaccination and health-education campaigns; and program design for both the development of human resources and the provision of specific medical services, among other things.[2] Early cooperation agreements were bilateral, but over time Cuba also became a party to multilateral aid agreements and began to provide assistance to other Third World countries under the auspices of various United Nations agencies and regional organizations.

The first beneficiary was Premier Ahmed Ben Bella's newly independent Algeria, to which Cuba sent a group of fifty-six physicians and other health workers for fourteen months in 1963.[3] This was done despite the fact that half of Cuba's physicians emigrated (mostly to the United States) shortly after the revolution, reducing the number of Cuba's physicians from about six thousand to three thousand. Interestingly, this first program of medical assistance was known as the "Plan Fidel," presaging Castro's later daily involvement in and concern for health care.[4] The growth of medical diplomacy and other civilian aid programs increased dramatically beginning in the mid to late 1970s, so much so that Cuba had in 1985 what *The New York Times* called "perhaps the largest Peace Corps style program of civilian aid in the world," with approximately sixteen thousand doctors, teachers, construction engineers, agronomists, economists, and other specialists serving in twenty-two Third World countries.[5] In fact, Cuba had more doctors working abroad then (fifteen hundred in twenty-five countries) than did WHO.[6]

Throughout the 1980s Cuban foreign policy dictates sent between two thousand and three thousand medical workers abroad each year for two-year stints; at least half of them were doctors.[7] In July 1991 over one thousand Cuban doctors were donating their services abroad, and up to that date more than ten thousand physicians had done likewise, as had another twenty thousand other health workers.[8] These medical personnel have served in over thirty-six countries on three continents, furthered Cuba's foreign policy goals, and contributed significantly to Cuba's symbolic capital.

According to an unsubstantiated but published Cuban source, the global reach of Cuban civilian aid expanded in the five-year period from 1985 to 1990, when Cuba supplied sixty countries with more than forty-six thousand civilian aid workers per year, primarily doctors, teachers, and construction crews. These workers served in thirty-seven African and Middle Eastern countries, thirteen Asian and Oceanian countries, and ten Latin American and Caribbean countries. A Cuban official claimed that over a twenty-five-year period ending in January 1990, more than half a million Cubans provided civilian assistance abroad, a figure equivalent to approximately 10 percent of Cuba's economically active population at that time.[9] These numbers appear to be high in light of other, better-known estimates.

Symbolically even more significant, by January 1985 Cuba had one civilian international aid worker for every 625 inhabitants and by January 1990 one civilian aid worker for every 228 inhabitants. In 1985, on the other hand, the United States had only one Peace Corps or Agency for International Development (AID) worker for every 31,023 inhabitants and in 1990 one for every 35,760 inhabitants.[10] Whereas U.S. Peace Corps workers often work alone, Cubans generally work in teams or brigades, which makes their presence more visible. Moreover, Cuba has often sent more highly skilled personnel than the United States has. According to the Agency for International Development, "In general, the Peace Corps supplies technical assistance at a much lower level in terms of expertise and experience than the technical assistance provided by other donors."[11]

The large number of international aid workers sent by Cuba compared with that sent by the United States not only signifies Cuba's emphasis on civilian aid as a foreign policy tool but also makes Cuba appear to provide more humanitarian aid than the United States despite the latter's much greater financial assistance. Recognizing this visibility problem, the General Accounting Office has suggested that the United States decrease the number of projects it finances and concentrate on larger, more visible ones to improve its image. This visibility problem is particularly important because in the early 1980s, the United States ranked seventeenth among the eighteen Development Assistance Committee member countries of the Organization for Economic Co-operation and Development (OECD) in foreign aid as a percentage of gross national product.[12] By 1988–89

Table 11: Communist Economic Technicians in LDCs, 1976, 1977, 1979, and 1981

	1976		1977		1979		1981	
	N	%	N	%	N	%	N	%
Total	70,145	100	89,345	99.9	107,300	99.9	118,760	100
USSR & E. Eur.	45,345	64.6	58,755	65.7	80,830	75.3	95,685	80.6
China	20,415	29.1	24,015	26.8	12,860	11.9	—	—
Cuba	4,385	6.3	6,575	7.4	13,610	12.7	23,075	19.4

SOURCES: Calculated from Central Intelligence Agency, *Communist Aid Activities in Non-Communist LDCs, 1979 and 1954–1979* (Washington, D.C.: CIA, April 15, 1980), 10, 21; CIA, *Communist Aid Activities in Non-Communist LDCs, 1978* (Washington, D.C.: CIA, 1979), 9; and CIA, *Communist Aid Activities in Non-Communist LDCs, 1977* (Washington, D.C.: CIA, 1978), 9.

the United States was tied with Ireland for last place, providing only 0.18 percent of its GNP in development assistance.[13]

Cuba, by contrast, when compared with its former allies and benefactors in the Soviet Union and eastern Europe, has sent a disproportionately large number of international economic technicians to developing nations. Cuba supplied 19.4 percent of the total Soviet, eastern European, and Cuban economic technicians abroad in 1979, as table 11 indicates,[14] yet Cuba's population was only 2.5 percent of the combined populations of these countries.[15] More importantly, Cuba was and still is the least developed of all these countries. Although the USSR and the eastern European countries had more economic technicians abroad than the Cubans, most were contract workers earning hard currency for their countries, whereas most of the Cubans were aid workers.[16] Once again, Cuba demonstrated its commitment to civilian aid as a means of improving its international relations.

Moreover, Cuba's development of doctors as an export commodity is unprecedented. The Soviet Union, the eastern European countries, and China have provided some medical assistance to developing nations, but it has been a small part of their aid programs and they did not train surplus doctors specifically for export as Cuba did. For example, China, the other communist country that has primarily provided aid, had almost four times the number of economic technicians abroad that Cuba did in 1977, but in 1979 Cuba provided slightly more economic technicians than did China. During that two-year interval, China had decreased its aid by 50 percent and Cuba had doubled its aid.[17] In medicine alone, Cuba also far outpaced China in the provision of international aid, sending almost as many health workers abroad from 1983 through 1985 (7,544) as China sent abroad between 1963 and 1986 (8,000).[18] This achievement alone has made Cuba a world medical power in the eyes of many international organizations officials and Third World intellectuals and policy-makers, and as a result it has contributed substantially to Cuba's symbolic capital.

Direct Provision of Medical Care in the Host Country

Difficulty in gaining access to information makes it somewhat problematic to separate out the different types of medical aid Cuba has provided to each country; however, the most symbolically significant aid has usually been direct medical care in the host country itself, because such aid acknowledges both that country's inability to care for its own people and Cuba's scientific superiority. Along with direct care, Cuba has generally provided on-the-job training for host-country medical workers and carried out sophisticated medical procedures on foreign patients in Cuba.

As the following list demonstrates, most of the recipients of medical aid have been countries with ideologies similar to or compatible with Cuba's. These thirty-two countries were receiving Cuban medical aid in November 1988 (most still were in July 1991) in the form of long-term direct provision of medical care. They are listed chronologically by the date that this aid began: Algeria (1963), Mali (1965), Congo (1966), Tanzania (1966), Guinea-Conakry (1967), Vietnam (1969), Democratic (South) Yemen (1972), Equatorial Guinea (1973), Laos (1973), Guinea-Bissau (1975), São Tomé and Príncipe (1976), Angola (1976), Guyana (1976), Cape Verde Islands (1976), Mozambique (1977), Benin (1977), Ethiopia (1977), Saharan Arab Republic (Western Sahara–Polisario guerrillas) (1977), Iraq (1978), Kampuchea (1979), Nicaragua (1979), Uganda (1979), Burundi (1980), Seychelles (1980), Ghana (1983), Kuwait (1985), Burkina Faso (1985), Zimbabwe (1986), Sri Lanka (1986), Maldives

(1988), and Botswana (1988).[19] Grenada (until October 1983) and Jamaica (until 1981) also received Cuban medical aid.[20] Zambia was later added to the list. Other countries have received and still receive Cuban medical aid but in different forms. Where direct patient care has been a part of that aid in other countries, it often has been ancillary to Cuban training programs or ministerial-level advisory services.

Cuba's civilian aid has been provided largely as a means of establishing ties with another country but has also accompanied military aid. It expanded considerably, therefore, when troops were deployed to Angola in late 1975 and then to Ethiopia in 1977. Figures for 1977 indicate that Cuba provided between 45 percent and 84 percent of the doctors in seven countries (six in Africa), and also sent 650 health-care workers to Libya, of whom 357 were physicians.[21] Cuba had 686 medical workers in Angola in 1981, of whom 335 were doctors and 12 were dentists. They saw about one million patients that year.[22]

Cuban medical teams provided health care in thirteen Angolan provinces until September 1987, when they retired from two provinces, Lunda Sul and Moxico. During 1986 they saw 1,280,787 medical and surgical cases and 17,160 dental cases. In 1987 Cuban doctors treated 1,051,892 cases, including surgical cases, and dentists attended 13,104 patients.[23] With the retirement of Cuban troops from Angola in 1990 in accordance with the peace accord and changing politics within Angola, the Cuban medical brigade began to shrink. Health workers were said to have withdrawn completely from one province, Benguela, where a medical brigade had been working for fifteen years. They were to be replaced by Bulgarians and Vietnamese (both of whom were less dogmatic than the Cubans at the time), probably because of growing political differences between the Angolan and Cuban governments as the Angolans moved away from Marxism-Leninism.[24]

In Ethiopia, Cuban medical personnel stationed in eleven out of fourteen provinces numbered over 300 in 1978 but 234 by 1984; 130 were physicians and dentists.[25] Between 1979 and 1981, Cuban doctors treated almost 1.5 million Ethiopian patients.[26] Precarious working conditions there because of the civil war and extraordinary poverty did not deter the Cubans from delivering as much medical care as possible. A European nurse who worked in Ethiopia in the late 1980s observed that the Cubans there worked extremely hard and were very effective and self-sacrificing, yet lived in squalid conditions like most Ethiopians and unlike other foreign aid workers, and did not complain about their lot.[27]

Despite their dedication and hard work, Cuban aid workers were not always appreciated by everyone in the host country. In January, 1990, a six-member medical brigade was captured in Assossa, Ethiopia, by the Oromo National Liberation Front, probably because the Cuban government supported the government of Haile Mariam Mengistu, against which the Oromos were fighting. The brigade was held captive in the Sudan and released between May and August 1990 after the Cuban government enlisted various African heads of state and the heads of the Organization of African Unity and the International Red Cross to intervene with the Sudanese government on the hostages' behalf.[28] By mid 1991, however, all Cuban medical personnel had returned from Ethiopia because of political change there.[29]

Elsewhere in the developing world, the Cuban medical brigade in the Cape Verde Islands provided 36,000 medical consultations and 1,500 surgical interventions during 1977.[30] In 1978 Cuban medical workers treated over 39,000 patients in outpatient clinics and 5,600 in hospitals, performed thirty major operations, and delivered more than 2,000 babies in rural areas of the People's Republic of the Congo. They attended 200,000 patients during a fifteen-month stay in Guyana.[31] Although Cuba sent only twelve physicians to Grenada in 1979, they had treated about half of Grenada's population by mid 1980 and tripled the number of physicians in Grenada.[32] Under the first Michael Manley administration in Jamaica, fifty Cuban doctors worked in Jamaica, of whom fourteen provided services in the hospital in Savana-La-Mar in Westmoreland province as of 1976.[33] Eighteen Cuban specialists worked in a hospital in the capital of Kampuchea in 1980.[34]

In 1987 the Cuban medical brigade in Nicaragua attended 856,000 patients, performed 7163 major operations and delivered 1704 babies.[35] With the electoral defeat of the Sandinistas in 1990, Cuba withdrew most of its civilian aid workers at the request of the new government, but a medical brigade of 167 workers remained.[36] In December 1990 there were 150 Cuban doctors working in various Nicaraguan provinces including the areas of Bluefields, Granada, Managua, and Masaya. In October alone they attended over 30,000 outpatients and expected to treat up to half a million people by the end of 1990.[37] Under specific agreements with the Violeta Barrios de Chamorro government, some new medical brigades have been sent. In mid 1992, over one hundred Cuban doctors were providing free medical care to Nicaraguans, many in areas where other doctors would not work.[38] Continued Cuban medical aid to Nicaragua despite the Barrios government's deep ideological differences with Cuba attests to the wisdom of this form of nontraditional diplomacy; without medical aid, it is unlikely that there would be any positive relations between the two governments.

During fifteen months from late 1984 through 1985, Cuban physicians in Iraq treated over one million patients on an outpatient basis, performed 1,743 operations, and assisted 3,700 births.[39] In 1986 there were 372 Cuban medical workers in various Iraqi cities, some of whom were orthopedists working at the Children's Orthopedic Hospital in Baghdad, a hospital that had been developed with Cuban assistance.[40] Sixty-seven Cubans staffed the orthopedic hospital in 1988, a year in which the total number of children the Cuban physicians had attended since 1980 exceeded 25,000 and in which the number of operations performed had reached approximately 10,000.[41] During the Persian Gulf War, a team of 182 medical workers, mostly women, remained in Iraq to continue providing medical aid in Iraqi hospitals. It was urgently needed then not just because of the war but also because other foreign health workers had left by January 1991. The Cubans returned home in April 1991, only after the war had ended and after completing their assignment in Iraq.[42]

These "proletarian internationalists," as they are called in Cuba, often work in remote areas, providing services that the host country's population has never experienced before.[43] In 1986 in Laos, 11 members of a Cuban medical brigade organized two medical posts in remote areas.[44] Two Cuban medical brigades worked in Mali in 1987; the larger one in a distant town, Segou, but the other in the capital, Bamako.[45] In the outlying town of Harar, Ethiopia, in 1985, the police hospital was staffed entirely by Cubans, both doctors and paramedical personnel, with the exception of one Ethiopian physician.[46] By 1988, a total of 706 Cuban doctors worked in five out of nine countries belonging to the South African Development Cooperation Council (SADCC). Fifty-seven percent of these doctors served rural areas. Since SADCC countries had only 4,200 physicians at that time, the Cubans increased their numbers by 17 percent.[47] Medical aid to Zambia in 1988 included an increase in the number of doctors to 143, of whom 80 were family doctors (recent graduates) and 43 were specialists. These physicians were slated to cover 60 percent of Zambia's medical needs.[48] Botswana's 1992–1993 cooperation agreement with Cuba also included an increase in aid as 27 Cuban physicians were dispatched there along with other aid workers in education and agriculture. Trade, of course, was also a part of the agreement.[49]

The geopolitical and ideological changes that began in 1989 as well as the economic crisis of the 1980s affected both the socialist world and the Third World and led Cuba to redouble its search for new allies and trade partners. Consequently its efforts at medical diplomacy expanded where possible. A 1991 supplement to the 1990 cooperation agreement between Cuba and Namibia increased the number of Cuban doctors working in Namibia to 50 from 19, with an increase in other health personnel as well. The additional doctors were specialists in obstetrics and gynecology, general surgery, neurosurgery, urology, orthopedics, comprehensive general medicine, internal medicine, pharmacology, radiology, nuclear medicine, and educational therapy.[50]

Cuba also bolstered its medical aid program with Guyana in 1990 by adding another 14 doctors, and in the same year discussed an expansion of cooperation in the health field with Iran as part of a renewed diplomatic effort.[51] Brazilian trade, investment, and travel to Cuba have increased steadily in the medical field, particularly since Cuba's 1988 donation of meningitis B vaccine, which led to its purchase thereafter.[52] Cooperation agreements also were signed in 1991 with the government of Ecuador, the Caracas [Venezuela] University Hospital, and the Andean Pact (Bolivia, Colombia, Ecuador, Peru, and Venezuela).[53] The agreement with Ecuador was quite wide-ranging and included assistance in medical education, research, science and technology, basic medicines and food hygiene, occupational medicine and environmental health, medicine and rehabilitation, control over vector-transmitted diseases, and integral and community-based family health.[54] Reunification of Yemen has led to increased medical aid there as well.[55]

Adverse political and economic changes have led to vastly decreased aid to Angola, Ethiopia, Iraq, and Nicaragua,[56] and adverse economic conditions have limited the possibility that host-country governments would help cover transportation costs and in-country expenses for Cuban medical-aid workers.[57] Cuba's own economic difficulties make it impossible to cover all the needs of its aid workers abroad; thus other forms of medical aid, such as that provided in Cuba itself, have become more prevalent.

Medical Care in Cuba

Cuban medical aid has often included free medical care in Cuba, particularly for very complex procedures or for those requiring high-technology medical equipment or facilities not available in the host country. For example, in 1983 Cuba agreed to provide hospital treatment for a specific number of Guyanese during that year as well as to extend for another two years the terms of the twenty-four Cuban doctors already serving in Guyana.[58] Later agreements called for the continued treatment of Guyanese in Cuba. About three hundred disabled FMLN Salvadoran guerrillas traveled to Cuba for treatment during the 1980s, but in May 1991, after they had been rehabilitated, they still awaited their government's permission for repatriation.[59] Nicaraguans requiring advanced medical procedures are still treated in Cuba. In 1987 a young Nicaraguan underwent a neural transplant in Cuba, and 20 Nicaraguan children underwent cardiovascular surgery.[60]

Free medical aid in Cuba is also provided on an individual basis to patients from capitalist countries that do not otherwise receive Cuban medical aid. From the 1986 opening of the William Soler [Pediatric] Cardiocenter until 1988, children from Bolivia, Chile, Colombia, Costa Rica, the Dominican Republic, Guyana, Nicaragua, Uganda, and Uruguay had cardiovascular surgery performed at no charge. Thirty-five children from Latin American countries and 2 from African countries were operated on in 1987, and in the following year, 17 Latin Americans and some Africans were operated on.[61] In December 1988 there were 2 Nicaraguan infants waiting for surgery, and 1 was recuperating.[62] By 1991 a total of 233 children from Chile, Costa Rica, the Dominican Republic, Nicaragua, Peru, Uruguay, and other Latin American countries had undergone cardiovascular surgery in the cardiocenter.[63]

Cuba's most sophisticated hospital, the Hermanos Ameijeiras Hospital in Havana, always has foreign patients. During a site visit I made in November 1988, 5 percent of the patients were nonpaying foreigners who had asked Cuban embassies in their countries for medical assistance or made their requests through labor unions, peasants' leagues, political organizations, or in some cases directly. The patients' case histories and laboratory and diagnostic analyses are sent to Cuba, where physicians determine whether successful treatment is possible and, if so, which institution can provide the best treatment. Patients in the Ameijeiras in November 1988 were from Bolivia, Brazil, Colombia, the Dominican Republic, Ecuador, Nicaragua, Panama, Spain, and Uruguay. One Nicaraguan woman, a guerrilla, had been there for two years undergoing rehabilitation and was preparing to return home. As the director of international relations for the hospital said, "We really can't afford to give any other type of aid."[64]

As the stature of the Cuban medical establishment has become better known, more people have inquired about medical care in Cuba. One Cuban exile working at an international organization in Santiago, Chile, has intimated that when people find out that he is Cuban they often ask him for aid in getting medical care there. He said that even some Chilean politicians with anti-Castro political views have gone to Cuba for medical treatment. After the baby of Andrés Alemán, one of the leaders of the Chilean right, fell into a pool, Castro invited Alemán to Cuba for an experimental treatment that saved the child. Since then, Alemán has supported improved relations with Cuba.[65]

In an impressive symbolic move, Castro offered at the end of 1989 to treat each year up to 10,000 children affected by radiation from the Chernobyl nuclear accident in 1986. He proposed to expand and remodel the José Martí Pioneer City (a seaside youth vacation camp) on the eastern outskirts of Havana to house 10,000 children and about 3,000 to 4,000 mothers. Approximately 6,000 voluntary workers labored on the facilities, which were completed in time to receive the first group of "Chernobyl children." Because not all the children would need to be there for long periods, Castro stated that about 30,000 children could pass through that facility each year based on an average stay of a few months for most. Some, however, would require longer-term care lasting six months to a year or longer.[66]

Castro contended that the costs would be minimal for Cuba because Cuba already had all of the medical staff necessary, the physical plant was in place, and the pioneer city staff was the same one that always worked there. The food would be better than that normally provided to pioneers. The only real expense would be medicines,

although Castro claimed that "it would be at the reach of our country. Therefore, that does not involve any sacrifice."[67]

The first 139 Chernobyl children and the 43 mothers accompanying them arrived in Havana on March 29, 1990, at which time
Castro corrected a reporter who called this medical aid; he said that
it was "not aid, it is a basic cooperation duty."[68] He explained that
Cuba had received three requests for medical cooperation from various organizations in the Soviet Union: one to treat the Chernobyl
children, one to treat Afghan war veterans, and one to take in Armenian earthquake orphans. The last proposal had been changed to
provide vacations for the orphans instead.[69]

Whether it was aid or "cooperation," by April 1991 a total of 3,591
Chernobyl children had been treated in Cuba, and by March 1991
about 400 Afghan war veterans had either undergone orthopedic
surgery, been fitted for prostheses, or pursued rehabilitation therapy in Cuba.[70] In 1991 Cuba agreed to care for 12,000 Chernobyl
children in 1991 and 1992.[71] By 1993 over ten million Chernobyl children from the Russian Republic and the Ukraine had flown to Cuba
for medical treatment.[72] Although the United States offered medical
expertise immediately after the Chernobyl disaster, the victims were
soon forgotten: a total of 10 were given vacations in California in
1991 by a private charitable organization.[73]

The benefits to Cuba of medical diplomacy go beyond repayment
of the debt of solidarity with the Soviets; they also provide clinical
and scientific experience for Cuban doctors in treating the effects of
nuclear radiation. Since Cuba has been developing nuclear power,
this benefit is not inconsequential. The symbolism of a developing
nation treating the ill who reside in a former superpower is truly
extraordinary, and Cuba has gained considerable prestige and influence from this experience.

Provision of Medical Education
and Training Abroad

Cuban medical-aid workers also help train the local
population, thereby producing their own replacements and reducing
the ratio of Cuban physicians to the indigenous physician population.
This has been the case in Yemen, Ethiopia, Guinea-Bissau, Angola,

and Nicaragua.[74] In Democratic (South) Yemen the Cubans constructed, equipped, and staffed the first medical school and provided direct medical care. The school opened in 1975 with 57 students and 7 Cuban professors, and by 1982, when the first doctors graduated, there were over 400 students, 24 Cuban professors, and 35 Cuban-trained Yemeni professors. In the seven years prior to 1982, a total of 101 Cuban medical professors had taught in Yemen.[75]

As of 1979 Cuban medical assistance to Ethiopia included professors for the medical school at the University of Addis Ababa.[76] In 1987 aid to Guinea-Bissau to establish a medical school included 19 experienced medical professors, one of whom was a founder of the premier postrevolutionary medical school in Cuba.[77] Cuba also helped Guyana construct and staff a medical school at the national university.[78]

Having trained local physicians in some countries, Cuban internationalists were able to dedicate their efforts to providing secondary and tertiary care and to providing further training for local physicians. Efforts such as this occurred in Ethiopia where in 1984 only 10 Cuban medical workers (including 6 doctors) out of 234 medical personnel delivered primary-care services in remote areas "as a symbol of the solidarity" of medical workers. The other 224 worked in 34 hospitals located in 12 of Ethiopia's 14 provinces.[79] This trend away from primary care was probably the result of an increase in both the number of Ethiopian doctors trained and the number of Cuban specialists available to do internationalist work.

Cuban medical professors and specialists also train doctors from and in other countries through lectures, workshops, courses or seminars, and regular teaching positions. For example, the Cuban National Institute of Oncology provides training for Ecuadoran doctors.[80] Moreover, a 1991–1993 agreement between Cuba and Ecuador calls for Cuban assistance in medical education, research, and science and technology, as well as in other areas.[81]

Additionally, Cuba has lent its foremost medical experts to other nations. As part of an agreement on Cuban cooperation with the Heart Institute of São Paulo, Brazil, in the field of cardiovascular surgery, the Cuban heart transplant specialist Dr. Noel González Jiménez and the children's heart surgery specialist Dr. Andrés Savio were in Brazil in September 1986.[82] Dr. Rogelio Marrero, from Cuba's Institute of Occupational Medicine, lectured on the prevention of occupational disease at the medical school in Valencia, Venezuela.[83] Two

Cuban pharmaceutical experts were sent to Peru to assist in the expansion of the pharmaceutical industry.[84] Orthopedist Dr. Rodrigo Alvarez Cambras, the director of the Frank País Orthopedic Hospital in Havana, has lectured and performed demonstration operations in many countries, both developing and developed, and he and his colleagues established an Iraqi pediatric orthopedic hospital and began training the staff in 1979.[85]

Cuban medical professionals have also advised other ministries of health on health-care organization and administration, staff training programs, scientific research, epidemiological surveillance, and "the acquisition, production and distribution of medicines, and maintenance for medical technology, among other things."[86] Working with local health ministries, they have jointly organized mass vaccination and health-education campaigns and scientific meetings.[87]

Scholarships to Study Medicine in Cuba

An important part of Cuba's international aid has been free education in Cuba. The large numbers of scholarships given makes Cuba one of the major influences on future generations of Third World leaders and professionals. Whereas the Reagan and Bush administrations decreased the number of government scholarships available to people from the Third World for study in the United States, Cuba has steadily increased the number of similar scholarships it offers. During the 1984–1985 academic year, there were 22,000 scholarship students from eighty-two developing countries studying in Cuba at various levels, from high school through university and postgraduate levels, and in 1990, there were 25,000 studying at elementary, secondary, pedagogical, and polytechnic schools.[88] By 1990 approximately 16,700 foreign students had graduated from Cuban schools, of whom 5,800 had graduated at the university level.[89]

In medicine alone at the end of 1984, Cuba had 1,800 scholarship students from seventy-five Third World countries studying in schools for intermediate-level medical technicians, in medical schools, and in postgraduate medical courses.[90] Scholarship students from seventy-one countries enrolled in Cuban medical schools during the 1985–1986 academic year included 825 medical students and 84 dental students.[91] In 1988–1989, there were approximately 2,000 scholarship students at these medical institutions, and the 1990–1991 enrollment was up to 2,219 for all levels of medical education.[92]

From 1981 to 1985, Cuban medical schools graduated 422 doctors and 67 dentists from other Third World countries. Since Cuba began offering medical school scholarships, 1,523 foreign doctors had graduated prior to the 1987–1988 academic year, another 355 doctors had completed postgraduate training, and 752 middle-level health technicians (including nurses) had graduated.[93] Data for 1990 could not be broken down according to specialization, but a geographic breakdown was available. A reported 3,587 doctors, residents, and health technicians graduated in 1990–1991. These graduates came primarily from the Americas (1,418) and sub-Saharan Africa (1,507), but also from North Africa (517), Asia and Oceania (92), and Europe (53).[94]

In 1982 the U.S. government funded only 9,000 scholarships for Third World students, and this number has been decreasing as funding for the program has been reduced.[95] Of all foreign students studying at the university level in the United States in 1985, the U.S. government funded only 6,840.[96] By 1990 the United States had given only 3,015 scholarships to foreign nationals.[97] These figures are for government funding only; private sources may very well provide more funding. Cuba also provided proportionally more scholarships than the Soviet Union, eastern Europe, and China. The latter three provided 55,345 in 1979.[98]

Foreign students in Cuba may not stay beyond their course of study, but must return to their own countries.[99] Various cohort studies indicate that, by contrast, between two-thirds and three-fourths of all foreign medical graduates who go to the United States to work or study never return to their home countries.[100] The medical brain drain has negative implications for the donor country and often for the recipient country as well. For example, foreign medical graduates, whose training is often considered inadequate by U.S. standards,[101] are overrepresented in U.S. hospital-based practices. Between 1970 and 1979, they accounted for 66 percent of the growth in full-time hospital-based physicians, 33 percent of the increase in physicians in general, and 20 percent of the yearly supply of active physicians.[102] Although their numbers declined to 15 percent of active physicians newly licensed in 1986,[103] state and local health officials have voiced considerable concern about the quality of care provided by foreign medical graduates.[104] Clearly, these concerns are valid; but more devastating is the donor countries' complete loss of both these medical personnel and the investment in their training.

Short-Term Crisis and Disaster Aid

Cuba has provided short-term crisis aid to many countries afflicted with natural disasters or epidemics irrespective of their political and economic orientations and has accumulated considerable symbolic capital in the process. Cuba's own success in domestic disaster relief (hurricanes) and epidemic control (dengue) has demonstrated the country's organizational and scientific ability in these fields, and it is therefore not surprising that Third World officials request Cuban assistance when disasters strike their countries. That the Cuban government repeatedly offers its services and experiences to other developing countries suggests that its concern for the amelioration of the human condition is genuine and that its use of medical diplomacy is well conceived.

Among the countries that have received significant medical aid from Cuba after suffering major natural or industrial disasters are Armenia, Brazil, El Salvador, Ethiopia, Honduras, Iran, Mexico, Nicaragua, Peru, and the former Soviet Union. Colombia and Venezuela also received aid recently.[105] As part of its earthquake relief for Peru in 1970, Cuba donated six rural hospitals that were shipped to Peru and constructed and equipped by Cuban workers, though Cuba and Peru did not have diplomatic relations then. The medical brigade that rendered direct attention to the Peruvian population included fifteen doctors, fifteen nurses, and ten hygienists.[106] After the 1986 earthquake in Peru, Cuba donated a one-hundred-bed field hospital complete with medicines.[107] Earthquake relief in 1986 for El Salvador, whose government Cuba opposed, was valued at half a million dollars and consisted of twenty-two tons of medicines and surgical materials.[108]

Nicaragua under Somoza received disaster-relief aid from Cuba just as it did under the Sandinistas and Barrios de Chamorro. In response to the 1972 earthquake that leveled Managua, Cuba dispatched doctors, paramedics, and one hundred tons of medicines and foods, despite Cuba's vehement opposition to the Somoza regime.[109] Likewise, within forty-eight hours of the Barrios de Chamorro government's request, Cuba sent a team of 28 doctors and six hundred tons of food to Nicaragua's Atlantic coast, which had been devastated by severe flooding, in spite of the rather frigid relations between the two governments.[110] Cuba also sent medical teams to Honduras in 1974, Ecuador in 1988 (105 health workers), and Brazil in 1991 to combat a dengue epidemic, and donated meningitis B vaccine to Brazil in 1988 to stem a meningitis epidemic.[111]

The 1991 cholera epidemic in Peru that then spread to other Latin American countries prompted significant Cuban medical aid despite the island's extremely difficult economic situation. Cuba donated twenty-seven tons of medications including antibiotics, intravenous fluid, oral rehydration salts, and other materials. A medical team composed of five specialists in microbiology, epidemiology, and hygiene was sent to Peru for two months to assist in the fight against the epidemic, primarily by training local doctors and nurses, developing a cholera control program, analyzing water quality, investigating bacteria in diarrhea cases, and isolating the causal agent, *vibrio cholerae,* in residues and popular fish species. The Cuban control program was implemented throughout Peru, and the results were scheduled for joint analysis by the two parties in September 1991.[112] Moreover, Cuban scientists began working on an improved cholera vaccine almost immediately.

In response to the earthquake that devasted Armenia in 1988, Cuban aid included tons of plasma, a field hospital, SUMA equipment for blood analyses, and a 150-member medical team.[113] In a symbolic gesture, Castro donated his own blood to kick off a major blood-donation drive to obtain plasma for the Armenians.[114] Cuban burn specialists worked in a Moscow burn unit applying Cuban-developed epidermal growth factor to patients burned in the chemical fire from a train accident in Siberia.[115] Leonid Abalkin, deputy chairman of the Soviet Union's Council of Ministers, commented on this Cuban aid to his country in May 1990:

Cuba was one of the first countries to come to the aid of Armenia when it was struck by the earthquake, and after the tragedy in Bashkiria [train accident and resulting chemical fire] the republic [Cuba] placed at the Soviet Union's disposal almost all its national blood reserves. They sent us some of the best, if not the best equipment for treating burns.[116]

Within a few hours of the Iranian earthquake of 1990, Cuba had already sent two planes with twenty-nine tons of medical cargo, including a field hospital, nineteen doctors, and twenty-one other medical personnel. A third plane full of medical supplies followed later. Again, Castro himself was the first to donate blood as an example to the rest of the population (21,500 people donated blood within seventy-two hours of the appeal and 40,595 during the first week) and as a symbol of his concern for the Iranians.[117] This aid was provided to the archenemy of Cuba's ally, Iraq.

One could speculate about the motives for this medical diplomacy conducted at a time when Cuba could ill afford to engage in it because of its own economic difficulties, but the symbolic capital gained from such an act probably outweighs all other considerations except humanitarian ones. Since Cuba supported Iraq in its war with Iran, this humanitarian gesture was a good way to begin to make amends and at the same time build up symbolic capital that may ultimately be converted into material capital, in this case oil. This angle was surely not missed by the Cuban leadership. It desperately has been seeking new trade partners, most particularly those with oil, because the Soviets were no longer willing or able to maintain the volume of oil they had delivered in the past.

In fact, Cuban aid resulted in vastly improved relations between Cuba and Iran. Cuba was able to convert its symbolic capital into material capital as trade followed aid later that year, when Iran and Cuba agreed to purchase medical products from each other. Cuba also agreed to send doctors to work in Iranian community hospitals and medical school professors to teach in the medical school in Teheran, and both countries agreed to exchange medical students to provide various types of training.[118] Because Iran is richer than Cuba, it is highly likely that the Iranians are paying for the Cuban physicians but at prices below those charged by doctors from capitalist countries.

Early in the following year (1991), Cuba and Iran signed an accord to cooperate in the development of sugarcane derivatives, an area in which Cuba has considerable experience and is in the forefront internationally. Cuba will train and assist the Iranians in this field, and both countries plan to cooperate in agricultural and industrial research on sugarcane.[119] It is difficult to know all Cuban motives for providing aid at a given time, but even if ulterior motives were absent when the decision was made to send medical aid to Iran, the consequences of this medical diplomacy have been very beneficial.

It is a both a duty and a matter of honor for Castro to provide medical aid to other countries, but most particularly to his longtime benefactor. He made that topic the centerpiece of his speech at the Soviet Embassy reception on May 8, 1990, to celebrate the thirtieth anniversary of the resumption of diplomatic relations between Cuba and the Soviet Union. In his speech Castro said that Cuba does not expect to be thanked for its aid because, for obvious reasons, it is the Cubans' obligation to do whatever possible to assist the Soviets under any circumstances. He further mentioned that because the Soviets "trust our doctors, our medicines, our workers . . . we consider it an honor that we are allowed to cooperate in that field."[120] Although he focused primarily on Cuban medical aid to the Soviet Union, Castro also indicated that "there has not been a tragedy in a Latin American country caused by hurricanes, earthquakes, or any other natural disaster, in which we have not offered cooperation."[121]

It is clear from Castro's words that his decision to provide medical aid and disaster relief to the Soviet Union in late 1988 was motivated both by humanitarianism and by the desire to repay Cuba's debt of solidarity. The consequences of this medical diplomacy cannot be overlooked, especially at a time when Cuba and the Soviet Union were at odds over domestic and foreign policy. Cuba's medical diplomacy made the Soviets more aware of the nonideological utility of their relationship with Cuba and of the potential benefits that could be reaped from relations with their less developed ally.

Donation of Medical Equipment and Supplies

Cuba also donates medical equipment, supplies, and complete medical facilities to countries with seriously underdeveloped medical infrastructures. One of the more fascinating cases of this type of medical diplomacy involved the donation of three fully equipped pediatric intensive care units to the Bolivian government (one each year in 1985, 1987, and 1989).[122] Just how Cuba conducts its medical diplomacy with a democratic capitalist country and the political outcomes in that country are demonstrated by the following detailed discussion of the Bolivian case from an interview with Dr. Javier Torres Goitia, then minister of health of Bolivia.[123]

When Bolivia redemocratized in 1982 and Dr. Hernán Siles Suazo ascended to the presidency, Bolivia reestablished diplomatic relations with Cuba after a twenty-year hiatus. Cuban medical diplomacy with

Bolivia began then as Cuba sent a delegation to Bolivia to reestablish diplomatic relations. During this visit Cuba offered technical assistance in creating an international relations office within the ministry of health. This assistance was to be conducted through the PAHO interregional cooperation program. Subsequently PAHO sent a Cuban physician to Bolivia for three months to organize such an office with the aim of teaching the Bolivians how to work with and get funding from international organizations.

The Cuban doctor also observed the terrible conditions of the hospitals, particularly the pediatric hospital. Through interviews with doctors and nurses there, she found that the majority of the children died because of the lack of intensive care facilities. Since Bolivian hospital-based doctors and nurses considered intensive-care units (ICUs) their greatest need, the Cuban doctor suggested that Cuba might be able to provide a pediatric intensive care unit. The hospital doctors, of course, were very pleased by this prospect and asked the Bolivian Ministry of Health to ask Cuba for an ICU. Torres Goitia held various meetings with the hospital staff to ascertain the appropriateness of the request, and then went to the Cuban embassy, where his petition for the ICU was quickly granted.

The Cuban government sent a delegation of architects and doctors to Bolivia to confer with Bolivian doctors on where to construct the ICU and install the equipment. Later Cuba sent a crew to construct the building with bricks and other supplies bought in Bolivia. Cuba paid all expenses for the project. At the same time, Cuban doctors organized a course for Bolivian doctors in intensive care and the use of the delicate and complex ICU equipment. The best prepared and most enthusiastic Bolivian personnel (one surgeon, one clinical pediatrician, and two nurses) were sent to Cuba for six to nine months of advanced training, paid for by the Cuban government. By the time construction was finished, the personnel had also been trained and had returned to Bolivia.

Upon completion of the construction, Cuba imported directly from Japan the most modern equipment available—valued at half a million dollars.[124] Because the pediatric hospital did not have a laboratory, Cuba included a diagnostic lab to serve both the ICU and the hospital in general. After the inauguration of services, a Cuban ICU medical team stayed in Bolivia for one year directing the ICU. The two Cuban doctors and the laboratory technician were department heads at the ICU and provided on-the-job training for their Bolivian staffs. Because the medicines for this type of service are very expensive, Cuba donated all of them, along with reagents for the laboratory. Cuba even donated special clothing for the workers. Torres Goitia classified the unit as a model service, truly first class ("primerísima clase").

When the Cubans departed after a year, they also left a one-year supply of medicines, but Bolivia had to find a way to get money for medicines after the Cuban supply had run out. This was very difficult because the poor could not pay; consequently the medicines and medical care were financed through social security insurance. This approach too was problematic, however, because the social security health services would attend children badly instead of remitting them to an expensive service. Finally, in order to guarantee sufficient money to maintain the ICU service, Torres Goitia insisted that social security send patients to the ICU and make contracts with the hospital to attend the poor without charge.

In recognition of Castro's contributions to Bolivian health, the nation awarded him its highest health honor, "La Gran Cruz de Salud," which had been given to only two people in Bolivia's entire history. When Torres Goitia gave him the medal, Castro said that although he had helped many countries, no one had thought to give him a medal, and that he was therefore the one who was thankful.

After learning that thirty children had been saved in the La Paz ICU after only three months of operation, Castro said that Bolivia should try to have ICUs in all regional capital cities. Cuba was not in an economic position to give much aid; nonetheless, Castro offered Bolivia two more ICUs in locations of their choice and instructed the Cuban Ministry of Public Health to begin the project immediately. Moreover, Castro directed the Cuban ambassador to Bolivia, who had accompanied Dr. Torres Goitia to Cuba, to begin expenditures for the project.

The development of the two new ICUs followed the same process as the first: there was advice in construction, training, equipment, and medicines. The third ICU, in Santa Cruz, was built after Siles Suazo left office, but in spite of political differences between Siles Suazo and his successor, Victor Paz Estenssoro, the project was continued following the initial plan.

Although Cuba provided Bolivia with three high-technology medical facilities that saved the lives of Bolivian children, it may not have been the most effective gift to accomplish those ends. Bolivia has had the highest rate of infant mortality in Latin America for some time (123 per 1,000 live births in 1989) and also high rates of death for children under the age of five.[125] For the Cubans, who assert that nothing is more important than the life of a child, this is a terrible state of affairs. But because the Cuban medical system is physician-based, and because cost was not a major issue before 1991, low-technology and nonmedical solutions to health problems may have been overlooked. In fairness to the Cubans, however, they probably recognized that the root of the problem is Bolivia's socioeconomic structure, but that some amelioration of the people's health can occur through specific measures and that these would not be threatening to the Bolivian government.

Low-technology solutions to Bolivian health problems might not have been logistically viable. It might have been more useful to provide Bolivia with large quantities of oral rehydration salts, basic medicines and vaccines, easily understandable health-education materials, and assistance in conducting public-health measures. But these would have required a well-established network of medical facilities and practitioners (even if only minimally trained community-health workers) to distribute them, and that was precisely what was lacking in Bolivia. It probably was not politically feasible for Cuba to offer or Bolivia to accept such labor-intensive assistance at that time.

Aid recipients and donors might concur on the type of aid that will be very beneficial to the recipients, but that will also provide the most political capital to each party. It was the Bolivian doctors who decided that they wanted an ICU, even if they were prompted by a Cuban doctor. Of course, asking any hospital-based doctor what is needed will invariably result in a request for more high technology. It is politically sound to accept a medical showpiece because it is useful and necessary and because it may be perceived as a monument to the existing government. For Cuba, the symbolism of providing high-technology ICUs is powerful and considerably greater than that of providing less visible yet also important aid, such as the large number of scholarships granted to Bolivians to study medicine and pursue paramedical careers in Cuba. Symbolism, though, was less the motivating factor for this aid than was the improvement of relations with Bolivia through medical diplomacy (read humanitarianism).

No matter how useful the aid, its acceptance may be problematic for the recipient country. The Bolivian government, for example, had financial difficulty in maintaining the ICUs. More importantly, dealing with Castro was not entirely popular, yet neither the U.S. Agency for International Development that worked in Bolivia, nor the political right, nor the church criticized the donation of pediatric ICUs by Cuba. In fact, all of these organizations attended the inauguration, and the Rotarians and the Lions Clubs not only attended but also contributed money for the maintenance of the ICUs later on. It would be perverse, after all, to oppose a gift of health. The Bolivian right, however, did criticize Torres Goitia for decorating Fidel Castro with the Gran Cruz de Salud, claiming that other countries had given more to Bolivia. Torres Goitia, in a fashion typical of Latin American officials familiar with Cuban health successes, responded that he wanted to recognize the person and the process in Latin America that had made the greatest contribution to health in Latin America: Fidel Castro and the Cuban revolution.

Host country domestic politics do affect Cuba's ability to use medical diplomacy. Bolivia provides both an example and a counterexample. The ICUs were not a serious political problem, but that was only because they did not adversely affect the finances of any group within the medical or pharmaceutical profession. Cuban medicines provided through PAHO, and later, directly by Cuba, threatened the livelihood of Bolivia's pharmaceutical importers. Independent of medical cooperation with Cuba, Torres Goitia established a policy of importing essential medicines in accordance with PAHO guidelines and decided to buy from PAHO about thirty or forty items of the highest necessity. In response, Bolivian medicine importers caused a very grave scarcity of medicines by taking their products off the market.

Because PAHO did not have sufficient stocks of all of the medicines ordered and because international orders take a long time to arrive in Bolivia, the government was obliged to look for ways to provide medicines more quickly. The Ibero-American Social Security Organization (OISS) in Spain and the government of Cuba assisted in this matter. The OISS bought medicines directly in Spain for Bolivia, and Cuba immediately supplied PAHO with the medicines needed to meet Bolivia's needs after the Bolivians directly requested Cuban assistance.

PAHO then sent Bolivia medicines from various countries, including Cuba, India, and Holland, but Bolivian importers claimed that the Cuban and other medicines were of bad quality and without guarantees. They were sold to Bolivia by PAHO, not by Cuba or any other country, and were therefore guaranteed by PAHO. The pharmaceutical importers criticized Torres Goitia and the Siles Suazo government as communists because they had acquired Cuban medicines both through PAHO and, subsequently, directly from Cuba. The only problem with any of the medicines was the price: one-tenth of that charged by the transnational pharmaceutical companies. Clearly, Cuban medicines were detrimental to the fiscal health of Bolivia's pharmaceutical importers.

With the new supplies, the ministry of health was able to install people's pharmacies (*farmacias populares*) that supplied medicines at affordable prices. At this point, the United States Agency for International Development directly donated enough medicines to supply the provinces they were aiding in primary health care, and sent the vehicles necessary to deliver them. Perhaps this is one of the very few cases in which the Cubans and the United States were working toward the same positive end: to improve a nation's health. It should have been an example of friendly competition (and cooperation) to see who could do the most toward that goal.

Cuba's medical diplomacy with Bolivia did result in some trade and medical exports, but the Cuban donations far exceeded any possible trade benefits. The initial payoff for Cuba has been primarily in greatly improved relations with Bolivia and in the accumulation of symbolic capital, not only with Bolivia but also with other countries and international organizations. Cuban donations to Bolivia and other countries are stunning examples of medical diplomacy with capitalist countries. They are effective because no one can fault aid that will save hundreds of lives.

International Medical Conferences and Scientific Exchange

Beyond direct medical assistance and training programs, Cuba has also shared its expertise through its sponsorship each year of numerous international medical and biotechnology conferences, bringing together experts from the western hemisphere as well as those from some of the developed countries, the former socialist countries, and international organizations. Many of these conferences have been cosponsored by regional professional associations or PAHO, and all have been attended by a considerable number of foreign delegates.[126] The Cubans have used these opportunities to show off their own health system through scheduled site visits and the presentation of scientific papers. On the whole, conference participants have been quite impressed with Cuba's accomplishments.[127]

A partial list of topics addressed at international medical scientific conferences held in Cuba since 1986 indicates the breadth of Cuban expertise: genetics and monoclonal antibodies; orthopedics, traumatology, and sports medicine; molecular and cell biology; general and pediatric surgery; digestive endoscopy; maxillofacial surgery; medical technology; gynecology; liver and bile duct surgery; nephrology; microbiology and parasitology; tropical medicine; interferon and biotechnology; cardiovascular surgery; endocrinology; angiology; and primary health care. The number and frequency of these conferences has increased notably since 1980, as have joint sponsorship and foreign participation.

Cuba scored an impressive coup in November 1988, when it hosted the prestigious commemorative conference for the tenth anniversary of WHO's Alma-Ata Declaration, "Health for All by the Year 2000," and the fortieth anniversary of the founding of WHO. This conference, called the "Second International Seminar on Primary Health Care, Family Physicians: A Response to Community Needs," was attended by 1,510 delegates, of whom more than 600 were foreign.[128] Fifteen ministers or vice-ministers of health from Europe, Africa, and Latin America attended, as did the directors-general of the WHO and PAHO, and other high level delegates from WHO, PAHO, UNICEF, and the Holy See.[129] Delegations from Latin America and Spain were very large. Honduras, for example, was represented by 116 doctors, nurses, and health administrators.[130] Venezuela, Brazil, Spain, Colombia, and Mexico had similarly large delegations. Nicaragua was represented by only a handful of delegates, probably because of their inability to release so many people even if Cuba provided special aid to them by paying their expenses.

Commemorating both the founding of WHO and the Alma-Ata conference, as well as recognizing Cuba's accomplishments in the health sphere, the directors-general of WHO, Dr. Hiroshi Nakajima, and of PAHO, Dr. Carlyle Guerra de Macedo, both sponsored and opened the conference. Additional sponsorship came from the Network of Community-Oriented Educational Institutions for Health Services (based in the Netherlands), and the Cuban Ministry of Public

Health. Panelists, presenters, and speakers came from all regions of the world, with only a few besides the Cubans from the socialist camp.

The Third International Primary Care Conference was also held in Cuba in March 1991, and cosponsored by PAHO, WHO, and the Network of Community-Oriented Educational Institutions. It was attended by three hundred foreign delegates from thirty countries. Once again, the directors-general of the WHO and PAHO touted the Cuban health system's accomplishments as extraordinary.[131] That Cuba was chosen as the venue for these conferences attests to PAHO and WHO support for and promotion of the Cuban health system.

Cuba has also promoted scientific exchanges in other ways. In July 1986 Cuba opened another major research facility, the Center for Biotechnology and Genetic Engineering (CIGB), with the explicit intention of fostering international collaboration. In addition to housing Cuban scientists, the facility is expected to accommodate over one hundred foreign researchers in the near future.[132] In June 1991 there were scientists at CIGB from Brazil, Chile, China, Colombia, Mexico, North Korea, Peru, Switzerland, and Venezuela but not in the numbers initially expected. Their visits lasted from a few months to two years depending on the program or course of study they pursued.[133] Because the Cubans have shared their knowledge and expertise with other developing countries, some United Nations agencies have reported that development aid to Cuba is a good investment precisely because of this multiplier effect.[134]

Multilateral Aid

Cuba's own aid programs led to the recognition of Cuban proficiency by international organizations that then contracted with Cuban experts to provide aid to third countries. WHO has contracted with Cuban physicians to train health workers, establish a statistical system, and control leprosy in Laos; advise African governments on campaigns to control tuberculosis; and provide epidemiological assistance to Angola and São Tomé and Príncipe. PAHO has employed Cuban doctors to train health technicians in Nicaragua and to work on an eight-year program to control malaria in Mexico.[135]

The Pedro Kourí Institute of Tropical Medicine in Havana was selected by PAHO to develop twenty-five teaching modules to be used throughout Latin American universities for undergraduate and postgraduate courses in tropical medicine, based on its experience in research and in the training of 351 professionals from fifty-four countries in Europe, the Americas, Africa, and Asia from 1979 to 1989.[136]

Recent multilateral cooperation has come under the rubric of what is called technical cooperation among developing countries, or TCDC, a term that implies reciprocity and exchange. TCDC was established in WHO (as well as in other United Nations organizations) in 1988, and a regional workshop was convened in Cuba in 1989 to institute programs of cooperation among the various subregions of the hemisphere. Within PAHO, the TCDC budget for 1990–1991 was a mere U.S. $4.7 million, of which Cuba received U.S. $53,000.[137] PAHO tries to promote collaboration among countries (regional integration), but since the budget is so limited and provides only travel funds, the political will of the governments involved determines whether cooperation becomes a reality. Because Cuba has such a highly developed medical-scientific-industrial complex, it, as well as Mexico, has been included in the Southern Cone region with Argentina, Brazil, Chile, and Uruguay, rather than in the Central American region, which includes the Dominican Republic.[138]

Accords exist between PAHO and Cuba for cooperation with (read "aid to") Belize, Bolivia, the Dominican Republic, Guyana, Nicaragua, Peru, and Venezuela; and still other accords were under discussion with Argentina and Brazil. The primary aim of this cooperation is training doctors and other health workers in the diagnosis of infectious diseases, maintenance of medical equipment, health technology, rehabilitation, nutrition, and development of health systems.[139] In 1991 an agreement was signed between PAHO, Cuba, and Ecuador for Cuba to provide assistance in training doctors, implementing community-based medicine and health, conducting rehabilitation, and providing health personnel for various projects.[140]

Explanations and Rewards for Cuba's Medical Diplomacy

Why does Cuba devote such a large portion of its financial and human resources to medical assistance abroad? First and foremost, Cuban medical diplomacy can be explained by a sincere concern for the betterment of people's lives. Second, the Cuban leadership sees as its duty the repayment of its debt to humanity for the aid they received, particularly in the early days of the revolution. Third, medical diplomacy improves relations among states and thereby lessens Cuba's sense of isolation in the international arena. Fourth, Cuba's domestic and international legitimacy is strengthened by its medical prowess. Fifth, Cuba's capacity to provide medical aid garners symbolic capital that ultimately can be converted into material capital in the form of trade with other countries and aid from international organizations. Sixth, Cuba's economic objective has been to earn hard currency through the development of a new export commodity, its human resources.[141]

Initially Cuban aid was nonrepayable.[142] Since 1977, however, Cuba has been charging on an ability-to-pay basis. Poor countries receive aid free. Wealthier nations, such as oil-rich Libya and Iraq, pay in hard currency, but at prices estimated to be considerably lower than those charged by the Soviet Union and eastern European countries, and far lower than Western rates.[143] Information on commercial contracts for international construction projects suggests which countries might be paying for medical assistance as well. Contracts existed with Libya, Angola, Iraq, Congo, and Algeria.[144] Available information indicates that all of those countries except Congo have at some point paid for medical aid. This list suggests that the Congo might have been paying as well.

In November 1988 the head of the International Collaboration Department of the Ministry of Public Health said that only Kuwait was paying at that time and that Libya was no longer receiving medical aid.[145] Other sources indicate that Algeria was paying for 65 Cuban medical specialists in 1989 and had done so since 1978. Algeria had received Cuban medical assistance at no charge from 1963 to 1978.[146] By mid 1991 neither Iraq nor Kuwait was receiving Cuban medical aid, although the Cuban medical team did remain in Iraq until the end of the 1990–1991 Gulf war. Because exact information on medical aid abroad is a state secret, this information may not be reliable. Moreover, the Cubans do not appreciate attempts to calculate their foreign exchange earnings from "aid."

When a country that pays for Cuban assistance has had economic difficulties, Cuba has continued to provide aid either at no charge or at a price that the country can afford.[147] The Iran-Iraq war disrupted Cuba's construction and other service contracts with Iraq, except for the contract for medical assistance, but as of July 1983 Cuba no longer charged Iraq for medical services. The war eliminated an important source of hard-currency earnings for Cuba, and, to make matters worse, Cuba had to absorb the payment of 120 percent of the medical team's salaries (the 20 percent is an overseas bonus) and all other expenses related to their mission. Cuba's medical mission to Iraq declined from 450 people in the first three months of 1982 to 100 in the first three months of 1983, as Iraq could afford to pay only a small amount for living expenses. The net cost to Cuba of its aid to Iraq from July 1983 to 1987 was calculated at approximately 2 million pesos.[148]

Angola paid in hard currency for much of its civilian assistance from the early 1980s, but with the deterioration of the economic and military situation there in 1984–1985, much of this aid reverted to grants.[149] The Iraqi case exemplifies the costs to Cuba of a large aid mission typical only of Iraq, Angola, Ethiopia, Libya, and Nicaragua. The cost to Cuba of a smaller, more typical aid mission, such as that to Tanzania—a country that has never paid for Cuban assistance—was 529,500 pesos in 1987–1988 for 41 civilian technical experts in six different fields including medicine.[150]

According to an advisor to Cuban vice president Carlos Rafael Rodríguez, Cuba has charged U.S. $1,100 per month (U.S. $13,200 per year) for a generalist medical doctor with eight years of experience. This is considerably less than charges levied by other bilateral or multilateral donors. Whether or not charges are levied, Cuba pays the salaries in Cuban pesos,[151] and the host country pays in-country living expenses and a small monthly allowance of approximately U.S. $30 in local currency. There are various arrangements for transportation of the Cuban aid workers to the host country. In some cases, Cuba flies the personnel to a European city into which the host country's national airline flies, and the host country then transports the Cubans to their final destination. In other cases, either the host country or Cuba pays all or half of the transportation costs, but this depends on the financial condition of the host country. In calculating either costs or earnings, the opportunity costs for tourism must be considered when Cubana Airlines space is used to transport aid workers.[152]

It has been estimated that Cuba earned approximately U.S. $50 million from work performed abroad by its civilian technicians in 1977 and an estimated U.S. $100 million in 1980.[153] These figures are for all types of technical expertise and skilled workers. There are no disaggregated data to assess how much of this total was paid for medical services, but data on international construction indicate that the bulk of the earnings were from that sector. For example, Cuba had a construction contract with Libya in 1979 for U.S. $115 million and another that year with Angola for U.S. $25 million.[154]

Nonetheless, one can estimate that if Cuba did charge Libya for the 357 physicians it supplied them in 1977, and if these physicians had eight years of experience and were billed at U.S. $1,100 per month each, then Cuba would have earned U.S. $4,712,400. By the same token, if Cuba charged Angola in 1981 for the 335 doctors it provided them that year, it would have earned U.S. $4,322,000 from the deal.[155] In both cases, a similar number of nurses and allied health workers were supplied as well, and earnings for them are only slightly less than for doctors.

Actual data for 1982 show earnings of U.S. $14,084,460 for Cuba's civilian assistance programs in Angola, of which U.S. $4,892,880 was for medical services rendered (U.S. $4,231,488 for the civilian health system and U.S. $661,392 for military health services).[156] Either the doctors sent to Angola did not have eight years of experience or Angola got a special price, because Cuban figures indicate that Angola paid the following amounts per year for Cuban medical aid workers: U.S. $5,760 for general practitioners and dentists, U.S. $6,552 for specialists, U.S. $5,160 for nurses and middle-level health technicians, U.S. $4,380 for support personnel, and U.S. $6,840 for the group leader.[157] (See table 12 for detailed information on the distribution of personnel across salary categories.)

Whether at U.S. $13,200 or U.S. $5,760 per year for a general practitioner, if these rates have been available to other countries that could afford to pay Cuba for its medical services, it would be irresponsible of a government not to take advantage of the offer. Nowhere else could a country get medical services at that price. The benefits to Cuba in potential and real earnings from the export of human resources are not inconsequential either, because it has had few opportunities to earn hard currency as a result of its trade dependence on the former Soviet Union and eastern bloc countries, the U.S. trade embargo, and Cuba's relative lack of export products in high demand. It also makes good diplomatic sense to provide assistance, minimally paid or gratuitous, particularly when a large pool of educated and skilled youth have been available to perform such duties.

Table 12: Cuban Medical Staff (Civilian) in Angola by Category and Salary, 1982

Category	Salary per year (U.S. $)	Number	Total Earnings (U.S. $)
General practitioner	5,760	91	524,160
Group leader	6,840	1	6,840
Medical specialists	6,552	294	1,926,288
Dentists	5,760	15	86,400
Nurses	5,160	167	861,720
Middle level technicians	5,160	155	799,800
Support personnel	4,380	6	26,280
Totals		729	4,231,488

SOURCE: Comité Estatal de Colaboración Economía, "Datos generales de los organismos," CECE internal document (report on review trip to Angola, 1982), 2.

Health Tourism

With the prestige gained from both their domestic health system and international medical services, the Cubans began to offer medical care to individuals from capitalist countries in an effort to capitalize on their previous investments. They have advertised "sun and surgery" and "health tourism" in Cuba, offering their medical services—including travel to and from Cuba and accomodations—to those who find prices at home to be considerably more than in Cuba.[158] According to a 1983 report in the journal *M.D.*, "Arterial grafts, including 20 days in the hospital, cost $3,363, a hysterectomy, $983, an abortion, $283, a new nose, $778," and consultation with university medical professors costs $60.[159] Neural transplants to treat Parkinson's disease cost only $14,974, and this price includes one week of tests and evaluation ($1,950) and three weeks of further evaluation, neural transplant, and recuperation, all fees included ($13,024). These are bargain prices, according to *M.D.*, with the potential to lure patients from the capitalist countries in the hemisphere as well as Europeans, to whom much of the advertising was addressed. (See appendix for a fuller description and comparative prices.)

Price is not the only lure. Many developing countries have neither the medical technology nor the highly trained specialists that Cuba has. Cuban physicians and medical scientists have also developed innovative cures, medical devices, and techniques largely unavailable elsewhere. One device, an external fixator claimed to lengthen bones, already had been applied by its developer, Dr. Alvarez Cambras, in thirty-four countries by 1988.[160] Dr. Alvarez Cambras's international reputation is extremely good, and he lectures and performs surgery all over the world, including western Europe. The prestige of his hospital is such that it was designated as the site for the Ibero-American School of Orthopedics and Traumatology. It therefore is not surprising that Venezuelan orthopedists regularly remit patients to Cuba for a variety of problems.[161] Because of the demand for Cuban orthopedics, the Frank País Orthopedic Hospital doubled the capacity of its forty-bed ward for foreigners.[162]

Dr. Alvarez Cambras and his colleagues perform innovative spinal cord surgery (revascularization of the spinal cord in cases of lesions) not available in the United States in early 1993 except on an experimental basis. Reports indicate that it has been effective in getting fresh sources of blood to the spinal cord to regenerate central nervous system tissue. In other cases where the spinal cord is severed, Dr. Alvarez Cambras performs advanced microsurgery (still on an experimental basis) to graft nerve tissue to the spinal cord. Eduardo Joly, a foreign observer of Cuban orthopedics and rehabilitation who is highly knowledgeable in that field, has suggested that patients with spinal cord lesions probably will come to Cuba for this surgery if they are made aware of its practice there.[163]

The number and nationality of patients at the Frank País Orthopedic Hospital has changed from 1980 to 1990. In 1980, when Cuba was not charging foreigners for medical care there, its patients included many war-injured Nicaraguans and Salvadorans. In 1990 there were many patients in Cuba from a variety of countries, some paying and others not. Those observed at the Frank País Orthopedic Hospital by Eduardo Joly from mid 1990 to mid 1991 included people from Argentina, Bolivia, Brazil, Colombia, Costa Rica, the Dominican Republic, Ecuador, El Salvador, Guyana, Mexico, Nicaragua, Panama, Peru, the United States, Uruguay, and Venezuela. In addition, there was an entire ward filled with Soviet veterans of the Afghan war.[164]

Doctors in the Dominican Republic refer patients to Cuba for specialized treatment unavailable in their country. They and their patients say that Cuban fees are about one-quarter to one-third of U.S. fees. Although most people pay for treatment in Cuba, some charity cases are accepted. The demand to travel to Cuba from the Dominican Republic for various reasons was so great that weekly charter flights were begun in early 1988 despite the absence of diplomatic relations between the countries. From then until the end of May that year, "At least 150 Dominicans have flown to Cuba for medical treatment."[165]

Brazilians have been going to Cuba for treatment of the skin disease vitiligo, for which Cuban medical scientist Dr. Carlos Miyares Cao discovered a cure that is sold under the name Melagenina. From September through December 1986, 3,000 Brazilians were expected to travel to Cuba for "sun and medical care."[166] By 1987 Dr. Miyares had successfully treated 800 patients from twenty-four countries (not including Cuba), 100 of whom were Venezuelans.[167] The number of those successfully treated or undergoing treatment reached 9,000 by the end of 1990. Between 1987 and 1990, Dr. Miyares's foreign-patient load increased from 15 patients per month from eight or nine countries to about 100 patients from seventy-five countries. Patients came from Europe, Asia, North Africa, Australia, and almost all of the countries in the western hemisphere.[168]

The popularity of the cure and of Dr. Miyares is evidenced by the establishment in many countries of patient support groups (twenty-eight in 1990) called Societies or Associations for the Cure of Vitiligo "Miyares Cao."[169] These associations, which arose spontaneously to organize group trips to Cuba for the cure, invite Dr. Miyares to lecture in their countries and provide emotional support for members. Sometimes they are led by medical professionals who also have vitiligo.[170]

Melagenina has been patented in twelve countries and is sold in Brazil, Spain, and Venezuela.[171] But because it is not available everywhere, patients from all over the world have gone to Cuba for treatment. Some have traveled from Algeria, Bahrain, Canada, Germany, Great Britain, India, Italy, Kuwait, Libya, Nicaragua, Oman, Saudi Arabia, and the Soviet Union.[172] Foreign demand for the vitiligo cure has been so great that the Cuban government has established an international Placental Histotherapy Center that treats foreigners two days a week.[173] It has also established a clinic in the Canary Islands specifically to treat European patients.[174] There are similar clinics in Madrid, Brazil, Mexico, and Venezuela, in addition to a "clinic ship."[175] Moreover, discussions are under way to open vitiligo clinics in the Dominican Republic, India (where five are planned), and Italy.[176]

The Iberian–Latin American Center for Neural Transplants and Nervous System Regeneration in Havana, which opened on February 26, 1989, under the direction of Dr. Hilda Molina, treats patients for Parkinson's disease, Alzheimer's disease, Huntington's chorea, neurological sequelae of strokes and brain and spinal cord injuries, and other diseases and conditions. In the first twenty months of operation, the center's staff treated 150 patients, some of whom came from the Dominican Republic, El Salvador, Ethiopia, Mexico, Spain, the Soviet Union, Uruguay, and Venezuela.[177] The transplantation of fetal neural tissue to treat Parkinson's disease is still experimental in the United States and has been blocked for some time by legislation prohibiting its use despite medical scientists' requests that it be made available. Cuba began this technique in 1985 with the aid of Mexican doctors working in that area, only three years after it was originated in Sweden.

A much publicized case in 1990 was that of a Spanish woman from the Canary Islands who, as the result of an automobile accident, had become, in the words of her father, "a vegetable." She was completely paralyzed and did not respond to treatment in Spain. Two months after surgery and rehabilitation at the Center for Neural Transplants, she was able to walk with crutches, do exercises, and say a few words.[178] This type of case produces enormous symbolic capital for Cuba, particularly because the patient came from a developed country and also because the procedure is highly sophisticated.

Dr. Orfilio Peláez has developed the first surgical procedure to halt and, in some cases, reverse, retinitis pigmentosa, an eye disease that leads to total blindness and whose symptoms are night blindness and tunnel vision. From November 1987 through January 1991, he had operated on 1,600 Cuban patients and 317 foreigners from twenty countries. He claims that 75 percent of his patients improved and that 20 percent have had "significant recovery." Again in highly publicized cases, a thirty-three-year-old West German woman with tunnel vision and an eight-year-old Spanish boy were operated on successfully.[179] Argentines who had been successfully treated by Dr. Peláez have created a foundation to fund treatment in Cuba for indigent Argentines.[180] Patients hospitalized for retinitis treatment at the Cira García Clinic in early 1991 were from Argentina, Bolivia, the Netherlands, India, Mexico, Norway, Peru, Spain, and Venezuela. One was the director of a hospital in Caracas, Venezuela, Dr. Lisandro López, whose father was the ophthalmologist who diagnosed his case. He and his three children, who also underwent operations in Cuba, had significantly better eyesight thereafter.[181]

The director of health tourism, Dr. Ricardo Martínez Rojas, said that as of 1988 more than 1,000 patients had gone to Cuba since health tourism was first conceived on a small scale in 1980. Eighteen hundred people went to Cuba for health tourism in 1990, leaving behind about U.S. $2 million in revenues. Approximately 1,000 were Latin Americans, who paid 30 percent less than the Europeans, who themselves paid prices lower than those charged by industrialized countries.[182] By June 1991, Dr. Martínez contended, the figure had increased to 2,000 for that year alone.[183] Not until mid 1986 did health tourism have its own organization and facilities.

Servimed (formerly Servimex), a division of Cubanacán, the umbrella company for a variety of tourist facilities and services, has produced glossy brochures (in English, French, and Spanish) offering a large variety of medical services from general checkups to neural and heart transplants, cosmetic surgery, stress-reduction regimens, and almost everything in between. The Cubans see other Latin Americans as their best market because Latin Americans have a history of traveling abroad for medical care. Most go to Houston, Miami, and other medical centers in the United States, but language and cultural similarities as well as price and quality persuade many Latin Americans to go to Cuba instead. In fact, Cuba already has accords with the social security institutions of the Dominican Republic, Ecuador, and Venezuela similar to the accords Cuba has had with countries in eastern Europe to provide health care in Cuba for their nationals.[184]

The Cira García Clinic, which is the base institution for health tourism, had only two rooms available out of forty-four in November 1988 and is almost always full. Among the 40 patients were 9 Yugoslavs being treated for retinitis pigmentosa; 9 Dominicans; 2 South Koreans; 2 Ecuadorans; 5 Soviets; 5 Bolivians; and 1 Brazilian, 1 Austrian, 1 Swiss, 1 Bulgarian, and 1 Kampuchean. The patients from communist countries and 1 South Korean were with either diplomatic or technical missions, and the other South Korean was a merchant marine injured in an occupational accident. The other patients were health tourists.[185]

Not all health tourism earns foreign exchange. The Cuban Ministry of Public Health reported that in 1987 they provided free medical treatment for 175 patients from forty countries, although they received 505 applications, up from 358 in 1986. Of the 505, a total of

316 were approved for treatment, and the remainder were still being processed. The charity cases were mainly from the developing countries, not all of which were regular recipients of Cuban medical aid, and they included most of the Latin American and African countries, and Algeria and Syria.[186]

One of Dr. Miyares's patients, an eight-year-old British girl, was, along with her mother, a guest of the Cuban government because the family was too poor to pay the costs of the trip and treatment.[187] The symbolism of a developing nation providing medical care to someone from, and previously treated unsuccessfully in, a developed country is rather extraordinary, and its propaganda value (read "symbolic capital accumulation") is enormous.

Symbolism aside, Cuba's international assistance contracts have become even more important as the price of sugar, Cuba's major export commodity, has plummeted to considerably less than its production cost. The decline of world oil prices also severely diminished Cuba's ability to earn hard currency through the reexportation of surplus Soviet oil, which was Cuba's major means of earning convertible currency in the mid 1980s but which was no longer an option by the late 1980s. Cuba's major export crops, which were severely damaged by Hurricane Kate in November 1985, were not expected to produce the previously planned amounts for some years. To make matters worse, since then Cuba has been plagued at inopportune times with either drought or heavy rains that have reduced agricultural yields. When heavy rains caused shortfalls in the 1989–1990 sugar harvest, Cuba was unable to supply contracted amounts to Bulgaria, East Germany, and Czechoslovakia.[188] Energy shortages and the scarcity of spare parts and lubricants during the 1990–1991 sugar harvest also diminished Cuba's sugar output.[189] Those same problems, coupled with drought followed by heavy rains, wreaked havoc on the 1991–1992 sugar harvest, which was only 7 million tons, and the 1992–1993 harvest, which is expected to yield less than 6.5 million tons.

Furthermore, as western European and Japanese currencies increased in value against the dollar, the cost of Cuba's imports from those countries increased, and the purchasing power of Cuba's dollar-denominated exports decreased. The Cubans estimated a loss of approximately U.S. $600 million in 1986 due to these factors, which rendered Cuba unable to pay the debt of U.S. $3.5 billion it then owed to the West.[190] Cuba's development plan for 1987 was implemented with "half the foreign exchange imports considered vital and with a fourth of the imports from the hard-currency area that were made in 1984."[191] The declining value of the dollar resulted in an increase in Cuban debt from 3.9 billion pesos for 1986 to 5.6 billion pesos for 1987.[192] By 1989 Cuban debt to the West had reached U.S. $6.6 billion, an increase over 1988 of 6 percent, primarily due to currency fluctuations.[193] The hard-currency debt had risen to U.S. $7.7 billion by 1991, and Cuba's debt to the Soviet Union was then pegged at between 15 and 24 billion rubles (the value of which in convertible currency is contested). Cuba had only U.S. $69 million left in hard-currency reserves in June 1990.[194]

Adding insult to injury, the Soviets reduced their subsidies to Cuba beginning in 1986 and paid less for Cuban sugar than previously, but failed to decrease their sales price for oil even though the world market price had declined.[195] When most Cuban trade with the Soviet Union except sugar was pegged to world market prices and denominated in dollars in 1991, the precarious nature of the Cuban economy became even more evident. Diplomats in Cuba then estimated 1991 losses from the curtailment of Soviet subsidies at approximately U.S. $150 million.[196] Castro himself stated that Cuba's purchasing power declined by over $1 billion because of less preferential prices agreed upon in the 1991 trade agreement with the Soviet Union.[197] Moreover, the Soviets delivered very little of the agreed-upon goods for 1991 apart from oil, and that too was reduced in quantity. By September 30, 1991, less than 50 percent of the grains had been shipped, and anywhere from zero to 50 percent of other contracted items had been shipped, with most pegged at less than 20 percent of the expected amounts.[198]

As a result of this economic malaise, the export of technical and skilled workers has become all the more important in filling the foreign exchange gap left by diminished traditional exports.[199] It had been argued in the early 1980s that further expansion of Cuba's human resource exports would be difficult because of cultural and political differences, particularly in language and ideology, and because of "the Reagan administration's policy of penalizing countries that receive island aid."[200] But this argument did not hold up during the 1980s because of the unfulfilled demand in developing nations for Cuba's expertise, particularly medical expertise, and the considerable overt and covert anti-Americanism in much of the Third World. Cuban aid may have been sought to symbolically counter the United States.

In 1978 Castro recognized the economic potential of exporting medical personnel and began to greatly increase the number of physicians Cuba produces specifically for that purpose. From 1978 through 1986, he argued, there were insufficient numbers of doctors to meet international demand, despite the requesting countries' willingness to pay hard currency for them.[201] Since Cuba has charged less than other socialist and capitalist countries for commercial contracts, with the exception of China (which has greatly reduced its aid program since the late 1970s),[202] it seemed likely then that Cuban doctors would win contracts on a purely competitive basis. In fact, both medical contracts and grant aid increased during the decade of the 1980s. Moreover, in most cases aid has led to trade if not to considerable income.

As Third World nations found themselves in dire economic straits in the 1980s, primarily because of the debt crisis and International Monetary Fund (IMF) structural adjustment policies, grant aid predominated. But as privatization moved forward at the IMF's behest and as governments were made to reduce their social expenditures, it became increasingly difficult for them to host Cuban doctors even when Cuba paid their salaries. Host governments could not even afford to pay the Cubans' living expenses (which were minimal because they lived like the local people rather than like other international aid workers). Moreover, the public sector medical infrastructure in many countries has been diminished or demolished. Cuban aid, therefore, began to dwindle in 1990 because of economic hardships in both the host countries and Cuba.[203]

Cuba's potential for expanding its aid programs at different times has been both improved and diminished by a changing geopolitical milieu. Improvement, for example, came shortly after the United States cut off aid to Zimbabwe. Cuba signed an agreement with the Mugabe government (July 12, 1986) for immediate cooperation (aid) in education and public health, and future cooperation in agriculture, construction, foreign trade, the sugar industry, and sports.[204] As part of a 1991 cooperation agreement, Namibia requested an increase in the number of Cuban scholarships awarded to its nationals beyond the eight hundred then offered.[205] Recent diplomatic efforts toward nonradical regimes such as Argentina, Bolivia, Brazil, Ecuador, Peru, and Venezuela have included medical aid and general scientific and cultural exchanges. The days of large-scale Cuban aid are over also because of the economic devastation Cuba itself has faced since the collapse of the socialist bloc and, to a lesser extent, because of the ideological hegemony of the United States now that the Cold War has ended.

Cuba's role in multilateral technical cooperation agreements, however, has increased as its ability to provide bilateral aid abroad has decreased. Cuba is still in a position to provide medical education and training both in Cuba and abroad, scientific exchange, medical treatment in Cuba and more limited treatment abroad (depending on the host country's ability to cover local expenses), and some donations of equipment and supplies, particularly of Cuban-made products, of which there are a large number that might be attractive to other countries. What is clear in 1991 is that large-scale medical missions like those sent to Angola will be the exception rather than the rule. Medical missions will persist but on a smaller scale and probably at a higher level of specialization. Certainly more cost-effective for Cuba and quite promising is the provision of medical care in Cuba as either aid or health tourism. With a considerable medical infrastructure which can be used for both domestic health care and health care for foreigners, it seems likely that this will be a priority area henceforth.

Moreover, ideological differences generally do not present an insurmountable obstacle to those seeking education abroad. A 1977 Central Intelligence Agency report indicated that Third World nationals who have studied in communist countries have obtained responsible positions on their return to their native lands despite their own government's hostility to communism. According to the CIA report, Third World countries' increased development efforts coupled with their critical shortage of highly skilled and educated workers should accelerate the trend among their nationals to seek education in communist countries.[206] It previously was reasonable to conclude that Cuba's potential for increased education of foreign nationals would be good because the demand still exists, but Cuba no longer has the capacity to support large numbers of foreign students at its own expense when food and energy shortages are so grave.

The Cuban government has recognized that establishing a model health care system at home and providing international aid demonstrate the humanitarian nature of the revolution. Influence (symbolic capital) garnered from these endeavors has aided in the dissemination of Cuba's socialist ideology. But rather than a fifth column advancing the socialist revolution, Cuban medical aid has had the potential to win converts through a more subtle but nonetheless important demonstration effect. The democratic changes that swept the Soviet Union and Eastern Europe, however, have left little drawing power for socialist ideology. Nonetheless, Cuban medical aid has created both friends (and allies) and influence abroad, and both of these are important goals of medical diplomacy. The symbolic capital gained in this endeavor has also led to trade as well as to aid from international organizations (U.S. $210 million from five United Nations agencies for 1976–1991 and U.S. $1.2 million from PAHO alone for 1991).[207]

Part of the payoff of medical diplomacy has been increased sales of medical and pharmaceutical products. In 1980 Cuba exported 1.166 million pesos in medical and pharmaceutical products and 888,000 pesos in medicines. There was a steady increase in exports in both categories in the 1980s until 1988, when there was a slight decline. But in 1989, with the addition of biotechnology exports, Cuba had quintupled the 1987 amount of exports in each category: 55.370 million pesos in medical and pharmaceutical products and 54.289 million pesos in medicines.[208] These amounts are significant for Cuba and demonstrate conversion of symbolic capital into material capital, which is the economic payoff of medical diplomacy.

7

Conclusions

Early on, the Cuban revolutionary government made health a high priority and invested in health as an end in itself, as a means of socioeconomic development, and as a way to achieve domestic legitimacy. A prerevolutionary history of HMO-type health facilities, the participation of many doctors in the revolutionary war, and the guerrillas' encounter with the abject poverty of the peasants led the government to place a high priority on health. From the outset of the revolution, the people responded positively to the promise and provision of various social services, particularly health care.

As the domestic health system developed and the diseases of underdevelopment were eradicated, Castro recognized the broader symbolic significance of success in the medical sphere both at home and abroad, and health became an even higher priority. By the end of 1977, he called for greater numbers of doctors to meet international demand; this growth in turn led to an even more aggressive use of medical diplomacy than in previous years. Thus as Cuba became a major player in African affairs, large numbers of doctors also became available for international aid work there and elsewhere in the Third World and were deployed abroad as medical ambassadors and medical missionaries.

In the 1980s, media coverage of health issues and Cuban sponsorship of international health conferences increased dramatically, reflecting Cuba's drive to become a world medical power and the real and symbolic importance given to health. The success of the Cuban health system and of the international conferences has made Cuba a destination de rigueur for Third World health officials and international organization representatives. As a result, Cuban medical diplomacy increased still further and led to more trade with aid recipients (often barter) and aid from international organizations. Moreover, not only did Cuba win contracts to provide medical services for countries that had more resources than it had, but Cuba also began to promote "sun and surgery," or health tourism for people from capitalist countries. Both of these endeavors resulted from the conversion of symbolic capital into material capital and thereby provided Cuba with sorely needed hard currency.

Cuba's entry into the biotechnology marketplace has further enhanced its symbolic capital and thus its ability to conduct medical diplomacy. Although Cuba is quite advanced in that field, it is primarily a copier rather than an innovator. This strategy, one could argue, is how Japan got to be number one, but it means that Cuba's participation in the scientific-technological revolution is limited and that its potential for making breakthroughs will depend on whether Cuban scientists can go beyond being technicians and become true scientists and discoverers of new products and techniques. This endeavor, in turn, depends on the establishment of strong curricula and research projects in structural molecular biology that have no end other than basic science. In the current political and economic climate, this is highly unlikely, despite aid from international organizations, to keep Cuba's scientific efforts afloat. But irrespective of these difficulties, Cuba is so far beyond other Third World countries in this field that considerable symbolic capital has been generated by this enterprise.

Costs and the Cuban Model: The Politics of Symbolism

Although Cuba's health system receives considerable praise from all quarters, it is not a plausible model for most developing nations primarily because physician-based, high-technology systems are costly compared with paramedic-based, low-technology systems. Further, few governments have central control over the economy, and thus the ability to allocate resources equitably. Nonetheless, attributes of the Cuban system are emulated in a variety of contexts. Countries such as Angola, Brazil, Ecuador, Ethiopia, Grenada (prior to October 1983), Guinea-Bissau, Mexico, Mozambique, Nicaragua, the former Soviet Union, and Uruguay, among others, have adapted or are adapting aspects of the Cuban health model, in some cases in a specific geographic area and in others on the national level.[1]

Moreover, the Cuban model is symbolically important in that it indicates that developing nations can aspire to and achieve First World rather than only Third World health-care systems. This achievement, along with Cuba's international medical aid program, its training of foreign students, and its sponsorship of international conferences, contributes significantly to Cuba's symbolic capital (political prestige) in the international arena, particularly in international organizations where symbolic capital (influence) accumulated in one forum may be carried over to another.

Although comparative costs are difficult to calculate because of different accounting methods, some general observations can be made about strict economic costs, disregarding momentarily the political and symbolic benefits. First, the cost of training and employing doctors is considerably less in Cuba than in capitalist countries, because in Cuba physicians' salaries are held constant and are in the midrange of salaries, not much higher than those of teachers or engineers, and medical schools are state-owned. Although the initial investment in medical schools may have been high, Cuba now has more than sufficient capacity to produce large numbers of doctors, dentists, and nurses without further capital investment. Second, as the sole employer and purveyor of health services, the state can justify the costs of health care and preventive medicine by pointing to the long-term savings that have resulted from greater and longer worker productivity and to the lower cost of prevention compared with treatment and rehabilitation. Third, domestic production of most pharmaceuticals and many basic health devices, supplies, and high-technology equipment is much cheaper than importing them.

Apart from the obvious direct costs of a health-care system, indirect opportunity costs appear in the form of diverted investment that might be better used in less developed sectors such as housing, and in the diversion of human resources from direct production to health services and from domestic to international health-care provision.

The diversion of medical personnel from domestic to international services is less of a problem than the others because Cuba has such a good ratio of physicians to population that, if anything, Cuba is an overmedicalized society.

Although it is difficult to measure human capital investment by strict cost-benefit analysis, from a long-term perspective Cuba's investment strategy makes sense given its objectives of societal transformation and symbolic capital accumulation. From a narrow economic perspective, that is, without regard to other governmental objectives, more investment would have been justified in sectors other than health. Although it seems obvious that the Cuban people would prefer a different allocation of national resources that would improve the quantity and quality of housing, transportation, food, and consumer goods, this cannot be stated definitively since survey research and opinion polling by foreigners are prohibited in Cuba. The Cubans themselves do very little opinion polling, and what is done is conducted by government agencies or the party. Questions generally deal with microeconomic rather than macroeconomic choice and generally do not broach sensitive political issues. Moreover, results of surveys are not easily obtainable.

Personal interviews I conducted in the course of this research indicate, however, that although the Cuban people are quite pleased with the success of their health-care system, most would much prefer greater investments in less developed sectors, such as housing, transportation, and food production and distribution.[2] They nevertheless also want better health service, as do the majority of Americans and Britons as well as a very large number of Canadians and Soviet peoples.[3] The desire for better health service should not be misunderstood. Public satisfaction is a relative concept and depends a great deal on expectations. In Cuba, expectations are raised constantly with extensive media coverage of medical advances.

If the Cuban government were concerned solely with the people's well-being or with achieving balanced and harmonious socioeconomic development, then other sectors, such as housing and transportation, would have been given priority over further investments in the health sector. Because the Cuban government has long since met the people's basic health needs, the populace can and does seek improvements in other sectors. Likewise, in the post–Cold War world, one could argue that the investment in biotechnology is probably not fully appreciated by a population that had to stand in line every day for a half-pound of bread (one roll) in 1991 and for only a quarter-pound of bread as of March 1992.

The priority Cuba places on health-care investments despite the costs is partially accounted for by the government's striving for legitimacy in an adverse geopolitical situation. Because they are not freely elected, socialist governments rely on their ability to meet the socioeconomic needs of their populations to legitimize their regimes.[4] The Cuban government recognizes this fact, as is evident in Castro's statement that

In the field of health, . . . we have been guided from the outset by a number of basic criteria. The first is to prioritize public health as one of the vital services for human society. Moreover, it is what the people value more than anything else. I can't understand how politicians do not understand that.[5]

This public preference for health services also is reflected in recent survey results from nearly identical polls taken in the United States, Canada, and Great Britain, where a majority of those polled cited health care as one of their two top priorities for government spending and suggested the need for an overhaul of their health systems. This sentiment was echoed as well in a Soviet survey conducted by the State Committee on Labor and also released in early 1989.[6]

Taking the public preference for health services to its logical conclusion, Castro places such high priority on health that he takes a daily interest in the operations of the health-care system and is thought by many to be the real minister of health.[7] Indeed, he has made health indicators the true test of government efficacy and the health of the individual a symbol of the health of the "body politic."

Castro himself has accumulated symbolic capital through his concern for health. The Ecuadoran Minister of Health, Dr. R. Yepez, publicly praised Castro in 1988 as the only head of state he had ever seen attend a health conference during his many years of attending international meetings, and he lauded Castro's considerable knowledge of medical issues and his participation in the proceedings. In fact Dr. Yepez indicated that if other heads of state took the same interest in health as Castro did, the WHO goal of "Health for All by the Year 2000" would become a reality rather than remain a dream.[8] Foreshadowing Dr. Yepez's praise, WHO conferred on Castro its highest honor, a medal for outstanding work in the health field.[9] This award generally goes to medical scientists or physicians like Dr. José

R. Jordan (also of Cuba) who won the WHO Child Health Foundation Award for his contribution to the eradication of childhood diseases.[10]

The praise Cuba receives for its domestic and international medical work has increased its prestige and influence (symbolic capital) in international forums and contributed to Cuba's election to leadership positions in many international organizations from the late 1970s to the present. Among the nonmedical organizations were the Non-Aligned Nations Movement, the United Nations General Assembly, the United Nations Council for Social, Humanitarian, and Cultural Affairs, UNESCO, the International Atomic Energy Agency, the Council of the Latin American Economic System, and the United Nations committees on Budget and Finance and Science and Technology. Medical organizations in which Cuba has held leadership roles include the executive committees of the World Health Organization and the Pan American Health Organization, the Latin American Pediatric Association, and the Latin American Genetics Association.[11]

Even more important, with the unanimous support of the Latin American nations, Cuba was elected to the United Nations Security Council for a two-year term than began in January 1990. The last time Cuba had made a bid for the Security Council seat, in 1979 (while chairing the Non-Aligned Nations Movement), the United States pressured nations to vote against Cuba, so that the balloting in the United Nations General Assembly went to 160 rounds before Colombia finally got the position. In 1989 no such opposition to Cuba was possible.[12]

Also symbolically significant, the Cuban jurist Miguel Alfonso was elected vice president of the United Nations Human Rights Commission in late 1989 despite increased U.S. efforts beginning with the Reagan administration to denounce Cuba in every session of that forum.[13] In fact Cuba was elected to a second term on the Human Rights Commission partly because of its very good record of meeting basic needs, particularly in health, education, and other social services that are considered to be basic human rights under the United Nations Covenant on Social, Cultural, and Economic Rights, and because of its record of providing medical and other aid to Third World countries. Although Cuba fares very well according to that conception of human rights, it does not fare well under the other United Nations Covenant on Civil and Political Rights, and in 1991 and 1992 was asked by the commission to account for reported abuses of civil and political rights.

Cuba's investment in health differs from its investment in other sectors because the creation of a national health system is in itself a material, psychological, and symbolic monument to socialism. The revolution created numerous "health monuments," ranging from rural dispensaries and family doctors' offices that dot the cities, towns, and countryside to specialized high-technology research institutes. Cuban medical diplomacy has also created health monuments abroad such as donations of equipment and facilities. These health monuments are symbols of Cuban socialism and the priority it places on health.

The revolution also created "human health monuments" in the form of tens of thousands of doctors, dentists, nurses, and allied health workers whose daily contact with the people both in Cuba and abroad is a constant reminder of what the revolution has done for all. These human health monuments are what differentiate investments in health and education from other government programs and from services such as housing, sewage disposal, potable water, electricity, and so on, and partially explain why there is greater investment in health than in these other sectors: human health monuments reinforce the values of the revolution through continual contact with the population. Recognizing this, Castro has even called the new family doctors "symbols of the Revolution."[14]

Before the collapse of communism elsewhere, the revolution provided a sense of security, a freedom from fear of illness and the financial devastation it can bring, because people knew that if they became ill, they would be given the best possible care without prejudice or charge. Now, although health care is still free, the scarcity of medicines and medical supplies has vastly reduced the quality of care available. The population's sense of well-being was increased by the knowledge that the government was also attempting to prevent illness through the promotion of general health education, public health and medical measures, and socioeconomic development. Even if these efforts were not appreciated by the beneficiaries (which is not the case), the investment in health would not be wasted, because the objective outcome is the human capital development necessary for the individual's own development and for societal transformation.

The symbolic importance of Cuba's investment in health has been explained by Castro: "Public health became a challenge and a battleground between imperialism [the United States] and ourselves, ... and this multiplied our efforts. That is why we have developed this field and are striving to become a medical power with the best possible health indices."[15] Elsewhere he has stated that if Cuba eventually surpasses the United States in the public health field, this would be Cuba's "historical revenge" for decades of hostility, and particularly for the U.S.–initiated economic embargo which includes medicines, medical technology, and medical information.[16] Thus, the economic dislocations resulting from the priority set on health are the costs of symbolic politics.

Since the accumulation of symbolic capital is always costly, Cuba's general civilian international-aid programs have had high direct and indirect economic-opportunity costs such as decreased efficiency and productivity.[17] Although the costs might outweigh the economic benefits,[18] in political terms "the international benefits still appear to outweigh the costs," despite limits on Cuba's influence over its aid recipients.[19] The provision of aid has led to trade and increased aid for Cuba from international organizations, yet it is still unclear whether Cuba's conversion of the symbolic capital gained in this endeavor into material capital would, in fact, have made medical diplomacy economically profitable in the short term had the geopolitical changes beginning in 1989 not taken place. In the long term, it seems that the investment would have paid off.

Cuba's actual costs are impossible to know, since even the Cubans themselves probably do not know them. They have only recently begun to do cost accounting, and even then they fail to include all of the inputs that would be included in the capitalist world (all of the fixed, variable, and opportunity costs, externalities, and costs of training). Castro, however, provided a clue to the costs when he stated in 1985 that it would cost an international organization over one billion dollars per year to provide the type and amount of civilian assistance that Cuba has granted other nations.[20] Clearly, costs for Cuba are less than for others because the state controls the economy, but this figure does suggest that if true costs were calculated the amount would be significant.

Problems and Prospects

Although Cuba has achieved health indices comparable to those of the developed countries, has developed a large physician pool, practices high-technology medicine, has developed biotechnology and genetic engineering, and has provided considerable international medical aid, many problems persist in the health sector, and they are getting worse because of the disintegration of the socialist world. Construction difficulties, lack of labor discipline, and inadequate basic supplies, the major problems before 1990, have become much more acute. Insufficient pharmaceutical supplies long ago led Cubans living in the United States to send medicines to their relatives on the island, but only in small quantities because of the U.S. economic embargo against Cuba. The situation has only become worse in the 1990s.

The construction industry, government-run like all else, can be blamed for some of the serious problems in Havana's hospitals because it either failed to complete certain projects or did such shoddy work that some hospitals have been unable to use their full capacity (hundreds of beds). For example, some of the areas of expansion of the Frank País Orthopedic Hospital were under construction for over a decade. "A simple hydromassage room under construction for seven years was only a third complete" by the end of 1986, leading Castro to speculate that it would take another fourteen years to complete at that rate.[21] The implications of this example are startling considering that the Frank País was designated as the site of the Ibero-American School of Orthopedics and Traumatology because of the high-quality medicine practiced there and because its director is on the Central Committee of the Communist Party. One must wonder what the situation might be in other, less prestigious institutions whose directors have less political clout. The shortages of construction materials, equipment, spare parts, and energy since 1990 have only exacerbated this long-standing problem.

Problems of labor discipline are common among nurses as well as among physicians. Absenteeism is high among the nurses, and some doctors have refused to go on call. Nurses also have been cited for pilfering resources and violating technical standards.[22] A selection of complaints from various health facilities throughout Holguín province in 1987 suggests that in some areas doctors were not on duty when they should have been, the numbers of specialists were insufficient, some physicians were ill-trained, patients may have been ill-treated, some facilities were in disrepair, resources were insufficient (some were sold on the side) and drugs were in short supply, hospital food, service, and care were sometimes poor, and sexual harassment was reported.[23] There is no information about the source or the circumstances of the complaints, but there is no reason to believe that they are not legitimate, particularly since the party has had to involve itself with similar problems in the health sector in Havana province.

My personal observations (both as a researcher and occasionally as a patient) in numerous Cuban health facilities over a fifteen-year period lend credence to some of the complaints brought forward in Holguín: inefficiency, labor indiscipline, shortages of medicines or other resources, equipment and facilities sometimes in disrepair, and sexual harassment. Although instances that would not warrant criticism far outnumbered those that would, these complaints cannot be dismissed. Moreover, the "special period" has led to greater labor indiscipline and shortages in all sectors, as workers everywhere try to meet their basic needs by taking whatever they can from the workplace or taking time off to stand in line for food. Medical workers are no exception.

The Cubans spend hundreds of millions of dollars on nuclear magnetic resonance equipment, CAT scanners, intensive care wards, and so on, yet there is still a shortage of such basic items as hospital bed linens, detergents, and cleaning agents. Such shortages may seem less important than the need to accumulate sophisticated diagnostic equipment that obviates the need for surgery through early and precise detection of disease, but basic hygiene is critical in order to avoid hospital-induced infections.

Complaints about hospital service by the population of Havana led to extraordinary meetings between provincial party officials and party members working in hospitals, as well as between party officials and hospital administrators and other personnel. The results have included greater party involvement in the supervision of hospital work, a better work attitude on the part of the staff, and improved care, which together have led to a considerable decrease in complaints.[24] The problems must indeed have been great, for Castro has stated that "for some years the provincial Party secretary will have to hold monthly meetings with the Party secretaries in the hospitals until everything runs smoothly . . . quite likely within ten years no monthly meetings will be necessary, but only when every hospital runs like clockwork."[25] What we have then is a health-care system that is in many ways impressive and successful in critical sectors but that fails to provide the standard of service and care that might be expected given its level of development. This is not unlike the health care situation in the United States, the country with which Cuba is competing.

It should be noted that party supervision of hospital work did not single out this sector for special treatment, since as part of the general process known as "rectification of errors" and the 1987 austerity plan, the municipal and provincial party committees were charged with overseeing all production units and services within their jurisdictions in an effort to improve efficiency, decrease waste, and improve the quality of products and services.[26] Given the Cuban government's control over all aspects of the economy and society, it has a greater chance of making positive changes than do countries where government intervention is considerably less or minimal.

Rectification in the construction industry led to the reorganization of work methods and the reestablishment of microbrigades to quickly complete many long-delayed construction projects, including the expansion of the Frank País Orthopedic Hospital (November 1988) and other health facilities. The microbrigades were made solely responsible for the construction of family doctors' home offices, which they have completed within two to three months. Shortages of supplies and energy in the 1990s have halted new construction except for the highest-priority facilities, and contingents have replaced microbrigades as the country's major builders.

There are, however, limits to the rectification program. The Cuban people have been asked to make material sacrifices for over three decades. In this time of increasing domestic economic hardship and ideological crisis because of the crumbling of the communist world, the Cuban government's exhortations to sacrifice for the millennium are much less persuasive than during the early years of the revolution; in fact, they may not be persuasive at all.

My observations while conducting field research in Cuba since 1978 suggest that many people are unwilling to work harder without a substantial increase in material incentives.[27] Moreover, material incentives are much less feasible now than before because of the economic crisis, and the government is consequently in a bind: without more goods and sufficient money to purchase them, people are unlikely to work hard and thus to produce the material wealth necessary for domestic consumption and export. Past exhortations have not been terribly successful over time, and the weakness of moral incentives has been confirmed by data from Cuba, the Soviet Union, the former eastern bloc, and China. Some people do respond positively to exhortations, of course, but their numbers are likely to be insufficient to achieve the Cuban government's long-term goals.

Moral incentives are unlikely to resolve all of the subjective problems; only greater enforcement of labor discipline will remedy absenteeism, shoddy work, and indifferent treatment of the public. Objective problems such as the lack of sufficient bed linens may persist because these items are less publicly noticeable and therefore less symbolically important than a new construction project or a piece of high-technology equipment. Taking these problems into account, Cuba cannot be considered a world medical power using criteria broader than its own. Nonetheless, Cuba's health-care system was, until recently, still capable of providing world class health care despite its problems and should be lauded for its achievements.

The Cuban leadership goes beyond providing world class health care to developing world class research and development capabilities. One of the hallmarks of the Cuban system is the ability to quickly mobilize resources to implement its priority policies and achieve real and symbolic victories. For example, Castro said in 1982 that "we're not a bunch of 'Indians in frock coats' as many people used to think, or as some people seem to think even now."[28] Almost as if to prove this, when the United Nations Industrial Development Organization (UNIDO) took too long to decide where to build a biotechnology and genetic engineering research center for which Cuba was in the running, Castro had a center built in Cuba following UNIDO's plans.

The result, the Center for Genetic Engineering and Biotechnology (CIGB), is a spectacular facility not just because of its size (it is one of the largest laboratories in the world) but also because of its equipment and physical beauty.[29] The symbolic capital accumulated through this act is remarkable even if the facility itself may prove to be underutilized. It is hard to imagine any developing country building and equipping a high-technology research center of a magnitude that only an international organization would conceive as a multinational project. The CIGB's scientific infrastructure and the dedicated and hard-working researchers stand as "biotechnology monuments" and symbols of the revolution's development.[30]

In sum, the Cuban government has embarked on a program to become a world medical power for humanitarian, political, economic, and symbolic reasons. Although meeting the population's basic health needs is the primary reason for this extraordinary effort, the accumulation of capital, both symbolic and financial, plays an important role in Cuba's plans. On the political level, the need for legitimacy, both at home and abroad, and a desire for international prestige and influence further account for Cuba's endeavor. Finally, Cuba's economic straits and the need for convertible currency have made the further development of international services and medical diplomacy a necessity.

Although Soviet aid to health and other sectors allowed the Cubans to divert more funds to health care than would otherwise have been possible, it has not been the determining factor in Cuba's success in the health sphere. Cuba's health-care system has succeeded through the political commitment to allocate significant fiscal, physical, and human resources to this sector. Mass participation in the implementation of health projects has considerably extended resources and made their impact much greater. Cuba's achievements are significant objectively and symbolically. For a resource-poor developing country to provide and share its First World health-care and research and development capabilities is indeed remarkable.

Whether Cuba can be considered a world medical power is ultimately less important than the symbolic capital Cuba accumulates in the process of aspiring to that status. By heralding its own work and making it available and visible to those from other developing countries and international organizations, Cuba is determining the health agenda for many who look to it for leadership precisely because of its achievements. By naming and defining its social world (to recall Bourdieu's terms), Cuba is setting the standards by which it wants to be judged. Reports from those attending international conferences in Cuba verify that Cuba has been successful in this endeavor; thus Cuba has accumulated considerable symbolic capital.

Attempting to become a world medical power is symbolically significant in that it suggests Cuba's ability to project an image of itself as a scientifically capable and developed country despite an underdeveloped economic base. It also is a measure of the self-confidence of a society that has survived and achieved considerable success against all odds. World medical power status confers legitimacy, prestige, and influence (three types of symbolic capital) on the Cuban government in both domestic and international forums, particularly because Cuba shares its expertise. This symbolic capital is ultimately convertible into material capital (commercial contracts, trade agreements, or aid from international organizations or developed countries) and can be spent or reinvested symbolically to further Cuba's political ends.

What can the developed countries learn from Cuban medical diplomacy? Medical diplomacy is an important foreign policy tool that could and should be utilized by all now that the Cold War has ended. Cooperation among countries to improve the living conditions of the developing nations would tend to further world peace and political and economic stability. This, in turn, would be economically beneficial to the developed countries because it would increase their markets. It is, in fact, in their best (economic) interests to foster development because only through development will developing countries be able to acquire the developed countries' products. Human capital investment, as the Cubans have shown, is a necessary condition for economic development.

Moreover, developed countries and developing countries alike should note that preventive medicine significantly reduces costs in the health sphere. In the context of the current debate over cost containment and the crisis of health care in the United States, an examination of the Cuban model is in order; even though it is highly unlikely that this country would adopt socialized medicine, lessons can be learned. If the United States were ever to normalize relations with Cuba, it would not be inconceivable for Cuba to provide reimbursable medical care just as some European countries do for others. This cost-containment measure might be acceptable to insurers seeking to decrease their expenses.

The end of the Cold War is a momentous time because it truly allows us to turn swords into plowshares, to concentrate our resources on development rather than destruction. It requires us to reassess and redesign the very nature of our foreign policy. Although it is too soon to bury ideology, we can bury enmity. Now that East-West relations can and should be based on mutual benefit and cooperation, competition for political allies in the Third World should give way to joint efforts to ameliorate social, economic, and environmental conditions worldwide, irrespective of politics. Despite their own need for material and technical aid, the countries of the former eastern bloc can still provide scientific expertise to others through multilateral aid projects.

The real issues facing humankind today are health in the broadest sense, development, the environment, and population growth. Without good health, both individual and societal development are limited. Demographic growth and environmental degradation place increased strain on already scarce resources in the developing world, leading to economic and politicial instability. In one way or another, environmental degradation affects everyone's health and quality of life, as well as the potential for sustainable development.

Certainly the technology is available to tackle the problems at hand, but the scientific-technological revolution is leaving developing countries even farther behind and with no hope of catching up. It is imperative, therefore, that the developed countries restructure their foreign policies and assistance programs to cooperate in meeting these challenges. Global interdependence necessitates it.

Much can be learned from the Cuban experience of promoting health and medicine in foreign relations as well as in domestic affairs. Medical diplomacy, defined as "collaboration between countries on health matters for the purposes of improving relations with one another," is a key factor in Cuban foreign policy.[31] The developed countries would do well to emulate Cuban medical diplomacy and Cuba's focus on domestic health programs to improve individual and thereby societal development.

Despite the changes that have swept the eastern European countries and the former Soviet Union, Castro and some other Cuban leaders remain committed to "socialism or death." But to those who have to live within those changes, a current Cuban joke goes, "What is the difference?" Priorities for economic and social development have not changed in recent years and will continue as before, but the ability to implement projects has greatly diminished. These priorities are import substitution; the continuing development of tourism, biotechnology, medicine, and other nontraditional exports; the completion, where possible, of social projects already under construction; housing construction for agricultural centers; and the current priority, a food program to assure food supplies given the failure to receive food shipments from the former socialist countries.

The Cuban government continues to promote medical, pharmaceutical, and biotechnology research to find solutions to domestic problems and to develop export products. In health-care delivery, emphasis is on tasks that can be accomplished with human resources rather than material resources: health promotion, disease prevention, and the monitoring of the population's health.

What have changed are Cuba's increased efforts to free itself from the strictures of past integration into the CMEA. Even before the fall of the Berlin Wall, Cuba had been seeking new trade partners, usually through countertrade and barter, particularly with other developing nations. Indeed, Cuba has been at the forefront of the promotion of south-south trade. More important for my analysis is the fact that Cuba is vigorously promoting biotechnology and medical products as important nontraditional exports.

Also changed are Cuba's prospects for continuing its social achievements in the face of geopolitical and hence economic adversity. Without democratization, economic salvation is unlikely because of the tightening of the U.S. embargo that, one could argue, is only now truly beginning to take effect thirty-two years after its imposition. Studies of both economic development and regime change in Latin America suggest that economic crisis leads to political change.

Because Castro has equated the health of the body politic with the health of the people, the body politic has fallen ill. Inadequate food and hygiene, resulting from decreased aid and trade, have affected the health of the Cuban population. Some of the more sensitive indicators of the decline in the standard of living—the maternal mortality rate, the percentage of babies born with low birth weight, the mortality rate from infectious and parasitic diseases, and the rate of patient visits for diarrhea and acute respiratory disease—have increased slightly from 1990 to 1991.[32] Data for 1992 can only indicate a further deterioration in the Cuban people's health.

The inability of the Castro government to provide adequate food and other basic consumer goods during this time of adversity has led many to question the legitimacy of his rule. Nonetheless, prior success in meeting basic needs helps to explain why this government has survived so long after the fall of the Berlin Wall.

Despite the Cuban government's best efforts, economic and political survival seem unlikely in the current geopolitical context, irrespective of the best efforts of Cuba's medical and scientific sector. It is indeed unfortunate that the medical edifice built by Cuba is unlikely to withstand the economic tremors of the post–Cold War world.

Appendix
Health Tourism in Cuba

Cubanacán, the agency that handles health tourism, has produced various color brochures in Spanish, English, and French to advertise the Cira García Clinic, the Center for Placental Histotherapy, and the Topes de Collantes health, rest, and recreation center. An accompanying 1988 price list for travel agents includes the following procedures (among others) with prices in U.S. dollars:[1]

1. The destruction of kidney stones through extracorporeal lithotripsy, $4,034 for one kidney and $5,020 for both. The price includes two weeks in the clinic, clinical history and all physical examinations, three simple abdominal x-rays, three abdominal ultrasounds, anesthesia, operating room, lithotripsy, and physicians' fees.

2. Open-heart surgery, $8,897. This includes twenty-one days in the clinic, clinical history and examinations, operation, operating room, anesthesia, surgical materials, sutures, medicines, extracorporeal circulation equipment, physicians' fees, and medical faculty report.

3. Ophthalmological microsurgery to correct myopia, $900 for one eye and $1,500 for both, all inclusive for one- and two-week clinic stays respectively.

4. Neural transplant to treat Parkinson's disease, $14,974. This price is for one week of tests and evaluation ($1,950) and three weeks of further evaluation, neural transplant, and recuperation, all fees included ($13,024).

5. Treatment for psoriasis, $727 (group rate per person in double room) for twenty-eight days, twenty treatments, medical consultations, airport transfers, and one clinic transfer. The price does not include medications the patient should take home to continue the treatment.

6. Treatment for vitiligo, $215 (group rate per person in double room) for seven days, three treatments, medical consultations, airport transfers, and one transfer to the clinic. Medicine the patients should take home is not included in the price.

7. Pacemaker installation, $4,613, all inclusive.

Most laboratory tests, x-rays, and ultrasound examinations are under $50 and the majority are less than $25. CAT scans are $200 each, and nuclear magnetic resonance (NMR) tests are $250. Abdominal ultrasound runs $33, most x-rays are about $9, and simple blood tests cost $2.20.[2] Also, an accompanying person can stay in the clinic and get three meals a day for an additional $16 per day. These prices are very attractive by U.S. standards.

For comparative purposes, prices at the University of Michigan's University Hospital in 1989 were about $2,000 per day just for the hospital stay, exclusive of physicians' fees for any major procedure such as a coronary bypass or any type of transplant. A coronary bypass costs about $21,000 for hospital and physicians' fees; a heart transplant runs about $50,000 to $100,000, plus another $10,000 to $15,000 in physicians' fees, depending on the circumstances.[3] Although the procedures are very different, contrasting these fees with the approximately $15,000 for a neural transplant in Cuba illustrates the potential economic lure of Cuban medicine.

Abbreviations

The following are Cuban entities unless otherwise noted:

AID	U.S. Agency for International Development
ANAP	National Association of Small Farmers
CDRs	Committees for the Defense of the Revolution
CECE	State Committee for Economic Cooperation
CIB	Center for Biological Research
CIGB	Center for Genetic Engineering and Biotechnology
CIMAB	Center for Molecular Immunology
CIPA-ICLD	U.N. Council on International and Public Affairs–International Center for Law and Development
CMEA	Council for Mutual Economic Assistance (eastern bloc)
CNIC	National Center for Scientific Research
CTC	Confederation of Cuban Trade Unions
EPI	Expanded Immunization Program (PAHO)
FAO	U.N. Food and Agriculture Organization
FEEM	Federation of Middle School Students
FEU	Federation of University Students
FMC	Federation of Cuban Women
ICEM	Cuban Medical Equipment Industries
MINSAP	Ministry of Public Health
NACSEX	North American–Cuban Scientific Exchange
OMS	World Health Organization (Spanish acronym)
OPP	Organs of People's Power
OPS	Pan American Health Organization (Spanish acronym)

PAHO	Pan American Health Organization
PCC	Cuban Communist Party
PNUD	U.N. Development Program (Spanish acronym)
RETOMED	Medical Equipment Factory of Santiago de Cuba
SADCC	Southern Africa Development and Cooperation Council
TCDC	Technical Cooperation among Developing Countries (U.N. programs)
UEPEM	Union of Medical Equipment Producing Companies
UJC	Union of Communist Youth
UNDP	U.N. Development Program
UNIDO	U.N. Industrial Development Program
WHO	World Health Organization

Notes

Introduction

1. República de Cuba, Ministerio de Salud Pública, *Salud para todos: 25 años de experiencia cubana* (Ciudad La Habana: MINSAP, July 9, 1983), 35. Unless otherwise noted, all references to government documents are Cuban. Further citations of Cuban documents will be listed under the name of the issuing agency but can be found in the bibliography under "República de Cuba," followed by the agency and department names.

2. Fidel Castro, *2nd Period of Sessions of the National Assembly of People's Power. Closing Speech* (La Habana: Political Publishers, 1978), 39–41; *Granma,* July 31, 1981, 1, 3; *Granma,* December 10, 1981, 1; *Bohemia,* September 15, 1978; and *Granma Weekly Review,* March 11, 1984, 4.

3. The Soviet Union, Czechoslovakia, and Hungary provided free health care for everyone as an entitlement. Poland and Romania had comprehensive social insurance, the former providing universal free service and the latter providing it for a majority of the population. The German Democratic Republic had a social insurance scheme similar to that of the Federal Republic of Germany, in which the employee pays for the bulk of the insurance. China's health-care financing varies from total subsidy by factories for their employees to 50 percent payment for their families to total payment by the patient. Rural communes have prepaid health plans for their members, but other rural workers must pay in full for their health care. See Michael Kaser, *Health Care in the Soviet Union and Eastern Europe* (Boulder, Colo.: Westview Press, 1976), 102–3, 115, 147–8, 156, 213, 248, 272; and

Victor W. Sidel and Ruth Sidel, *Serve the People: Observations on Medicine in the People's Republic of China* (New York: Josiah Macy, Jr. Foundation, 1973), 75.

4. For example, the Soviet Union was the only industrialized country to experience a decline in life expectancy and an increase in infant mortality over the past two decades. U.S. Congress, Joint Economic Committee, *Soviet Economy in the 1980s: Problems and Prospects,* part 2, "Issues in Soviet Health Problems," by Murray Feshbach (Washington, D.C.: U.S. Government Printing Office, December 31, 1982), 203-8. See also comments by the Soviet Minister of Health, Yevgeny I. Chazov, in "Delegates' [to the Communist party conference] Views: On Health, Wealth and Work," *New York Times,* July 1, 1988, 4; "Red Medicine," *Wall Street Journal,* August 18, 1987, 1, 27; and Constance Holden, "Health Care in the Soviet Union," *Science* 213 (September 4, 1981): 1090-92.

5. L. Frances Millard, "Health Care in Poland: From Crisis to Crisis," *International Journal of Health Services* 12, no. 3 (1982):497-515; U.S. Congress, Joint Economic Committee, *Soviet Economy in the 1980s;* Richard E. Weinerman with Shirley B. Weinerman, *Social Medicine and the Education of Medical Personnel in Czechoslovakia, Hungary, and Poland* (Cambridge: Harvard University Press, 1969), 160-79; Teh-wei Hu, "Health Services in the People's Republic of China," in *Comparative Health Systems: Descriptive Analyses of Fourteen National Health Systems,* ed. Marshall W. Raffel (University Park: Pennsylvania State University Press, 1984), 133-52; Norma K. Raffel, "Health Services in the Union of Soviet Socialist Republics," in *Comparative Health Systems,* 488-519.

6. Sidel and Sidel, *Serve the People,* 28-29.

7. Jorge F. Pérez-López, "Cuban-Soviet Sugar Trade: Prices and Subsidy Issues," *Bulletin of Latin American Research* 7, no. 1 (1988):132.

8. For an excellent analysis of the Cuban-Soviet sugar trade and subsidies, see Jorge F. Pérez López, *The Economics of Cuban Sugar* (Pittsburgh: University of Pittsburgh Press, 1991), particularly pp. 135-72.

9. *Granma International,* November 3, 1991, 20-21.

10. Ibid., 25.

11. Pan American Health Organization, *Evaluation of the Strategy for Health for All by the Year 2000. Seventh Report on the World Health Situation, vol. 3, Region of the Americas* (Washington, D.C.: Pan American Health Organization, 1986), 7, 10-12; Brian Abel-Smith, "The World Economic Crisis, Part 1: Repercussions on Health," *Health Policy and Planning* 1, no. 3 (September 1986): pp. 210-11, tables 3, 4, 5; and C. Arden Miller et al., "The World Economic Crisis and the Children: United States Case Study," *International Journal of Health Services* 15, no. 1 (1985):123-31.

12. Michael Ryan, *The Organization of Soviet Medical Care* (Oxford: Basil Blackwell & Mott, 1978), 130; Raffel, "Health Services in the Union of Soviet Socialist Republics," 488-519; U.S. Congress, Joint Economic Committee, *Soviet Economy in the 1980s,* 203-8; and *Wall Street Journal,* August 18, 1987, 1, 27.

13. *Granma Weekly Review,* March 24, 1991, 5.

14. Norman Hicks and Paul Streeten, "Indicators of Development: The Search for a Basic Needs Yardstick," *World Development* 7 (1979): 578–79.

15. There is no clear enunciation of their criteria, but these have been culled from various official statements over the years since the topic was first mentioned publicly. The 1987 statements allude only to the infant mortality rate and life expectancy at birth, and 1988 statements suggest that world medical power status means that Cuba can provide health care comparable to that provided by the developed capitalist countries, specifically the United States.

Chapter 1

1. In international relations research, small generally refers to state capacity (political-military and economic) rather than geographic size. One of the most important capabilities is "the ability of the small state to mobilize forces and resources of the international system in favour of its policy." See Wilhelm Christmas-Möller, "Some Thoughts on the Scientific Applicability of the Small State Concept: A Research History and a Discussion," in *Small States in Europe and Dependence,* The Laxenburg Papers, ed. Otmar Höll (Boulder, Colo.: Westview Press, 1983), 44–45; and Raimo Vayrynen, "Small States in Different Theoretical Traditions of International Relations Research," in *Small States in Europe,* 100–101.

2. Otmar Höll, "Towards a Broadening of the Small States Perspective," in *Small States in Europe,* 14; and Hans Vogel, "Small States' Efforts in International Relations: Enlarging the Scope," in *Small States in Europe,* 55.

3. Peter Shearman, *The Soviet Union and Cuba,* Chathman House Papers no. 38 (London: Routledge & Kegan Paul, 1987), 33; Jorge I. Domínguez, "Political and Military Limitations and Consequences of Cuba's Policies in Africa," *Cuban Studies/Estudios Cubanos* 10, no. 2 (July 1980): 2.

4. Jorge I. Domínguez, "Cuba in the 1980s," *Foreign Affairs* 65, no. 1 (Fall 1986): 130.

5. Domínguez, "Political and Military Limitations," 2.

6. On the Cuban policy of proletarian internationalism, see *Constitución,* Article 12, La Habana: Departamento de Orientación Revolucionaria del Comité Central del Partido Comunista de Cuba, (1976), 18–20; on Soviet and Eastern European aid to the Cuban Revolution, see Silvia N. Pérez, "La participación de Cuba en la comunidad socialista y su ejemplo para el Tercer Mundo," in *Cuba y Estados Unidos: Un debate para la convivencia,* comp. Juan Gabriel Tokatlian (Buenos Aires: Grupo Editor Latino-Americano, 1984), 115; on Cuban aid to other developing countries and national liberation movements, see Martínez Salsamendi, "Cuba en América Central, El Caribe y Africa," in *Cuba y Estados Unidos,* 135.

7. On similarities and differences between Cuban and Soviet foreign policy, see Jorge I. Domínguez, "Cuban Foreign Policy," *Foreign Affairs* 57 (Fall

1978): 83–108; Id., *To Make a World Safe for Revolution: Cuban Foreign Policy* (Cambridge: Harvard University Press, 1989); Carmelo Mesa-Lago and June S. Belkin, eds., *Cuba in Africa* (Pittsburgh: University of Pittsburgh Press, 1982); W. Raymond Duncan, *The Soviet Union and Cuba: Interests and Influence* (New York: Praeger, 1985); Peter Shearman, *The Soviet Union and Cuba;* Jacques Levesque, *The USSR and the Cuban Revolution: Soviet Ideological and Strategic Perspectives, 1959–1977* (New York: Praeger, 1978); on Cuban influence on Soviet foreign policy, see Domínguez, "Cuba in the 1980s," 134.

8. *Die Zeit* (West Germany), September 9, 1988, Dossier p. 6.

9. William M. LeoGrande, "Cuban-Soviet Relations and Cuban Policy in Africa," *Cuban Studies/Estudios Cubanos* 10, no. 1 (January 1980): 34; Nelson P. Valdés, "Cuba's Involvement in the Horn of Africa: The Ethiopian-Somali War and the Eritrean Conflict," *Cuban Studies/Estudios Cubanos* 10, no. 1 (January 1980): 49–80; Domínguez, "Political and Military Limitations," 9–10; Sergio Roca, "Economic Aspects of Cuba's Involvement in Africa," *Cuban Studies/Estudios Cubanos* 10, no. 2 (July 1980): 61; Cole Blasier, "The Cuban–U.S.–Soviet Triangle, Changing Angles," *Cuban Studies/Estudios Cubanos* 8, no. 1 (January 1978): 1.

10. In 1965, Puerto Rico received $262.7 million and Cuba received $102 million in non-repayable aid from the U.S. and the Soviet Union respectively. In 1970, Puerto Rico got $559.8 million and Cuba had a negative subsidy of $75 million. That is, the terms of trade were such that Cuba lost money rather than gained it. In 1975, Puerto Rico got $1,817.7 million and Cuba got $478 million. In 1980, Puerto Rico received $3,707.9 million and Cuba received $2,983 million. In 1985, Puerto Rico got $4,847.7 million and Cuba got $3.5 million. Calculated from data in National Foreign Assessment Center, Central Intelligence Agency, *The Cuban Economy: A Statistical Review* (Washington, D.C.: C.I.A., 1984), p. 40; Richard Turits, "Trade, Debt and the Cuban Economy," *World Development* 15:1 (January 1987), Table IV, p. 167; U.S. Department of Commerce. *Economic Study of Puerto Rico.* Volume I. (Washington, D.C.: U.S. Government Printing Office), December 1979, pp. 13–14; and U.S. Commerce Department. Bureau of Census. *Federal Funds Report Fiscal Year 1985* (Washington, D.C.: U.S.G.P.O., March 1986), pp. 76–77; *Fiscal Year 1984,* pp. 76–77; and *Fiscal Year 1983,* pp. 76–77.

11. On socioeconomic development in Puerto Rico, see U.S. Department of Commerce, *Economic Study of Puerto Rico* (Washington, D.C.: U.S. Government Printing Office, 1977), 313, 680; Estado Libre Asociado de Puerto Rico, Oficina del Gobernador, Junta de Planificación, *Compendio Estadísticas Sociales 1981* (San Juan: Junta de Planificación, October 1982), 150, 152, 159, 165; and Richard Weisskoff, *Factories and Food Stamps: The Puerto Rico Model of Development* (Baltimore: Johns Hopkins University Press, 1985). Puerto Rico began a regionalized, hierarchically organized public health system in 1953, more than a decade prior to Cuba's similar efforts. However, the Puerto Rican system never crystallized completely and was partially dismantled whenever the opposition PNP gained power. Further, Puerto Rico's public health system always existed alongside private practices

that drained medical personnel from the public system. See Guillermo Arbona with Annette B. Ramírez de Arellano, *Regionalization of Health Services: The Puerto Rican Experience* (Santurce, Puerto Rico: Talleres Gráficos, 1977).

12. Domínguez, "Political and Military Limitations," 3–4; LeoGrande, "Cuban-Soviet Relations," 34; Levesque, *The USSR and the Cuban Revolution;* Duncan, *The Soviet Union and Cuba;* and Shearman, *The Soviet Union and Cuba.*

13. Domínguez, "Cuba in the 1980s," 123–26. Susan Eckstein argues that the rectification process was "not categorically anti-market, but only selectively so." Eckstein, "The Rectification of Errors or the Errors of the Rectification Process in Cuba?" *Cuban Studies* 20 (1990): 68. Free markets run by peasants, the most important market mechanism introduced, were closed.

14. *New York Times,* October 17, 1988, 1.

15. On Soviet limitation of foreign entanglements, see Shearman, *The Soviet Union and Cuba,* 83; on Soviet ties with capitalist countries, see Shearman, 80–81.

16. Tad Szulc, *Fidel: A Critical Portrait* (New York: William Morrow, 1986), 585.

17. Jorge F. Pérez López, "Nuclear Power in Cuba after Chernobyl," *Journal of Interamerican Studies and World Affairs* 29, no. 2 (Summer 1987): 108.

18. Domínguez, "Political and Military Limitations," 4.

19. Robert A. Pastor, "Cuba and the Soviet Union: Does Cuba Act Alone?" in *The New Cuban Presence in the Caribbean,* ed. Barry B. Levine (Boulder, Colo.: Westview Press, 1983), 204.

20. Andres Oppenheimer, *Castro's Final Hour: The Secret Story Behind the Coming Downfall of Communist Cuba* (New York: Simon and Schuster, 1992), 369.

21. Hugh O'Shaughnessy, *Grenada* (New York: Dodd, Mead, 1984), 150–51, 189–90.

22. Domínguez, "Political and Military Limitations," 34; Susan Eckstein, "Structural and Ideological Bases of Cuba's Overseas Programs," *Politics and Society* 11 (1982): 121; and Michael H. Erisman, *Cuba's International Relations: The Anatomy of a Nationalistic Foreign Policy* (Boulder, Colo.: Westview Press, 1985), 5–8, 11.

23. On nationalism as an explanation for Cuba's foreign policy, see Erisman, *Cuba's International Relations,* 9–12; on the strategic value of Angola and Ethiopia as an explanation for that policy see Pamela S. Falk, "Cuba in Africa," *Foreign Affairs,* 65, no. 5 (Summer 1987): 1079–80; on revolutionary experience as an explanation for that policy, see Falk, *Cuban Foreign Policy: Caribbean Tempest* (Lexington, Mass.: Lexington Books, 1986), 106.

24. Roca, "Economic Aspects of Cuban Involvement," 60–67; and Eckstein, "Structural and Ideological Bases," 105–8.

25. Domínguez, "Political and Military Limitations," 28; and Eckstein, "Structural and Ideological Bases," 109.

26. Eckstein, "Structural and Ideological Bases," 105.

27. The sugar market declined over 23 percent in the two years from 1988 (16 cents per pound) through June 27, 1990 (12.67 cents per pound). The world market price for sugar was only 8.55 cents per pound on November 17, 1992, and futures through March 1994 (quoted on that date) were at 8.99 cents per pound. See *New York Times,* June 28, 1990, C15; November 26, 1991, D16; and November 18, 1992, C14.

28. On Cuba's ideology, see *Constitución,* 18–19; and Partido Comunista de Cuba, *Programa del Partido Comunista de Cuba* (La Habana: Editora Politica, 1987), 52; on Cuba's symbolic threat to U.S. hegemony, see Carla Anne Robbins, *The Cuban Threat* (New York: McGraw-Hill, 1983), 310–11; on the value of an external threat to Cuba's social cohesion, see Jorge I. Domínguez, "Cuba: Domestic Bread and Foreign Circuses," in *Cuban Communism,* ed. Irving Louis Horowitz, 5th ed. (New Brunswick, N.J.: Transaction Books, 1985), 478.

29. U.S. Senate, *Alleged Assassination Plots Involving Foreign Leaders,* 94th Cong, 1st Sess. (Washington, D.C.: U.S. Government Printing Office, November 20, 1975), 71–180; Warren Hinckle and William W. Turner, *The Fish Is Red: The Story of the Secret War Against Castro* (New York: Harper and Row, 1981); and Peter Wyden, *Bay of Pigs: The Untold Story* (New York: Simon and Schuster, 1979).

30. On the longstanding mistrust between Cuba and the United States, see Philip Brenner, *From Confrontation to Negotiation: U.S. Relations with Cuba* (Boulder, Colo.: Westview Press, 1988); Lynn-Darrell Bender, *Cuba vs. United States: The Politics of Hostility,* 2nd ed. (Hato Rey, Puerto Rico: Inter American University Press, 1981); *Agresiones de Estados Unidos a Cuba 1787–1976* (La Habana: Editorial de Ciencias Sociales, 1978); Tokatlian, *Cuba y Estados Unidos;* and Wayne S. Smith, *The Closest of Enemies: A Personal and Diplomatic Account of U.S.–Cuban Relations Since 1957* (New York: Norton, 1987); on Cuba's love-hate relationship with the United States, see Carlos Alberto Montaner, "The Roots of Anti-Americanism in Cuba: Sovereignty in an Age of World Cultural Homogeneity," *Caribbean Review* 13, no. 2 (Spring 1984): 13.

31. "Letter to Célia Sánchez, June 5 [1958]," quoted in Carlos Franqui, *Diary of the Cuban Revolution* (New York: Viking Press, 1980), 338.

32. Interviews conducted in Cuba, 1978, 1979, 1980–1981, 1988, 1990, 1991, and 1992.

33. See Michel Foucault, *The Order of Things: An Archaeology of the Human Sciences* (New York: Vintage Books, 1973), 3–16.

34. Ibid.

35. On the roles of myth in society, see George Sorel, *Reflections on Violence* (London: Allen and Unwin, 1925), 32; and David E. Apter, "Ideology and Discontent," in *Ideology and Discontent,* ed. David E. Apter (New York: Free Press of Glencoe, 1964), 17; the quotation on myth as a symbol system is from Richard R. Fagen, *The Transformation of Political Culture in Cuba* (Stanford, Calif.: Stanford University Press, 1969), 233n.17, citing Apter, "Ideology and Discontent."

36. Fagen, *Transformation of Political Culture*, 11. Fagen's observation is for the first decade of revolution but was still accurate in 1988 (the end of the third decade of revolution).

37. C. Fred Judson, "Continuity and Evolution of Revolutionary Symbolism in *Verde Olivo*," in *Cuba: Twenty-Five Years of Revolution*, ed. Sandor Halebsky and John M. Kirk (New York: Praeger, 1985), 242.

38. Ibid., 234.

39. Andrew Zimbalist, "Incentives and Planning in Cuba," *Latin American Research Review* 24, no. 1 (1989): 65–94.

40. Fagen, *Transformation of Political Culture*, 41.

41. Ibid., 246.

42. On the symbolism of Che Guevara, see Judson, "Continuity and Evolution of Revolutionary Symbolism," 244–45; on the symbolism of the Cubans who died in Grenada, see Judson, 246n.3 citing Castro in *A Pyrrhic Military Victory and a Profound Moral Defeat* (Havana: Editorial Politica, 1983), 18–19.

43. Ibid., 244.

44. On Castro's statement about Television Martí, see "Castro Holds News Conference," Foreign Broadcast Information Service, *Latin America Daily Report*, FBIS-LAT-90-065, April 4, 1990, 18–19; on Cuban jamming of Television Martí, see "Havana Reports Jamming 1 Apr," Foreign Broadcast Information Service, *Latin America Daily Report*, FBIS-LAT-90-063, April 2, 1990, 6.

45. Smith, *Closest of Enemies*, 264–65.

46. Armando Valladares, *Against All Hope: The Prison Memoirs of Armando Valladares* (New York: Knopf, 1986).

47. Personal communication from German delegate, Bruno Simma, September 10, 1988. For contrasting views on Cuban human rights, see Institute for Policy Studies, *Preliminary Report of U.S. Delegation to Cuba. Institute for Policy Studies–National Union of Cuban Jurists. Joint Commission on the Conviction and Treatment of Prisoners in the United States and Cuba. February 26–March 5, 1988* (Washington, D.C.: Institute for Policy Studies, March 1988) (mimeographed); Organization of American States, *The Situation of Human Rights in Cuba*, Seventh Report (Washington, D.C.: OAS, 1983); and Cuban Committee for Human Rights, *Political Executions and Human Rights in Cuba: Annual Report, December 10, 1987* (Washington, D.C.: Of Human Rights [Georgetown University], 1988).

48. On Bishop and Castro at the United Nations, see Robbins, *Cuban Threat*, 241; on Angola as Cuba's Vietnam, see Robbins, 225.

49. On symbolism and substance in the 1988 presidential campaign, see Elizabeth Drew, "Letter from Washington," *New Yorker*, October 31, 1988, 102; *New York Times*, September 5, 1988, 1; and *New York Times*, August 27, 1988, 1; on symbolism and substance at the Reagan-Gorbachev summit, see Drew, "Letter from Washington," *New Yorker*, July 4, 1988, 77. See also *New York Times*, May 22, 1988, sec. 4, p. 1; and *New York Times*, May 19, 1988, 12.

50. For example, see the analysis of Ligachev's absence from various photos of the Soviet Politburo, *New York Times,* November 8, 1988, 4.

51. *New York Times,* March 14, 1985, p. 7.

52. *New York Times,* November 4, 1987, 1.

53. *New York Times,* January 30, 1988.

54. David E. Apter and Nagayo Sawa, *Against the State: Politics and Social Protest in Japan* (Cambridge: Harvard University Press, 1984).

55. Ibid., 5.

56. Ibid., 3.

57. Ibid., 108–9.

58. Ibid., 109.

59. See C. Fred Judson, *Cuba and the Revolutionary Myth: The Political Education of the Cuban Rebel Army, 1953–1963* (Boulder, Colo.: Westview Press, 1984).

60. Fagen, *Transformation of Political Culture,* 54.

61. Foreign Broadcast Information Service, *Latin America Daily Report,* FBIS-LAT-90-065, 4 April 1990, 18.

62. David E. Apter, "The New Mytho/Logics and the Specter of Superfluous Man," *Social Research* 52, no. 2 (Summer 1985): 269–70.

63. Apter and Sawa, *Against the State,* 108.

64. Pierre Bourdieu, "The Social Space and the Genesis of Groups," *Theory and Society* 14, no. 6 (November 1985): 727.

65. Karl Marx, *The German Ideology,* in *The Marx-Engels Reader,* ed. Robert C. Tucker (New York: Norton, 1972), 136.

66. Bourdieu, "Social Space," 728.

67. Ibid., 729.

68. Karl Marx, "Theses on Feuerbach," in *The Marx-Engels Reader,* ed. Robert C. Tucker, (New York: Norton, 1972), 109.

69. Apter, "The New Mytho/Logics," 273.

70. Ibid., 273.

71. Pierre Bourdieu, *Outline of a Theory of Practice* (Cambridge: Cambridge University Press, 1987), 177, 180.

72. Ibid., 181.

73. FAO, OMS, PMA, PNUD, UNESCO, "Informe de las agencias de las Naciones Unidas representadas en Cuba," (November 1989): 2, 7 (typescript).

74. Bourdieu, *Outline of a Theory of Practice,* 183.

Chapter 2

1. *Constitución,* Articles 8 b, 48 and 49, pp. 17, 36–37; and Ministerio de Salud Pública, *Subdesarrollo económico principal enemigo de la salud: como lo combate la revolución cubana. 19 meses de labor del MINSAP* (La Habana: MINSAP, n.d. [probably late 1961]), 3.

2. Osvaldo Castro Miranda, "Situación actual y perspectiva de la salud pública en Cuba," *Revista cubana de administración de salud* 7, no. 2 (1981): 103.

3. Ministerio de Salud Pública, *Subdesarrollo económico,* 4.

4. Fidel Castro Ruz, *History Will Absolve Me* (Havana: Guairas Book Institute, 1967), 83.

5. Ibid., 72–73.

6. Ministerio de Salud Pública, *Subdesarrollo económico,* 1. This position is also taken by the Pan American Health Organization. See *Evaluation of the Strategy for Health for All by the Year 2000. Seventh Report on the World Health Situation, vol. 3, Region of the Americas,* (Washington, D.C.: Pan American Health Organization, 1986), 12.

7. One can argue that labor is still exploited under socialism, but by the state rather than by the capitalists. A Cuban joke attests to this view: "What is the difference between capitalism and socialism?—Under capitalism man exploits man. Under socialism it is the reverse."

8. Despite economic diversification, Cuba was still dependent on sugar production for both foreign exchange earnings and trade and barter within the Community for Mutual Economic Assistance until its demise, but not to the same extent as before the revolution. Cuba had developed numerous new industries, but sugar remained king. See Claes Brundenius, *Revolutionary Cuba: The Challenge of Economic Growth with Equity* (Boulder, Colo.: Westview Press, 1984): 61–78; Andrew Zimbalist, "Cuban Political Economy and Cubanology: An Overview," in *Cuban Political Economy,* ed. Andrew Zimbalist, 5–8; and Carmelo Mesa-Lago, *The Economy of Socialist Cuba: A Two-Decade Appraisal* (Albuquerque, N. Mex.: University of New Mexico Press, 1981), 82–84.

9. Beginning in 1980 there was some unemployment as the result of an effort to increase efficiency, but unlike in the prerevolutionary days workers were paid 70 percent of their salaries and provided with free retraining if necessary. The economic crisis of the early 1990s led to many layoffs because of a lack of industrial inputs and insufficient fuel to keep factories running at capacity, but once again workers were given other employment in agriculture or paid compensation. This approach, however, has not been particularly appealing to many who would rather maintain their city jobs than do agricultural labor.

10. On Cuba's performance in meeting basic human needs see Brundenius, *Revolutionary Cuba.*

11. Ministerio de Salud Pública, *Subdesarrollo económico,* 1.

12. Ministerio de Salud Pública, *Informe anual 1976* (La Habana: MIN-SAP, 1977), 9–11.

13. Ruth Leger Sivard, *World Military and Social Expenditures 1987–88* (Washington, D.C.: World Priorities, 1987), 47; and The World Bank, *World Development Report 1990* (New York: Oxford University Press, 1990), 233, 244–45.

14. Ministerio de Salud Pública, *Fundamentación para un nuevo enfoque de la medicina en la comunidad* (La Habana: MINSAP, 1977), 27.

15. Mario Escalona Reguera, *La participación popular en la salud* (La Habana: MINSAP, Instituto de Desarrollo de la Salud, 1980), 57; Sergio R. Ledo Duarte, "Participación popular en salud," *Revista cubana de administración de salud* 10, no. 3 (July–September 1984): 220–25; and interview with Rogelia Rojas Requena, municipal health director, La Lisa, City of Havana province, February 26, 1981.

16. Interview with Cosme Ordóñez Carceller, Director of the Policlínico "Plaza de la Revolución," Havana, December 28, 1978.

17. Interview with Osvaldo Castro Miranda, head of planning department, Viceministerio de Economía, MINSAP, Havana, June 13, 1991, and with Francisco Rojas Ochoa, vicerrector de investigaciones, Instituto Superior de Ciencias Médicas-Habana (Girón), Havana, June 17, 1991.

18. Ministerio de Salud Pública, *Evaluación estrategias de salud para todos en el año 2000: Informe de Cuba 1990* (La Habana: MINSAP typescript, January 1991), 8–9.

19. Ross Danielson, *Cuban Medicine* (New Brunswick, N.J.: Transaction Books, 1979). See especially 76–78; and interview with Mario Escalona Reguera at the Instituto de Desarrollo de la Salud, Havana, December 1978.

20. Danielson, *Cuban Medicine,* 120–21.

21. Ministerio de Salud Pública, *Subdesarrollo económico principal enemigo de la salud: como lo combate la revolución cubana: 19 meses de labor del MINSAP* (La Habana: MINSAP, n.d. [probably late 1961]), 2; Roberto Hernández Elias, "Desarrollo de la salud pública en Cuba," in *Teoría y administración de salud* (La Habana: MINSAP, 1980), 63–64; and on poverty see Agrupación Católica Universitaria, "Encuesta de los trabajadores rurales 1956–1957," *Economía y desarrollo* 3, no. 12 (July–August 1972): 188–213.

22. Sally Guttmacher and Ross Danielson, "Changes in Cuban Health Care: An Argument Against Technological Pessimism," *International Journal of Health Services* 7, no. 3 (1977): 389.

23. Roberto E. Capote Mir, "La evolución de los servicios de salud y la estructura socioeconómica en Cuba," *Saúde em debate* (Rio de Janeiro), no. 14 (1982): 53.

24. Hernández Elias, "Desarrollo de la salud pública," 63–64. The Chinese did the same during their revolutionary war but failed to provide much rural health service until after 1965. Joshua S. Horn, *Away With All Pests: An English Surgeon in People's China, 1954–1969,* (New York: Monthly Review Press, 1969), 128; and Sidel and Sidel, *Serve the People,* 21, 29.

25. Roberto Hernández Elias, "Princípios de la salud pública socialista," in *Teoría y administración de salud,* (La Habana: MINSAP, 1980), 25.

26. Jorge Aldereguía Henríques and Osvaldo J. Castro Miranda, "Lo sviluppo della salute pubblica nell'esperienza cubana," *The Practitioner (Edizione Italiana)* (Milano) 103 (June 1987): 32.

27. Roberto E. Capote Mir, "La evolución de los servicios de salud y la estructura socioeconómica en Cuba," (La Habana: Instituto de Desarrollo de la Salud, 1979), 14 (mimeographed).

28. Escalona Reguera, *La participación popular,* 61.

29. Ibid., 61; and Danielson, *Cuban Medicine,* 144. The Czechs had the best health system and health indicators among the eastern bloc countries both before and after World War II, which made theirs the most attractive model for Cuban adaptation.

30. Capote Mir, "La evolución de los servicios de salud," 15.

31. Vicente Navarro, "Health, Health Services, and Health Planning in Cuba," *International Journal of Health Services* 2, no. 3 (August 1972): 413.

32. Roca, "Economic Aspects of Cuba's Involvement in Africa," 56–57.

33. Hernández Elias, "Desarrollo de la salud pública en Cuba," 66.

34. Milton I. Roemer, *Cuban Health Services and Resources* (Washington, D.C.: Pan American Health Organization, 1976), 44.

35. Interview with Mario Escalona Reguera, Instituto de Desarrollo de la Salud, La Habana, December 1978.

36. Navarro, "Health, Health Services, and Health Planning," 418–19. In 1986 there was one medical school in every province except Ciudad de la Habana, which had eight; Santiago de Cuba, which had two; and La Habana, which had none because of its proximity to Ciudad de la Habana. Ministry of Public Health, *Public Health in Figures, 1986* (Havana: MINSAP, 1987), 63.

37. On political and economic reforms see Carmelo Mesa-Lago, *Cuba in the 1970s: Pragmatism and Institutionalization,* rev. ed. (Albuquerque, N. Mex.: University of New Mexico Press, 1978); Max Azicri, "The Institutionalization of the Cuban Revolution: A Review of the Literature," *Cuban Studies/Estudios Cubanos* 9, no. 2 (July 1979): 63–78 with commentaries pp. 78–84. On health sector reforms see República de Cuba, Ministerio de Salud Pública, *Fundamentación para un nuevo enfoque,* 21–26.

38. Mario Escalona Reguera, "La medicina en la comunidad," in *Teorías y administración de salud,* (Havana: MINSAP, 1980), 112–23.

39. Roca, "Economic Aspects of Cuban Involvement," 70, 72.

40. Ministerio de Salud Pública, *Informe anual.* See each year from 1976 to 1991.

41. Castro, *2nd Period of Sessions of the National Assembly,* 39–41.

42. Jeffrey L. Fox, "Cuba Plans a Century of Biology," *American Society of Microbiology* 52, no. 5 (1986): 245.

43. See Castro's speeches dated September 12, 1981, and November 6, 1982, and cited in Ministerio de Salud Pública, Vicerrectoría Desarrollo ISCM-H, "Algunas ideas vertidas en diferentes discursos pronunciados por el Comandante en Jefe Fidel Castro que tienen que ver con la formación del médico a egresar de la educación médica superior y con la especialidad de medicina general integral y que sirvieron de base para la elaboración del nuevo plan de estudio de medicina (1981–1984)," 1, 12 (mimeographed).

44. Ibid.

45. MINSAP began to study and promote the cultivation and use of herbal remedies in the early 1980s and published a booklet on the proper use of medicinal plants as remedies for minor ailments. Family doctors were encouraged to plant herb gardens in response to the needs of their patients and the characteristics of the soil in their locales. Interview with Miguel

Figueras, adviser to the President of the Comité Estatal de Colaboración Económica, Havana, June 14, 1991; Luis Foyo, Programa de Medicina Familiar, Viceministerio de Asistencia Médica, Havana, June 17, 1991; and Rosa Ana de la Torre, Facultad de Medicina Salvador Allende, Havana, June 22, 1991.

46. *Granma Weekly Review,* August 5, 1990, 4.

47. Unlike the Soviets, the Cubans invested heavily in health care and sought greater equality and, at a minimum, equity in the delivery of services.

48. On the requisites of regionalization see Arbona, with Ramírez de Arellano, *Regionalization of Health Services,* 8–12.

49. Interview with Mario Escalona Reguera, director of education, Instituto de Desarrollo de la Salud, Havana, February 1981.

50. Prior to the Family Doctor Program, basic primary care in rural areas was provided by resident physicians, dentists, nurses, and technicians and by specialists from the municipal hospital of the nearest municipality, who rotated regularly through the rural health facilities.

51. "El médico de la familia: una experiencia cubana." Address by Abelardo Ramírez, vice-minister of health for Medical Care. 2nd International Seminar on Primary Health Care, Havana, November 15, 1988.

52. Vicente Navarro, "Health Services in Cuba," *New England Journal of Medicine* 287, no. 19 (November 9, 1972): 955; and Margaret Gilpin and Helen Rodríguez-Trias, "Looking at Health in a Healthy Way," *Cuba Review* 7: no. 1 (March 1978): 9.

53. Ministerio de Salud Pública. *Fundamentación para un nuevo enfoque,* 32–33.

54. Cosme Ordóñez Carceller, "La medicina en la comunidad," in *Medicina en la comunidad.* (La Habana: MINSAP, 1976), 18.

55. Ministerio de Salud Pública, Dirección Nacional de Planificación de Salud, *Programas básicos del área de salud y su evaluación* (La Habana: MINSAP, 1977).

56. Ibid.

57. Interview with the Pan American Health Organization's statistical chief, Hans Bruch, Washington, D.C., October 1982.

58. Funding for automated information systems has come from the Pan American Health Organization and the United Nations Population Fund. UNICEF, UNFPA, OPS/OMS, MINSAP, *El plan del médico de la familia en Cuba* (La Habana: UNICEF, 1991), 43–44.

59. Observation of system demonstration and sample printout by Mario García Ibarra of the Buro Conjunto de Ingeniería Cubano-Bulgaro para la Aplicación de las Técnicas de Computación Electrónica at the 2nd International Seminar on Primary Health Care in Havana, November 1988.

60. Ordóñez Carceller, "La medicina en la comunidad," 12.

61. Ibid., 12–13; see also Galaz Góngora, Robna R. et al., "Análisis de las actividades del policlínico integral docente 'Plaza de la Revolución,'" Trabajo en equipo, Asignatura: Administración de Salud del Curso Internacional de Salud Pública. (La Habana: Instituto de Desarrollo de la Salud, March 1979), 14 (typescript).

62. Estela Ramírez López et al., "Conocimiento de una comunidad urbana a través del Policlínico Comunitario Docente 'Plaza de la Revolución'" (La Habana: Instituto de Desarrollo de la Salud, trabajo en equipo, October 21, 1978), 8 (typescript).

63. Mario Escalona Reguera, "Panel informativo; 'La medicina en la comunidad,' 'El policlínico': presente y futuro," in *Medicina en la comunidad* (Havana: MINSAP, 1975), 25; and Sarah Santana, "The Cuban Health Care System: Responsiveness to Changing Population Needs and Demands," *World Development* 15, no. 1 (January 1987): 117.

64. Ramírez, "El médico de la familia," 3.

65. These problems were not new despite the ministry's attempts to ameliorate the situation. Most can be found in critiques of the system before medicine in the community. See Ministerio de Salud Pública, *Fundamentación para un nuevo enfoque* and *Medicina en la comunidad.*

66. Observations of family doctor offices in San Miguél del Padrón, City of Havana province, and Baracoa, Guantánamo province, November 16 and 27–28, 1988; and *Granma,* January 17, 1984.

67. Ramírez, "El médico de la familia," 3, and *Granma,* January 17, 1984.

68. Problems have arisen as some doctors have chosen not to live in the home offices built for them. *Granma,* January 17, 1984; and *Granma Weekly Review,* April 19, 1987, 10.

69. Interview with Dr. Maria de los Angeles Batista Peña, the family doctor in Cagüeibaje and Palma Clara, Guantánamo province, November 27, 1988.

70. Interview with Luis Foyo, June 17, 1991.

71. Ministerio de Salud Pública, *Programa de trabajo del médico y enfermera de la familia, el policlínico y el hospital* (La Habana: MINSAP, March 1988).

72. José García Rodríguez, Raúl Mazorra Zamora, and Omar Morell Rodríguez, "Plan de actividades físicas que debe realizar el médico de la familia," *Revista cubana de medicina integral* 3, no. 1 (1987): 109–12.

73. Observations of exercise classes in Havana and discussions with senior citizens of the "Alegrías de la vida" Grandparents' Club in the Vedado section, 1988 and 1990, and interview with their family doctor, Dr. Loida Zúnga Aguirre, from the Policlínico Comunitario Héroes de Corynthia, January 22, 1990.

74. This is confirmed by informal interviews in Havana, 1988, 1990, 1991, and 1992.

75. *Granma,* October 22, 1984, 2.

76. Ministerio de Salud Pública, *Informe anual 1989,* 74.

77. Ibid., 8.

78. *Granma Weekly Review,* March 29, 1987, 3; *Granma,* October 16, 1986, 1; and personal observations of family doctors in remote areas of Guantánamo province, November 27–28, 1988.

79. Data for 1987 were calculated from "Cifras de Médicos de la Familia, según el lugar donde prestan sus servicios, desglosadas por provincias. Noviembre de 1987," *Revista cubana de medicina general integral* 4, no. 1 (January–March 1988): 78.

230 NOTES TO PAGES 42–46

80. *Granma Weekly Review,* September 9, 1988, 12, and September 2, 1990, 9.

81. Interview with Osvaldo Castro Miranda, June 13, 1991, and Luis Foyo, June 17, 1991.

82. Ministerio de Salud Pública, *Evaluación estrategias de salud para el año 2000: Informe de Cuba* (La Habana: MINSAP, January 1991), 5.

83. Interview with Otto Machado, Dpto. Programa Materno-Infantil, Vice-ministerio de Asistencia Médica, Havana, June 14, 1991.

84. Interview with Osvaldo Castro Miranda, June 13, 1991.

85. Ramírez, "El médico de la familia," 15.

86. Interview with Osvaldo Castro Miranda, June 13, 1991, and with Marco A. Montano Díaz, profesor, Facultad de Ciencias Médicas de Pinar del Río, in Pinar del Río, June 18, 1991.

87. Ramírez, "El médico de la familia," 16.

88. UNICEF, UNFPA, OPS-OMS, MINSAP, *El plan del médico de la familia,* 23.

89. Interview with Marco A. Montano Díaz, June 18, 1991.

90. Ministerio de Salud Pública, *Programa de trabajo del médico y enfermera de la familia,* 7.

91. Data on hospital emergency-room use since 1963 indicate a steady increase until 1987, the third year of partial implementation of the Family Doctor Program, when it decreased to a little below the 1985 level. In 1988, however, hospital emergency-room use increased again but decreased in 1989 to below the 1984 level. See Comité Estatal de Estadísticas, *Anuario estadístico de Cuba 1988,* (La Habana: CEE, 1989), 581–82, and Ministerio de Salud Pública, *Informe anual 1989,* 107.

92. Lilliam Jiménez Fontao and Enf. Mayra Zaldívar Lores, "Experiencia del médico de la familia en un consultorio de Plaza de la Revolución," *Revista cubana de medicina general integral* 3, no. 1 (1987): 135; *Granma,* May 26, 1986, 1–3; *Granma Weekly Review,* October 27, 1985, 8–9; and numerous papers presented at the 2nd International Seminar on Primary Health Care, Havana, November 14–18, 1988.

93. Ministerio de Salud Pública, *Informe anual 1989,* 127.

94. Interview with Osvaldo Castro Miranda, June 13, 1991; and Ministerio de Salud Pública, *Evaluación estrategias de salud,* 6.

95. Ministerio de Salud Pública, *Informe anual 1989,* 107.

96. *Granma Weekly Review,* October 27, 1985, 8–9; and UNICEF et al., *El programa del médico de la familia,* 36.

97. *Granma Weekly Review,* October 27, 1985, 8–9.

98. Ministerio de Salud Pública, *Programa de trabajo del médico de la familia,* 8–22.

99. UNICEF et al., *El programa del médico de la familia,* 31.

100. *Granma Weekly Review,* March 24, 1991, 5.

101. Interview with William Domínguez, provincial health director, Guantánamo province, Baracoa, November 28, 1988.

102. The Central Planning Board of Cuba calculated costs for building and equipping a family doctor's office in 1989 as 45,400 pesos (35,000 pesos

for construction and 10,400 pesos for equipment) and operating expenses per year at 6,528 pesos. Both initial investment and operating expenses are low, particularly when compared with those of hospitals. See UNICEF, et al., *El plan del médico de la familia,* 36.

103. Personal communication from George A. Silver, Professor Emeritus of Public Health at the Yale School of Medicine, March 27, 1984; and interview with Richard Cash, director of international health, Harvard Institute of International Development, and professor, Harvard School of Public Health, September 24, 1984.

104. Interviews with doctors from a number of Latin American countries and Spain, 1988, 1990, and 1991, and personal communications from Jorge Castellanos Robayo, regional adviser on health administration and health care, Pan American Health Organization, January 19, 1988. This is not only the Cuban opinion, but also that of those physicians from Latin America who have visited Cuba in recent years.

105. Organización Panamericana de la Salud, *Informe sobre medicina familiar* (Washington, D.C.: OPS, April 1984).

106. Ministerio de Salud Pública, *Evaluación estrategias de salud para todos,* 6.

107. Official pronouncements by and informal discussions with a variety of health officials from the hemisphere, international organizations, Canada, Scandinavia, and the former socialist bloc at the 2nd International Seminar on Primary Health Care, Havana, November 14–18, 1988.

108. Ministerio de Salud Pública, *Programas básicos.*

109. Navarro, "Health, Health Services, and Health Planning," 409.

110. Ministerio de Salud Pública, *Programas básicos,* 79.

111. Ibid., 79–85. In 1987 the national average number of prenatal care visits per pregnancy was 14.6, and 99.4 percent of childbirth took place in hospitals. Ministerio de Salud Pública, *Informe anual 1987* (La Habana: MINSAP, 1988), 79 and 105.

112. In 1979 the norm was 11 prenatal consultations; by 1984 it had risen to 12, and by 1989 to 15.1. Raúl Riverón Corteguera, José A. Gutiérrez Muñiz, and Francisco Valdés Lazo, "Mortalidad infantíl en Cuba, en el decenio 1970–1979," *Boletín de la Oficina Sanitaria Panamericana* 92, no. 5 (May 1982): 385; *Granma Weekly Review,* November 25, 1984, 3; Ministerio de Salud Pública, *Informe anual 1989,* 109.

113. Dirección Provincial de Salud, Organo del Poder Popular Ciudad de La Habana, Dpto. Provincial Educación para la Salud, Dpto. de Nutrición, *Nutrición* (La Habana: OPP, 1980) (mimeographed).

114. *Granma Weekly Review,* November 4, 1984, supplement, 3.

115. Interview with Lorenzo Heredia del Portal, director of the Centro de Inmunoensayos (Immunoassay Center), Havana, November 25, 1988.

116. Interview with Daniel Joly, Pan American Health Organization regional representative in Cuba, 1974–1981, Havana, October 18, 1980; and David Werner, "Health Care in Cuba Today: A Model Service or a Means of Social Control—or Both?" Unpublished manuscript, n.d. [probably late 1978 or early 1979], 27.

117. The length of stay is determined by the patient's need and can be months rather than weeks. Interview with Otto Machado, June 14, 1991. The number of these homes has increased dramatically from 22 in 1970, to 61 in 1975, to 67 in 1980, to 135 in 1987. Ministerio de Salud Pública, *Informe anual 1987,* 74.

118. Before returning to their homes, they may pass through the maternity home again briefly, but this is not the rule. Interviews with the nurses and patients at the Hogar Materno Provincial, Santiago de Cuba, April 7, 1981; and Hogar Materno Municipal, Baracoa, Guantánamo province, November 28, 1988.

119. There were 6701 (0.3 percent) housing units that did not fit any category, and these were probably very substandard housing. Comité Estatal de Estadísticas, Dirección de Demografía, *Encuesta demográfica nacional de 1979: Metodología y tablas seleccionadas. Parte 1* (La Habana: CEE, April 1981), p. 231, table 17.

120. Kosta Mathéy, "Recent Trends in Cuban Housing Policies and the Revival of the Microbrigade Movement," *Bulletin of Latin American Research* 8, no. 1 (1989): 68.

121. Personal observation and communication, Juan Antonio Blanco, Vedado resident, La Habana, 1980. Also see *New York Times,* June 23, 1985, p. 8.

122. Interview with Daniel Joly, October 18, 1980; and participant observation, 1990–1992.

123. José Gutiérrez Muñiz et al., "The Recent Worldwide Economic Crisis and the Welfare of Children: The Case of Cuba," *World Development* 12, no. 3 (March 1984): 247–260. See particularly p. 252. Discussions of the value of human capital investment appear in numerous World Bank Staff working papers, among them, Odin K. Knudsen, *Economics of Supplemental Feeding of Malnourished Children: Leakages, Costs, and Benefits,* World Bank Staff working paper no. 451 (Washington, D.C.: World Bank, April 1981); and Marcelo Selowsky, *Nutrition, Health, and Education: The Economic Significance of Complementarities at Early Age,* World Bank reprint series no. 218 (Washington, D.C.: World Bank, 1981).

124. Interview with Rogelio Rojas Requena, February 26, 1981.

125. Interview with William Domínguez, November 28, 1988.

126. Personal observation, Hospital Docente Octavio de la Concepción y de la Pedraja in Baracoa, Guantánamo province, November 28, 1988.

127. Interview with the pediatrician at the Policlínico Punta Brava, in La Lisa municipality, province of the City of Havana, March 4, 1981; and with the director of the Policlínico Comunitario Docente de Holguín, city and province of Holguín, April 2, 1981.

128. The ideal in the United States, but not the enforced norm as in Cuba, is also seven well-baby visits the first year, three the second, and one thereafter until about the age of six, after which there should be one visit every other year.

129. Personal observation of neonatal home visits by a pediatric medical team (pediatrician and pediatric nurse) from the Policlínico Elpidio Bero-

vides in San Augustín, La Lisa municipality, City of Havana province, March 12, 1981. In all cases, the physician examined the infants, discussed with the mother the baby's feeding habits and the proper diet to be followed, and inspected the premises for general hygiene and for the presence of vectors.

130. *Granma Weekly Review,* November 25, 1984, 3; and "Maternal-Infant Care in Cuba," 4.

131. Ministerio de Salud Pública, *Informe anual 1987,* 83.

132. Ministerio de Salud Pública, *Informe anual 1989* (La Habana: MIN-SAP, 1990), 90, 113.

133. Interview with Dr. Maria de los Angeles Batista, November 27, 1988; and the municipal director of health for Baracoa, Juan G. Capetillo, at the family doctor's office in Cagüeibaje, November 27, 1988.

134. Ministerio de Salud Pública, *Programas básicos,* 98–99.

135. Ministerio de Salud Pública, *Informe anual 1989,* 112–13.

136. Personal observations of a pediatric health team, Ricardo Cassván and Fiora Grisolía, making home and day-care center visits in the San Augustín neighborhood of La Lisa municipality, City of Havana province, March 12, 1981.

137. Ministerio de Salud Pública, *Informe anual 1987,* 87.

138. Ministerio de Salud Pública, *Informe anual 1989,* 117.

139. Interview with the pediatrician at the Policlínico Punta Brava, March 4, 1981.

140. Interview with Ricardo Cassván, Policlínico Elpidio Berovides in San Augustín, La Lisa municipality, province of the City of Havana, March 12, 1981.

141. According to James P. Grant, executive director of UNICEF, "The Cuban government and Fidel personally consider children's health as one of the country's most important matters." Quoted in *Granma Weekly Review,* November 25, 1984, 4.

142. For example, the president of the Cuban Planning Board, Humberto Pérez, in a speech on behalf of the Council of Ministers noted under achievements that "visits to the doctor per inhabitant were up 6.3 percent." See *Granma Weekly Review,* January 13, 1985, supplement, 13.

143. Ministerio de Salud Pública y Organización Panamericana de la Salud, *Informe final sobre la evaluación del programa ampliado de inmunización. República de Cuba,* OPS report PAI/81/002 (Washington, D.C.: Organización Panamericana Sanitaria, 1981). See anexo III, pp. 3–5 for a discussion of Cuba's success and pp. 21–23 for morbidity rates for the six vaccine-preventable diseases for the period 1959–1980.

144. Ibid., 26.

145. Interview with Mercedes Torres, Ministerio de Salud Pública, Dirección Nacional de Educación para la Salud, Havana, June 21, 1991.

146. Ministerio de Salud Pública, *Programas básicos,* 83.

147. Interview with Ciro de Quadros, director of the Expanded Program on Immunization in the Americas (Programa Ampliado de Inmunizaciones), Pan American Health Organization, Washington, D.C., April 12, 1984.

148. Ministerio de Salud Pública, *Informe anual 1989,* 75.

149. Ibid., 76, 77.

150. *Granma Weekly Review,* November 11, 1990, 3.

151. Organización Panamericana de la Salud, Programa Ampliado de Inmunización, *PAI Boletín Informativo* año II, número 6 (December 1980), 5; and año III, número 5 (October 1981), 5; and Pan American Health Organization, *Health Conditions in the Americas* (1990), Scientific Publication no. 524 (Washington, D.C.: Pan American Health Organization, 1990), 1, 81.

152. Chile's National Health Service began in 1952. See *Medicina Social en Chile,* ed. Jorge Jiménez de la Jara (Santiago de Chile: Ediciones Aconcagua, 1977), 90. Costa Rica's social insurance scheme providing health care began in 1941. A constitutional amendment passed in 1961 stipulated universal coverage by 1970. However, 1979 data indicate that coverage reached only 77 percent of the total population. See Carmelo Mesa-Lago, "Financing Health Care in Latin America and the Caribbean With a Special Study of Costa Rica," World Bank Population, Health and Nutrition Department, unpublished manuscript, March 1983, 54, 59.

153. Pan American Health Organization, *Health Conditions 1990,* 1, 79.

154. *New York Times,* July 10, 1991, A18.

155. Interview with Ramón Casanova, director of the Cardiocentro William Soler (Pediatric Cardiovascular Surgery Center), Havana, December 1, 1988.

156. "Maternal-Infant Care in Cuba," 7, 5.

157. Observation of home visits by an internal medicine team in Julio Antonio Mella neighborhood, sector 2, Policlínico Comunitario Docente Monte Carlo, city and province of Camagüey, April 10, 1981; and interviews with the director of the Policlínico Segundo Frente in Mayarí Arriba, Sierra Maestra, province of Santiago de Cuba, March 1980; and the director of the Policlínico Punta Brava, La Lisa municipality, province of the City of Havana, March 4, 1981.

158. Interview with Ana Teresa Farina, director of the Policlínico Elpidio Berovides, La Lisa municipality, province of the City of Havana, March 6, 1981. See also Ministerio de Salud Pública, *Programas básicos,* 117–21.

159. Interview with the director of Policlínico Punta Brava, March 4, 1981.

160. Ministerio de Salud Pública, *Informe anual 1989,* 91, 94, 96.

161. Ministerio de Salud Pública, *Informe anual 1991* (La Habana: MINSAP, 1992), 92.

162. *Informe del Gobierno de Cuba a la Organización Panamericana de la Salud sobre las condiciones de salud pública y los adelantos logrados en el intervalo transcurrido entre la XXI y XXII Conferencias Sanitarias Panamericanas. 1982–1986* (Washington, D.C.: Organización Panamericana Sanitaria, September 1986), 2; *Granma Weekly Review,* June 6, 1982, 4; September 16, 1984, 12; August 24, 1986, 3; October 26, 1986, 5; January 18, 1987, 3; May 10, 1987, 12; May 24, 1987, 3; March 31, 1991, 6; and May 12, 1991, 2; and *Granma,* January 4, 1986, 2; and December 30, 1986, 3.

163. *Granma,* July 30, 1986, 1; *Granma,* January 4, 1986; *Granma Weekly Review,* May 10, 1987, 12; *ABC News* (New Haven), March 8, 1986.

164. *Granma Weekly Review,* December 9, 1990, 3, and March 31, 1991, 6.

165. *National Public Radio News* (Middlefield, Conn.), July 6, 1987; and *Granma Weekly Review,* April 13, 1986, 3.

166. *Granma Weekly Review,* November 11, 1990, 3.

167. Personal communication from an Honduran pediatrician (who would like to remain anonymous because of political violence against physicians in his country), Havana, November 30, 1988.

168. See Pan American Health Organization, *Health Conditions 1990,* 1, 114–15 for the techniques. Richard S. Bierstock, an ophthalmological surgeon, assessed the techniques based on the information given in *Health Conditions.* Interview with Richard Bierstock, Rhinebeck, New York, January 15, 1991.

169. *Granma Weekly Review,* March 31, 1991, 6.

170. *Granma Weekly Review,* December 16, 1990, 3.

171. Interview with Eduardo Joly, a sociologist with expertise in rehabilitation and a frequent observer of work at the Frank País Orthopedic Hospital, Havana, June 22, 1991 and data from Department of Neurosurgery, Cleveland Hospital, April 26, 1993.

172. Interview with Daniel Joly, July 7, 1979; and discussions with Eduardo Joly, in Havana in 1978, 1979, 1980, and June 22, 1991, and in New York in 1985.

173. *Granma Weekly Review,* May 5, 1991, 3.

174. Personal observation in various cities throughout Cuba, 1980–1981, 1988, and 1991.

175. Interview with Dr. Rolando Villafuerte, head of the burn unit staff at the Hospital Clínico-Quirúrgico Provincial Abel Santamaria, Pinar del Río, June 18, 1991.

176. Interview with Zenobio González León, chief of public and international relations at the Hospital Hermanos Ameijeiras, Havana, November 30, 1988.

177. Ibid.

178. César Vieira, "PAHO/WHO Interoffice Memorandum HSP/84/242/88, 6 de abril de 1988," (Washington, D.C.: PAHO, 1988), 5 (typescript).

179. *Granma Weekly Review,* July 7, 1991, 8.

Chapter 3

1. Cubans identify with the struggle of Third World peoples, although they compare themselves with their Miami relatives. This view is confirmed by personal observations and discussions with many Cubans of all walks of life from 1978 through 1992.

2. Ledo Duarte, "Participación popular en salud," 224–25.

3. Ministerio de Salud Pública, *Programas básicos,* 120.

4. Personal observation of medical education dealing with the elderly and with the parents of newborns and imparted by physician and nurse teams meeting with patients in their homes. Policlínico Comunitario Docente Monte Carlo, city and province of Camagüey, April 10, 1981; and San Augustín, La Lisa, province of the City of Havana, March 12, 1981.

5. Interview with Dr. Maria de los Angeles Batista Peña, Cagüeibaje, and Palma Clara, November 27, 1988.

6. Interview with the director of the Policlínico Comunitario Docente de Holguín, April 2, 1981; and Ministerio de Salud Pública, Dirección de Educación para la Salud, *Temas populares de salud* (La Habana: MINSAP, 1976).

7. Interviews with the director of the Policlínico Comunitario Docente de Holguín, April 2, 1981, and the director of the Policlínico Punta Brava, March 4, 1981.

8. Interview with the director of the Policlínico Punta Brava, March 4, 1981.

9. As one polyclinic physician put it, the mass organizations' health liaisons help the polyclinic pursue patients until they are vaccinated. The Spanish word *perseguir* means to pursue as well as to persecute. Although there was no indication of persecution, one could speculate that being hounded by one's health liaison is both, despite the fact that it is for one's own good as well as that of the society as a whole. Interview with Ricardo Cassván, March 12, 1981.

10. Interview with Ana Teresa Farina, March 6, 1981.

11. Interview with Mercedes Torres, June 21, 1991; and Ministerio de Salud Pública, *Programa de trabajo del médico y enfermera*, 17.

12. Ibid.; and interview with the director of the Policlínico Comunitario Docente de Holguín, April 2, 1981.

13. Interview with Mercedes Torres, June 21, 1991, and population figures from Ministerio de Salud Pública, *Informe anual 1989*, 18.

14. Interview with Ana Teresa Farina, March 6, 1981.

15. Ibid.

16. Remarks by Victor Mironenko, head of the Komsomol (Communist Youth Organization), as reported in *Wall Street Journal*, August 18, 1987, 27.

17. Ministerio de Salud Pública, *Programa del trabajo del médico y enfermera de la familia*, 16.

18. Interview with Lázara Madem, director of the Clínica Estomatológica Elpidio Berovides, municipality of La Lisa, City of Havana province, March 11, 1981.

19. Psychoprophylaxis is the Soviet term for psychological preparation for pregnancy and childbirth, prenatal exercises (popularized by Lamaze in the West), and child-care education.

20. Physician and nurse teams from each health sector took turns at giving the lectures. Interview with the director of the Policlínico Comunitario Docente de Holguín, April 2, 1981.

21. Interview with Manlio López Pérez, director of the Policlínico Comunitario Docente Monte Carlo, Camagüey, April 10, 1981. See also Galaz Góngora, et al., "Análisis de las actividades," 14; and Ramírez López et al., "Conocimiento de una comunidad," 7.

22. Ministerio de Salud Pública, *Temas populares de salud.*

23. Interview with Mercedes Torres, June 20, 1991.

24. Observations during field research in Cuba, 1980–1981.

25. Interview with Lázara Madem, March 11, 1981.

26. Observation of several of the videos and interview with Manuel Peña Escobar, Pan American Health Organization consultant, Havana, December 1, 1988.

27. Observation of television programs in Havana, November 1988; January and March 1990; June 1991.

28. Interview with Reinaldo Gil, Viceministerio de Higiene y Epidemiología (AIDS), MINSAP, Havana, June 12, 1991.

29. *Bohemia,* Año 75, No. 5 (February 4, 1983), inside front cover and p. 36; Año 75 No. 6 (February 11, 1983), inside front cover; Año 75, No. 8 (February 25, 1983), inside front cover; and Año 76, No. 3 (January 20, 1984), inside front cover.

30. U.S. Senate, Committee on Labor and Public Welfare, Special Subcommittee on the National Science Foundation, *Chemical and Biological Weapons: Some Possible Approaches for Lessening the Threat and Danger* (Washington, D.C.: U.S. Government Printing Office, May 1969). For the symptoms of dengue see David M. Morens, John P. Woodall, and Raúl H. López-Correa, "Dengue in American Children of the Caribbean," *Journal of Pediatrics* 93, No. 6 (December 1978): 1049–50.

31. Personal observation of billboards, particularly in Camagüey province in 1981, depicting the need for greater physical activity. Also, interview with Daniel Joly, October 27, 1982. See Medea Benjamin, Joseph Collins, and Michael Scott, *No Free Lunch: Food and Revolution in Cuba Today* (San Francisco: Food First Books, 1984), 117.

32. Personal observation, November 1988.

33. Observation of judo lessons on the beach at Santa María del Mar, province of City of Havana, July 1979.

34. "La participación activa de la comunidad en Cuba," presentation at 2nd International Seminar on Primary Health Care, Havana, November 14–18, 1988. The one-hundred-year-old exercise leader stood and delivered a brief statement from the audience. Also, film on Grandparents' Clubs by Estela Bravo and personal observation of various daily exercise sessions in the Vedado district of Havana, January and March 1990.

35. *Granma,* November 18, 1988, 1.

36. Personal observations, 1978, 1979, 1980–1981, and 1988. And interview with Daniel Joly, October 27, 1982.

37. Ibid; Benjamin, Collins, and Scott, *No Free Lunch,* 117.

38. Ministerio de Salud Pública, *Para tu salud, corre o camina, Educación para tu salud* (Havana: Editorial Científico-Técnica, 1983), 14 quoted in Benjamin, Collins, and Scott, *No Free Lunch,* 117.

39. Television and print ads and interview with Eugenio R. Balari, president of ICIODI, Havana, November 24, 1988.

40. According to Daniel Joly, Cubans must eat a huge amount of rice three times a day to feel that they have eaten enough. Interview in Washington, D.C., October 27, 1982.

41. Agrupación Católica Universitaria, "Encuesta de los trabajadores rurales," 188–213.

42. Participant observation, 1978, 1979, 1980, 1981, 1988, and 1990. See also Benjamin, Collins, and Scott, *No Free Lunch,* 108; and Howard Handelman, "Cuban Food Policy and Popular Nutritional Levels," *Cuban Studies/ Estudios Cubanos* 11, no. 2/12, no. 1 (July 1981–January 1982): 142–3.

43. Interview with Ricardo Cassván, March 12, 1981.

44. Personal observations 1978, 1979, 1980–1981.

45. Participant observation at the workers' cafeteria at the Institute for Health Development, Havana, 1980–1981.

46. Ministerio de Salud Pública, Viceministerio de Higiene y Epidemiología, *Cuba: situación nutricional 1991.* (La Habana: Comité Estatal de Estadísticas, 1991), 10 (typescript).

47. Interview with Delia Placencia, Dirección de Nutrición, Viceministerio de Higiene y Epidemiología, MINSAP, Havana, June 13, 1991.

48. Handelman, "Cuban Food Policy," 143.

49. Benjamin, Collins, and Scott, *No Free Lunch,* 117. Cites a 1979 survey conducted by the Cuban Institute for Consumer Orientation and Internal Demand.

50. Quoted in Benjamin, Collins, and Scott, *No Free Lunch,* 117–18.

51. Ibid., 118.

52. Data provided at meeting of the Consejo de Dirección (executive committee) of *Opina* magazine to discuss the launching of the antismoking campaign, ICIODI, March 27, 1981. Interestingly, two members of the executive committee opposed having the mass organizations, particularly the CDRs, involved in the campaign, since they claimed that not all mass organizations would handle it correctly, and that the CDRs limit people's privacy. The latter statement is remarkable because although everyone knows this to be the case, it is not generally acknowledged officially.

53. Benjamin, Collins, and Scott, *No Free Lunch,* 32–33.

54. *Granma Weekly Review,* April 26, 1987, 12.

55. *Granma Weekly Review,* October 26, 1986, 5.

56. *Granma Weekly Review,* August 24, 1986, 3. Unfortunately, there were no data as to the magnitude of the increase in female smokers.

57. *Granma Weekly Review,* April 26, 1987, 12.

58. Nery Suárez Lugo (coordinator of the antismoking campaign), untitled draft internal report of ICIODI (La Habana: ICIODI, June 1991), table 10, p. 9.

59. Ibid.

60. Ibid., table 6, p. 7.

61. Nery Suárez Lugo, "Actividades antitabáquicas en Cuba" (La Habana: ICIODI para la Segunda Reunión de Intercambio de Experiencias, Campaña para Desestimular el Hábito de Fumar, November 1988), 3–4 (mimeographed).

62. Ibid, 19–21. As early as 1978, smoking was prohibited in the Policlínico Comunitario Docente in Holguín. Interview with the director, April 2, 1981.

63. Nery Suárez Lugo, "Actividades antitabáquicas," 19–20.

64. Interview with Nery Suárez Lugo, Havana, June 20, 1991.

65. Observation of a representative sample of these announcements on videotape at the office of Eugenio R. Balari, president of ICIODI, November 24, 1988.

66. According to Eugenio R. Balari, Sweden registered a 12 percent reduction after five years of its campaign, Finland had a 20 percent decline after eight years, and the U.S. had a 30 percent decrease in thirteen years. "Una campaña paradójica: el mejor productor de tabaco del mundo contra el hábito de fumar: entrevista con el Dr. Eugenio R. Balari por Gabriel Molina," La Habana: ICIODI pamphlet reprinted from *Opina* no. 94, February 1987, 1, 15–16.

67. *Granma Weekly Review,* October 26, 1986, 5.

68. Interview with Nery Suárez Lugo, June 20, 1991.

69. *Granma Weekly Review,* April 26, 1987, 12.

70. Interview with Nery Suárez Lugo, June 20, 1991.

71. Ibid.

72. Pan American Health Organization, *Community Participation in Health and Development in the Americas: An Analysis of Selected Case Studies.* (Washington, D.C.: PAHO Scientific Publication no. 473, 1984), ix, xi.

73. Ibid., 1–25 passim.

74. Ibid., 43–44.

75. Ledo Duarte, "Participación popular en salud," 221; and interviews with the directors of the following polyclinics: Policlínico del Segundo Frente, Mayarí Arriba (Sierra Maestra), province of Santiago de Cuba, March 1980; Policlínico Comunitario Docente de Holguín, April 2, 1981; Policlínico de Cruces, city of Cruces, Cienfuegos province, April 14, 1981; Policlínico Punta Brava, La Lisa, March 4, 1981; and Policlínico Elpidio Berovides, San Augustín, La Lisa, March 6, 1981, and March 12, 1981.

76. Interview with Cosme Ordóñez Carceller, December 28, 1978; and public discussion at the 2nd International Seminar on Primary Health Care, Havana, November 14–18, 1988.

77. Estela Ramírez López et al., "Conocimiento de una comunidad urbana a través del Policlínico Comunitario Docente, 8–9; Septimio González et al., "Descripción y análisis del sistema de atención primaria en el Policlínico Integral Docente 'Plaza de la Revolución,'" La Habana: Instituto de Desarrollo de la Salud, práctica-docente en la asignatura de Administración de Servicios de Salud, December 1978, 17; Robna R. Galaz Góngora et al., "Análisis de las actividades del Policlínico Integral Docente," 13; Interview with Cosme Ordóñez Carceller, Havana, December 28, 1978. In this interview Ordóñez Carceller stated that he made the decisions in the People's Health Commission but would prefer to have "active, informed, critical collaboration" from the mass organization representatives.

78. Escalona Reguera, *La participación popular en la salud,* 62.

79. Ministerio de Salud Pública. Dirección Municipal La Lisa. Cuidad La Habana. "Calendario y plan de trabajo del Director Municipal de Salud La Lisa." February 1981. La Habana: 4 (mimeographed).

80. Ministerio de Salud Pública y Organización Panamericana de la Salud, *Informe final sobre la evaluación.*

81. Ministerio de Salud Pública, *Programas básicos,* 171–77.

82. On duration of marriages see Comité Estatal de Estadísticas, *Anuario estadístico de Cuba 1988,* 78.

83. "Entire Cuban Population to Be Tested for AIDS, Official Says," *Cuba Update* 8, nos. 5–6 (Winter 1987): 10.

84. See *Granma Weekly Review,* January 31, 1988, 3.

85. *New York Times,* February 19, 1989, 4.

86. *Granma Weekly Review,* June 15, 1990, 3; and June 16, 1991, 6.

87. Interview with Reinaldo Gil, June 12, 1991.

88. Observation of a sanatorium, March 21, 1993; interviews with seven patients, March 21 1993; interview with Karen Wald, Havana, January 20, 1990; *New York Times,* February 6, 1989, 18; and *New York Times,* February 11, 1988, 25.

89. Interview with AIDS patients, Havana, January 8, 1990.

90. Interview with Reinaldo Gil, June 12, 1991.

91. Discussions with various health officials at the 2nd International Seminar on Primary Health Care, Havana, November 14–18, 1988.

92. Interview with Reinaldo Gil, June 12, 1991.

93. Observation of interviews with a cross section of the population on various television programs about AIDS aired in Havana in January and March 1990.

94. Sociedad Científica Cubana para el Desarrollo de la Familia (SOCU-DEF), *¿Qué es el SIDA?* La Habana: MINSAP Educación para la Salud, n.d. (obtained in November 1988).

95. Interview with Reinaldo Gil, June 12, 1991.

96. *Granma,* July 29, 1981, 3–4.

97. *Granma Weekly Review,* November 18, 1984, 2.

98. See inter alia, U.S. Congress, House Committee on Foreign Affairs, *Chemical-Biological Warfare: U.S. Policies and International Effects. Hearings before the Subcommittee on National Security Policy and Scientific Developments.* 91st Cong., 1st sess., November 18, 20; December 2, 9, 18, and 19, 1969; Robin Clarke, *The Silent Weapons* (New York: David McKay, 1968), 118; and Seymour Hersh, *Chemical and Biological Warfare: America's Hidden Arsenal* (Indianapolis: Bobbs-Merrill, 1968), 73.

99. *New York Times,* September 6, 1981, 5.

100. *Granma,* July 7, 1981, 1.

101. *Granma,* July 4, 1981, 3.

102. The farmers participated if the health area contained rural zones and the student organizations if there were student residences in the zone.

103. *Granma,* July 16, 1981, 3.

104. *Granma,* July 15, 1981, 2.

105. Cuba has a program called the "accompanying mother" (*madre acompañante*), in which the mothers of hospitalized children aid the nursing staff in the care of their children, and by their presence decrease the psychological trauma of hospitalization. See Manuel Alvarez Alonso et al., "Impor-

tancia de la madre acompañante en pacientes hospitalizados," *Revista cubana de pediatría* 54, no. 5 (September–October, 1982): 622–34. By the mid 1980s, there was also a program for the "accompanying father."

106. *Granma,* July 15, 1981, p. 1.

107. *Granma,* July 20, 1981, p. 3.

108. *Granma,* July 4, 1981, 3; July 6, 1981, 3; July 7, 1981, 1.

109. *Granma,* August 3, 1981, p. 1.

110. Personal observation, Habana Vieja, November 30, 1988.

111. *Granma Weekly Review,* November 18, 1984, 2.

112. *Granma,* August 3, 1981, 1.

113. According to Daniel Joly, the Cubans did an excellent job of handling the dengue epidemic, following the recommendations of PAHO. They overdid some things, such as the attempt to institutionalize every case, but the eradication campaign was very well executed, and care of those with complications was also superb. Interview on October 27, 1982.

114. See Emile Durkheim, *The Elementary Forms of Religious Life* (New York: The Free Press, 1954).

115. Interviews with Cubans, primarily in Havana, 1980–1981. The scars were clearly visible. One high school student mentioned that although she was a militant in the communist youth (UJC) and participated in denunciations of Marielitos and in the march of the *pueblo combatiente* (combative people), she did so only to avoid jeopardizing her admission to the university. Two of her brothers were Marielitos, and she could hardly discuss the issue without tears coming to her eyes.

116. Fagen, *Transformation of Political Culture,* 149–50.

Chapter 4

1. Halfdan Mahler, "Discurso pronunciado en la sesión inaugural de la conferencia 'Salud Para Todos': 25 años de experiencia cubana," La Habana, Cuba, July 3–9, 1983; Carlyle Guerra de Macedo, "Discurso pronunciado en la sesión inaugural de la conferencia 'Salud Para Todos'" (La Habana, Cuba, July 3–9, 1983). See articles in *Medical Tribune* 29, no. 27 (September 1988): 2, 22; *The Physiologist* 22, no. 1 (February 1979): 9–11, and 22, no. 6 (December 1979): 15–17; *Nursing Mirror* (Surrey, England) 153, no. 20 (November 11, 1981): 36–38; *Journal of the Medical Association of Georgia* 68 (February 1979): 99–100; *Pediatric Nursing* 6, no. 5 (September/October 1980): 51–53; *Science* 200, no. 4347 (June 16, 1978): 1246–49; *Western Journal of Medicine* 132 (March 1980): 265–71; *Obstetrics and Gynecology* 49, no. 6 (June 1977): 709–14; and the *Canadian Medical Association Journal* 111 (November 2, 1974): 991–1002, among others.

2. U.S. Congress. Joint Economic Committee. *Cuba Faces the Economic Realities of the 1980s,* by Lawrence Theriot. 97th Cong., 2nd sess. (Washington, D.C.: U.S. Government Printing Office, March 22, 1982), 5.

3. Sergio Díaz-Briquets, *The Health Revolution in Cuba* (Austin, Tex.: University of Texas Press, 1983), 113.

4. See Danielson, *Cuban Medicine;* Agrupación Católica Universitaria, "Encuesta de trabajadores rurales," 188–213; Pan American Sanitary Bureau, *Summary of Four-Year Reports on Health Conditions in the Americas, 1953–1956.* Scientific Publication no. 40. (Washington, D.C.: PSB, June 1958); Pan American Health Organization, *Health Conditions in the Americas, 1957–1960,* Scientific Publication no. 64 (Washington, D.C.: PAHO, 1962); Díaz-Briquets, *The Health Revolution in Cuba;* and Sergio Díaz-Briquets and Lisandro Pérez, "Cuba: The Demography of Revolution," *Population Bulletin* 36, no. 1 (April 1981): 5–6.

5. *Granma Weekly Review,* supplement, February 24, 1985, 3.

6. *Granma Weekly Review,* March 11, 1984, 4.

7. Ruth Leger Sivard, *World Military and Social Expenditures 1985* (Washington, D.C.: World Priorities, 1985), 39.

8. The data used in these comparisons are not always for the year stated but may be for any year close to that date for which comparable data are available. Ruth Leger Sivard, *World Military and Social Expenditures 1989* (Washington, D.C.: World Priorities, 1989), 51.

9. Disaggregation of U.S. data indicates an infant mortality rate for blacks of almost twice the national rate. U.S. Bureau of the Census, *Statistical Abstract of the United States, 1990* (110th edition), Washington, D.C.: U.S. Government Printing Office, 1990, p. 78, table 113; Ministerio de Salud Pública, *Informe anual 1990,* 33; and *Granma Weekly Review,* supplement, February 24, 1985, 3.

10. *Granma Weekly Review,* supplement, February 16, 1986, 4.

11. "Rise in Infant Mortality Rate," *Cuba Update,* 7, nos. 1–2 (Winter–Spring 1986): 7.

12. Ministerio de Salud Pública, *Informe anual 1989,* 33; and *Granma Weekly Review,* January 20, 1991, 4.

13. U.S. Dept. of Commerce, Bureau of the Census, *Statistical Abstract of the United States, 1987* (Washington, D.C.: U.S. Government Printing Office, 1986), 58; and *Statistical Abstract of the United States, 1990* (110th edition), p. 62; table 80, and p. 78, table 113; World Health Organization, *World Health Statistics Annual 1987* (Geneva: WHO, 1987), 80; and personal communication from Linda Washington of the National Center for Health Statistics, January 16, 1991.

14. Pan American Health Organization, *Health Conditions in the Americas* (1990 edition). Vol. 2 (Washington, D.C.: PAHO scientific publication no. 524, 1990), 57.

15. *Granma Weekly Review,* January 25, 1987, 4.

16. Sivard, *World Military and Social Expenditures, 1985,* 39, 41.

17. National Center for Health Statistics, *Vital Statistics of the United States, 1982.* Vol. 2, sec. 6, life tables. DHHS publication no. (PHS) 85-1104. Public Health Services (Washington, D.C.: U.S. Government Printing Office, 1985), 6; *New York Times,* March 23, 1985, p. 8; U.S. Department of Com-

merce, *Statistical Abstracts 1990,* p. 72, table 103; *Granma Weekly Review,* February 16, 1986, supplement, 4.

18. Ministerio de Salud Pública, *Informe anual 1989,* 23; Ministerio de Salud Pública, *Evaluación estrategias de salud para todos,* 26; and U.S. Bureau of the Census, *Statistical Abstract 1990,* p. 72, table 103.

19. Ministerio de Salud Pública, *Informe anual 1982* (La Habana: MINSAP, 1983); and National Center for Health Statistics, *Vital Statistics 1982.*

20. Pan American Health Organization, *Health Conditions* (1990), 1: 423, 428, 432, 435.

21. Sivard, *World Military and Social Expenditures 1985,* 35–36; and *World Military and Social Expenditures 1989,* 51.

22. Paul Streeten, "Basic Needs: Some Unsettled Questions," *World Development* 12, no. 9 (September 1984): 977.

23. Gordon Hatcher, Peter R. Hatcher, and Eleanor C. Hatcher, "Health Services in Canada," in *Comparative Health Systems: Descriptive Analyses of Fourteen National Health Systems,* ed. Marshall W. Raffel (University Park, Pa.: Pennsylvania State University Press, 1984), 90.

24. There are still some doctors in private practice in Cuba, but all are on the verge of retirement, and no new M.D.'s have been allowed to go into private practice since 1964. The 1981 census indicates that there were 178 self-employed medical workers; there was no disaggregation of data to indicate how many were physicians, although it is likely that all were. Even if all were doctors, the 178 would represent only 0.008 percent of the total physician pool in 1985. See Comité Estatal de Estadísticas, Oficina Nacional del Censo, *Censo de población y viviendas de 1981,* vol. 16, tomo 1 (La Habana: CEE, July 1983), 281.

25. Kenneth Hill, "An Evaluation of Cuban Demographic Statistics, 1938–1980," quoted in Paula E. Hollerbach and Sergio Díaz-Briquets, *Fertility Determinants in Cuba* (Washington, D.C.: National Academy Press, 1983); and Díaz-Briquets, "How To Figure Out Cuba," 10. See also Díaz-Briquets, *The Health Revolution in Cuba;* Santana, "Some Thoughts on Vital Statistics," 107–18; Carmelo Mesa-Lago, "Cuban Statistics Revisited," *Cuban Studies/ Estudios Cubanos* 9, no. 2 (July 1979): 61, and 10, no. 1 (January 1980): 99; Navarro, "Health, Health Services and Health Planning," 403. For a contrary view, see Nicholas Eberstadt, "Did Fidel Fudge the Figures? Literacy and Health: The Cuba Model," *Caribbean Review* 15, no. 2 (Spring 1986): 5–7, 37–38.

26. Interviews with Hans Bruch, October, 1982; and Myron Wegman, former assistant director of PAHO and dean emeritus of the University of Michigan School of Public Health, Ann Arbor, March 19, 1984.

27. Sarah Santana, "Some Thoughts on Vital Statistics and Health Status in Cuba," in *Cuban Political Economy: Controversies in Cubanology,* ed. Andrew Zimbalist (Boulder, Colo.: Westview Press, 1988), 107–18.

28. Because of negative trends, the Soviets stopped publishing statistics on infant mortality in 1974, life expectancy in 1971–1972, and a whole host of other statistics on mortality, resource distribution, and similar phenomena

in 1975 or earlier. See U.S. Congress, Joint Economic Committee, *Soviet Economy in the 1980s,* 205. For Cuban trends see Ministerio de Salud Pública, *Informe anual,* yearly. Some negative trends in the *Informe anual 1989* can be found on pp. 37, 52, 54, and 57; and in the *Informe anual 1991,* pp. 37, 53–55, and 79.

29. The only negative report was an erroneous analysis of data conducted by Nicholas Eberstadt of the American Enterprise Institute in "Did Fidel Fudge the Figures?" He argues that Cuban infant mortality data are always provisional and cites one instance of a change. Since corrections are made in most countries, this is not proof of doctoring the figures. The data are provisional for a year or two after the printing of the statistical reports but are rarely changed thereafter.

30. C. Arden Miller et al., "The World Economic Crisis and the Children: United States Case Study," *International Journal of Health Services* 15, no. 1 (1985): 95–134 (see especially pp. 123–32).

31. U.S. Bureau of the Census, *Statistical Abstract 1990,* p. 77, tables 110, 111.

32. Postneonatal mortality is generally associated with environmental factors such as poverty, although some argue that with the widespread availability of neonatal intensive care units, some infants who would have died in the first month are dying later during the first year. *New York Times,* January 4, 1986, 11; February 24, 1985, 1; and *International Herald Tribune,* January 18–19, 1986, 3.

33. U.S. Bureau of the Census, *Statistical Abstract 1990,* p. 66, table 87.

34. Ministerio de Salud Pública, *Informe anual 1989,* 109.

35. Ibid., 20.

36. Ministerio de Salud Pública, *Informe anual 1989,* 132.

37. *New York Times,* February 27, 1985, 8.

38. U.S. Congress, Joint Economic Committee, *Cuba Faces the Economic Realities of the 1980s,* 5.

39. Pan American Health Organization, *Health Conditions 1990,* 1:193.

40. Handleman, "Cuban Food Policy and Popular Nutritional Levels," 142.

41. Benjamin, Collins, and Scott, *No Free Lunch,* 99.

42. Pan American Health Organization, *Health Conditions in the Americas, 1977–1980* (Washington, D.C.: PAHO Scientific Publication no. 427, 1982), 102.

43. Pan American Health Organization, *Health Conditions 1990,* 1:187; and 2:112.

44. Pan American Health Organization, *Health Conditions 1977–1980,* 102, 243.

45. Pan American Health Organization, *Health Conditions 1990,* 1:393.

46. Personal observations in Cuba in 1978, 1979, 1980–1981, 1988, 1990, 1991, 1992. On how rationing works in Cuba, see Benjamin, Collins, and Scott, *No Free Lunch,* especially pp. 27–39.

47. Austerity measures enacted in late 1987 did not affect these programs. *Granma,* December 31, 1987, 1.

48. *Granma Weekly Review,* October 26, 1986, 3.

49. *Granma Weekly Review,* January 20, 1991, 4; and March 24, 1991, 5.

50. *Granma Weekly Review,* January 25, 1987, 4.

51. United Nations, *Living Conditions in Developing Countries in the Mid-1980s, supplement to the 1985 Report on the World Social Situation* (New York: United Nations, 1986), 11.

52. Interview with Ramón Casanova, December 1, 1988.

53. PAHO-sponsored international seminar lecture by Luis Heredero, provincial director of genetics, City of Havana, PAHO consultant, and president of the Latin American Genetics Association, November 22, 1988, Havana.

54. Personal observation of Home for Physically and Mentally Impaired Children, Santiago de Cuba, April 6, 1981.

55. Interviews with Roberto Capote Mir, a ranking Cuban physician and public health professor employed as a regional adviser for health systems and hospital administration at the Pan American Health Organization, Washington, D.C., April 21, 1987; Luis Heredero, provincial director of genetics for the City of Havana, November 22, 1988; and Lidia Rodríguez, municipal director of genetics for the City of Havana, November 22, 1988, Havana.

56. Ministry of Public Health, *Annual Report 1986,* 18; Ministerio de Salud Pública, *Informe anual 1989,* 90; *Evaluación estrategias de salud para todos,* 8; and *Granma Weekly Review,* September 9, 1990, 9.

57. This conservative estimate is based on a population projection using *Life Tables for Developing Countries* (the Latin American table) with ten million as the population baseline in 1985 and with the number of physicians in the year 2000 pegged at the conservative estimate of 65,000. A more optimistic calculation results in one physician for every 190 inhabitants by taking the number of physicians in 1984 (20,545) plus 50,000 that are to be trained by the year 2000, and subtracting the 3,267 physicians aged 45 or over in 1979. United Nations, Department of Economic and Social Affairs, Population Studies, *Model Life Tables for Developing Countries,* no. 77 (New York: United Nations, 1982); *Granma Weekly Review,* September 16, 1984, 3, and November 18, 1984, 3; and *Revista cubana de administración de salud* 8, no. 1 (January/March 1982):119.

58. Calculated from 247 M.D.'s per 100,000 population. U.S. Department of Health and Human Services, Public Health Service, Human Resources Administration, Office of Graduate Medical Education, *Report of the Graduate Medical Education National Advisory Committee to the Secretary, Department of Health and Human Services, Volume 2.* DHHS Publication No. (HRA) 81–652 (Washington, D.C.: U.S. Government Printing Office, 1981), vol. 2, p. 274, table V.3. This report is generally referred to as the GMENAC report.

59. *Granma Weekly Review,* July 24, 1983, 3.

60. *Granma Weekly Review,* May 13, 1984, 3.

61. *Granma,* July 30, 1986, 3. The dropout rate was close to 50 percent when the initial estimate was revised downward by 10,000 to a total of 65,000 M.D.'s by the year 2000. But since then the dropout rate has decreased. See *Granma Weekly Review,* September 20, 1987, 5; and interview with Francisco Rojas Ochoa, June 17, 1991.

62. Calculated on the basis that 50 percent of the population was served by 11,882 family doctors in September 1990, when 73.4 percent of the graduating class was incorporated into the program. There were 27,924 students enrolled in medical school in the 1989–1990 academic year and 24,629 in 1986–1987. If about 4,000 graduate per year (the term of study is six years) and 75 percent, or 3,000, become family doctors, then by the 1994 graduation (September) another 12,000 family doctors will enter the system for a total of about 23,900. If 11,882 doctors cover half of the population, then 23,900 should cover the whole population. If the total population of Cuba for 1989—estimated at 10.6 million—is divided by 23,900, the result is 443.5 inhabitants per family doctor, a figure considerably lower than that projected recently by the ministry as the population to be served (600–700) but only slightly lower than the initial projection of 500. The 1995 graduating class would add to the total, to account for those working in schools, factories, homes for the aged, ships, and day-care centers. Calculations made from data in Ministerio de Salud Pública, *Informe anual 1989,* 17, 152; *Informe anual 1987,* 110, 116; and *Granma Weekly Review,* November 18, 1984, 3; September 2, 1990, 9; and September 9, 1990, 9.

63. Ramírez, "El médico de la familia," 15; and interviews with Osvaldo Castro Miranda, June 13, 1991; and Francisco Rojas Ochoa, June 17, 1991.

64. Rodolfo Rodríguez, "Informe viaje a Cuba," PAHO/WHO Interoffice Memorandum HSI/84/2.1 (53/90), May 2, 1990, 2.

65. In theory the former Soviet Union and Czechoslovakia, as well as other former eastern bloc countries, provided sabbaticals for their physicians, but often there were insufficient numbers of physicians to allow them to grant the sabbaticals when due. Personal communication from George A. Silver, March 24, 1986.

66. Ministerio de Salud Pública, *Informe anual 1987,* 61, and *Informe anual 1989,* 102; and 1990 figures calculated from Ministerio de Salud Pública, Area de Docencia, "Recursos humanos en salud." La Habana: MINSAP, December 1990, 1 (typescript).

67. Pan American Health Organization, *Health Conditions in the Americas, 1981–1984* (Washington, D.C.: PAHO, 1986), 150, 153–54; and Ministerio de Salud Pública, *Informe anual 1987* (La Habana: MINSAP, 1988), 61.

68. Ministerio de Salud Pública, *Evaluación estrategias de salud para todos,* 8–10.

69. Ibid., 145, 151.

70. Ibid., 146, 152.

71. Juan Vela Váldes (rector del Instituto Superior de Ciencias Médicas de La Habana), untitled paper presented at the Conferencia Integrada Universidad Latinoamericana y Salud de la Población, La Habana, June 3–7, 1991, 25.

72. Data are only for the Instituto Superior de Ciencias Médicas de La Habana and may or may not be generalizable to the entire country. Interview with Dr. Francisco Rojas Ochoa, June 17, 1991.

73. Interview with Osvaldo Castro Miranda, June 13, 1991.

74. Interview with Francisco Rojas Ochoa, June 17, 1991.

75. Calculated from Ministerio de Salud Pública, Area de Docencia, "Recursos humanos," 1, 5.

76. Interview with Francisco Rojas Ochoa, June 17, 1991.

77. Quoted in "Una conquista: la salud," *Cuba Internacional,* no. 103 (May 1978): 35.

78. Castro, *2nd Period of Sessions of the National Assembly,* 39–41.

79. *Granma Weekly Review,* May 27, 1984, 4; and July 24, 1983, 3.

80. Calculated from Ministerio de Salud Pública, *Informe anual 1989,* 19, 90.

81. Calculated from Comité Estatal de Estadísticas, *Guía estadística 1985* (La Habana: CEE, 1986), 8; and Ministry of Public Health, *Public Health in Figures 1986,* 55.

82. Osvaldo Castro Miranda, "Recursos humanos en salud en Cuba," *Educación médica y salud* (Washington, D.C.: PAHO) 20, no. 3 (1986): 376–77.

83. Ministerio de Salud Pública, *Public Health in Figures, 1986,* 6, 32, 33.

84. *Granma Weekly Review,* January 31, 1988, 9.

85. Ministerio de Salud Pública, *Informe anual 1989,* 23, 34.

86. U.S. Commerce Department, *Statistical Abstract of the United States, 1987,* 91; and *Statistical Abstract of the United States, 1990,* p. 101, table 155.

87. *New York Times,* April 4, 1986, p. B4.

88. Castro Miranda, "Recursos humanos en salud," 376–77; Ministry of Public Health, *Public Health in Figures 1986,* 55; and Pan American Health Organization, *Health Conditions in the Americas 1981–1984,* 150, 153, 154.

89. U.S. Department of Health and Human Services, *Report of the Graduate Medical Education National Advisory Committee,* 274.

90. Giorgio Solimano et al., "Health For All in Cuba: Policies and Strategies" (New York, n.d. [probably 1986]) 21 (typescript).

91. Pan American Health Organization, *Health Conditions 1990,* 2:115.

92. Personal communication from George A. Silver, September 20, 1989.

93. Rodríguez, "Informe de viaje a Cuba," anexo, 5.

94. See table 5 and U.S. Bureau of the Census, *Statistical Abstract 1990,* p. 77, table 110.

95. U.S. Bureau of the Census, *Statistical Abstract 1990,* p. 66, table 87.

96. *Granma Weekly Review,* December 9, 1990, 3.

97. Rodríguez, "Informe de viaje a Cuba," anexo, 5, 6.

98. These speeches, dated September 12, 1981, and November 6, 1982, were cited in Ministerio de Salud Pública, Vicerrectoría Desarrollo ISCM-H, "Algunas ideas vertidas en diferentes discursos pronunciados por el Comandante en Jefe Fidel Castro que tienen que ver con la formación del médico a egresar de la educación médica superior y con la especialidad de medicina general integral y que sirvieron de base para la elaboración del nuevo plan de estudio de medicina (1981–1984)," 1, 12 (mimeographed).

99. Ibid.

100. Ministerio de Salud Pública, Instituto Superior de Ciencias Médicas de La Habana, *La formación del médico general básico como médico de la familia: Plan de estudio de la carrera,* n.d. [probably prepared for the November 1988 primary care conference], 4–5.

101. Ibid., 10–12, 17.

102. See *Annals of Community-Oriented Education* (the Netherlands), yearly.

103. Fidel Ilizastigui Dupuy, *La educación médica superior y las necesidades de salud de la población* (La Habana: MINSAP, 1988), 6.

104. Interview with anonymous source 65, 1988.

105. *Atención primaria de salud* (Geneva and New York: Organización Mundial de la Salud y Fondo de las Naciones Unidos para la Infancia, 1978).

106. Thomas McKeown, "Determinants of Health," *Human Nature* (April 1978): 66.

Chapter 5

1. David E. Apter, ed., *Ideology and Discontent* (New York: Free Press of Glencoe, 1964), 23–30.

2. Fox, "Cuba Plans a Century of Biology," 243.

3. Robert N. Ubell, "High-Tech Medicine in the Caribbean: 25 Years of Cuban Health Care," *New England Journal of Medicine* 309, no. 23 (December 8, 1983): 1471.

4. *Granma Weekly Review,* August 5, 1990, 4.

5. Marcel Roche, "Cuba: El Centro de Investigaciones Biológicas," *Interciencia* (Buenos Aires, Argentina) 10, no. 6 (November–December 1985): 300; and interview with Harvey Bialy, research editor, *Bio/Technology,* Red Hook, New York, September 15, 1990.

6. Interview with Harvey Bialy, February 15, 1991.

7. Interview with Luis Herrera, November 25, 1988.

8. *Granma Weekly Review,* August 14, 1983, 1.

9. Interview with Leonardo Cabezas, deputy director, National Center for Laboratory Animal Science (CENPALAB), Havana, June 20, 1991.

10. "Recombinant Alpha-2 IFN Cloned in Havana, Faces Animal Testing, Questions," *Newswatch,* March 17, 1986, 4.

11. Jon Beckwith, "Cuba Report: Science and Society Are Inseparable," *Science for the People* 17, no. 5 (September/October 1985): 21; Fox, "Cuba Plans a Century of Biology," 245; Julie Ann Miller, "Cuba's Commitment to Genetic Engineering Grows in Size and Scope," *Genetic Engineering News* (May 1986): 22; and Marcel Roche, "Cuba: el Centro de Investigaciones Biológicas," 299.

12. See advertisements in *Biotecnología aplicada* (Cuba) 7, no. 2 (1990).

13. Interview with Harvey Bialy, February 15, 1991.

14. Tim Beardsley, "Cuban Biotechnology: Progress Despite Isolation," *Nature* 320 (March 6, 1986): 8.

15. Harvey Bialy, "Cuban Biotechnology: Interferon As a Model," *Bio/Technology* 4, no. 4 (April 1986): 265.

16. Ibid., 265; and interview with Harvey Bialy, February 15, 1991.

17. Daniel J. Goldstein, *Biotecnología, universidad y política* (México: Siglo veintiuno editores, 1989), 206. The quotation is from an interview with Harvey Bialy, February 15, 1991.

18. *New York Times,* August 16, 1990, C17.

19. "Cuban-Made Interferon Reaches out for World Markets," *Newswatch,* March 17, 1986, 3.

20. Interview with Osvaldo Vela, deputy director of MediCuba (for many years the primary Cuban medical export-import firm), Havana, January 16, 1990, and June 13, 1991.

21. *New York Times,* August 16, 1990, C1, C17.

22. Ibid.

23. Ibid.

24. Telephone interview with Harvey Bialy, June 17, 1991.

25. *New York Times,* August 16, 1990, C1, C17.

26. *Granma Weekly Review,* August 5, 1990, 4; and interview with Miguel Figueras, advisor to the president of the Comité Estatal de Colaboración Económica (CECE), Havana, June 14 and 21, 1991, and José Luis Rodríguez, subdirector of the Centro de Investigación de la Economía Mundial (CIEM), Havana, June 19, 1991.

27. Calculating the exchange rate is rather tricky since the official Soviet and Cuban rates do not reflect reality. There were three official rates in the Soviet Union, ranging from 6 rubles per dollar for noncommercial exchanges to 0.65 rubles per dollar for certain types of trade. The Cuban peso is considerably overvalued as well. The rate was negotiated for a whole package of items traded. Interview with José Luis Rodríguez, Smith College, February 8, 1991, and Havana, June 19, 1991; and interview with Miguel Figueras, June 21, 1991.

28. Foreign Broadcast Information Service, *Latin America Daily Report,* FBIS-LAT-91-014, January 22, 1991, 3.

29. Foreign Broadcast Information Service, *Latin America Daily Report,* FBIS-LAT-91-014, January 22, 1991, 3; and interview with Miguel Figueras, June 21, 1991.

30. Interview with José Luis Rodríguez, Pittsburgh, April 27, 1992.

31. Interview with Igor Nit, economic advisor to Boris Yeltsin, president of the Russian Republic, the Jerome Levy Economics Institute, Bard College, October 27, 1991.

32. Interview with José Luis Rodríguez, Pittsburgh, April 27, 1992.

33. Robert N. Ubell, "Cuba's great leap," *Nature* 302 (April 28, 1983): 746.

34. Comité Estatal de Estadísticas, *Anuario estadístico de Cuba 1989* (La Habana: CEE, 1991), 48, 303.

35. Ibid., 746; and interview with Luís Herrera, November 25, 1988. Herrera spent three months working in the laboratory of Mark Ptashne at Harvard and also studied briefly in Houston, San Francisco, and Washington, D.C.

36. Beardsley, "Cuban Biotechnology," 8.

37. Fox, "Cuba's Century of Biology," 244; Issar Smith, "Report on NACSEX 1/28–2/7/90 Trip [to Cuba]," NACSEX internal document; interview with Luis Herrera, November 25, 1988; and telephone interview with Issar Smith, NACSEX, New York, September 1990.

38. Beckwith, "Cuba Report," 21.

39. Gerardo Trueba González, "Política científica y biotecnología en Cuba: 5a curso de planificación de C & T en América Latina," La Habana, Cuba: unpublished typescript, March 1991, 8. Trueba González is the director of the Instituto de Investigaciones Económicas of the JUCEPLAN (Central Planning Board).

40. "Educación: Un instituto preuniversitario diferente," *Cuba internacional* (9/85): 53–57.

41. Smith, "Report on NACSEX 1/28–2/7/90 Trip [to Cuba]," n.d., 4–6 (typescript).

42. Trueba González, "Política científica," 8.

43. Interview with Víctor R. Jiménez, J'Dpto. de Química, División de Proteínas y Hormonas, at CIGB, Havana, June 19, 1991.

44. Beckwith, "Cuba Report," 21. See also Miller, "Cuba's Commitment to Genetic Engineering," 22; and Fox, "Cuba Plans a Century of Biology," 248.

45. Beckwith, "Cuba Report," 21.

46. Ibid.

47. Personal observations at CIGB, Havana, November 25, 1988, and June 19, 1991; and interview with Victor R. Jiménez, June 19, 1991.

48. Telephone interviews with Daniel J. Goldstein, October 16, 1990, and January 7, 1991. See also Goldstein, *Biotecnología, universidad y política;* Id., "Latin American Pseudobiotechnology: A Pathway to Underdevelopment, Misery, and More Trade Deficit," paper presented at an international conference on "Biotechnology and International Trade: 1992 and Beyond," Maastricht, the Netherlands, June 20–22, 1990; and Id., "The Strategic Meaning of Structural Molecular Biology in Biotechnology: X-Ray Crystallography, Nuclear Magnetic Resonance and Protein and Nucleic Acid Engineering," unpublished manuscript, 1990.

49. Interview with Harvey Bialy, February 15, 1991.

50. Interview with Harvey Bialy, September 15, 1990. This view was corroborated in "Biotechnology and Economic Development: Introduction," *Economic Bulletin for Europe* (Journal of the United Nations Economic Commission for Europe) 38, no. 1 (March 1986): 7.

51. Mario González Pacheco, "Informe de Viaje 27–31 mayo de 1989," Washington, D.C.: Pan American Health Organization internal document [unnumbered], n.d., 1.

52. Interview with Luis Herrera, November 25, 1988.

53. Issar Smith, "Report on NACSEX," 2–4.

54. Telephone interview with Issar Smith, New York, September 1990. The president of the Cuban Academy of Sciences, Rosa Elena Simeon, has stated that 17 percent of Cuban scientific research is basic research. However, the Cuban definition of basic research differs from the norm in that it presupposes that an end product will result from the endeavor; Cuban research thus cannot be considered as true basic research. Foreign Broadcast Information Service, *Latin America Daily Report,* FBIS-LAT-91-007, July 10, 1990, 4.

55. Ubell, "Cuba's Great Leap," 746.

56. Interview with Luis Herrera, November 25, 1988.

57. Julie Ann Miller, "For Cuba, the Key is Bioresearch," *Chemical Week,* May 7, 1986, 71.

58. Ubell, "Cuba's Great Leap," 747.

59. Ministry of Public Health, *Annual Report of the Minister 1986,* 10.

60. Trueba González, "Política científica," 3.

61. Simeon Negrín, Rosa Elena, "Science and Technology, Their Role in the Development of Cuba," typescript, n.d. [probably 1988 or 1989], 11.

62. Personal observation at the CIGB library, June 19, 1991; and interview with Luis F. Lorenzo-Luaces, J'Dpto. de Automatización de Procesos, CIGB, Havana, June 19, 1991.

63. Interview with Miguel Figueras, April 6, 1991; and Miguel Alejandro Figueras, "Cuba en los 80: retos económicos para los 90," draft manuscript, June 19, 1991, 28.

64. Comité Estatal de Estadísticas, *Anuario estadístico 1989* (La Habana: CEE, 1991), 260, 269; interview with Miguel Figueras, June 21, 1991; and *Granma Weekly Review,* May 26, 1991, 8.

65. Ana María Granda Mir, "2a industria de equipos médicos en Cuba. Estado actual y perspectivas," Instituto Superior de Relaciones Internacionales, Trabajo de diploma, La Habana, November 1989.

66. Ubell, "Cuba's Great Leap," 746; Fox, "Cuba Plans a Century of Biology," 243–48; and Roche, "Cuba: El Centro de Investigaciones Biológicas," 299–300.

67. Interview with Lorenzo Heredia del Portal, director of Immunochemistry, Centro de Imunoensayos (Immunoassay Center—CIE), Havana, November 25, 1988. See also Fox, "Cuba Plans a Century of Biology," 244; and Miller, "Cuba's Commitment to Genetic Engineering," 22.

68. Interview with Lorenzo Heredia del Portal, November 25, 1988.

69. Harvey Bialy, "Cuba to Market an Ultra-Microelisa System," *Bio/Technology* 5, no. 7 (July 1987): 663.

70. *Granma Weekly Review,* August 5, 1990, 12; and observation at SUMA display, Biotecnología 92 international conference, Havana, July 11, 1992.

71. *Folha de São Paulo* (Brazil), April 6, 1988, A17, cited in Ulysses B. Panisset, "Health Diplomacy in Latin America: A Case Study of Health Technology Cooperation between Brazil and Cuba," unpublished manuscript, 1989, 114.

72. *Granma Weekly Review,* August 5, 1990, 12.

73. Interview with Miguel Figueras, June 21, 1991.

74. Cuba has made technology transfers in other sectors, particularly agriculture and the sugar industry.

75. Organización Panamericana Sanitaria, "Reunión operativa interpaises OPS/OMS en cooperación técnica entre paises (CTPD/CTP) en el contexto del presupuesto programa de la OPS/OMS 1990–1991," La Habana, November 1989.

76. "Cuban-made interferons reach out for world markets," *Biotechnology Newswatch* 6, no. 6 (March 17, 1986): 3.

77. Ibid.

78. World Health Organization (Geneva) internal memorandum BLG–B3/449/7, July 31, 1989, 1.

79. Pan American Health Organization, internal memorandum HSD/MGP/92.18, August 17, 1989, 1.

80. Anonymous source no. 51, July 20, 1990.

81. EFE cable, February 25, 1991; and anonymous source no. 51, May 1991.

82. Interview with Cuahtemoc Valdés Omedo, UNAM, Filosofía y Letras, Campinas, Brazil, July 6, 1990.

83. Pan American Health Organization, internal document HSP–C/28/2CUB, December 1990, 5.

84. Ibid., 5.

85. Interview with anonymous source no. 87, 1991.

86. José Luis Rodríguez, "La economía cubana ante un mundo cambiante," paper presented at the XVI Congreso de la Asociación de Estudios del Caribe and at the XVIII Congreso de la Asociación Latinoamericano de Sociología, La Habana, May 1991, 20; "Brasil: Ministro de Salud critica duramente a Cuba," EFE wire service, December 11, 1990; "Brasil-Cuba: Ministro critica excesivo precio de vacunas cubanas," Reuters wire service, December 11, 1990; *Jornal do Brasil,* May 21, 1991, 12; and anonymous source no. 87, August 8, 1991.

87. *Granma Weekly Review,* August 16, 1987, 3.

88. Ibid., and *Cuba Business* (London) 4, no. 1 (February 1990): 2.

89. Chamber of Commerce of the Republic of Cuba, *Foreign Trade* 4/90 (1990): 61.

90. *Jornal do Brasil,* May 21, 1991, 12; and *Granma Weekly Review,* June 30, 1991, 10.

91. *O Estado de São Paulo,* June 21, 1991, 10, cited in Foreign Broadcast Information Service, *Latin America Daily Report,* FBIS-LAT-91-138, 43–44.

92. Anonymous source no. 87, July 29, 1991.

93. Anonymous source no. 87, August 8, 1991, and July 13, 1992.

94. Anonymous source no. 87, July 13, 1992.

95. Interview with David R. Gómez Cova, ex-president of the Latin American and Caribbean Public Health Association, and professor, School of Public Health, Universidad Central de Venezuela [Caracas], Campinas, Brazil, July 6, 1990; and interview with anonymous source no. 51, a Latin American health expert, 1990.

96. Anonymous source no. 51, 1990.

97. Anonymous source no. 87, August 8, 1991.

98. *Jornal do Brasil,* May 21, 1991, 12.

99. Anonymous source no. 51, 1990; and anonymous source no. 87, 1991.

100. *Cuba Business* 4, no. 1 (February 1990): 2.

101. *Granma Weekly Review,* June 30, 1991, 10.

102. Pan American Health Organization, internal document HSD/BIO program, May 1989, 1, 3.

103. Anonymous source no. 87, August 8, 1991.

104. Pan American Health Organization, internal document, May 1989, table [unpaginated].

105. *Granma Weekly Review,* November 19, 1989, 5.

106. CIGB proposal to PAHO attached to PAHO/WHO interoffice memorandum DRC/ICP/RPD-020-534-89, dated 10-VIII-89.

107. Anonymous source no. 87, July 13, 1992.

108. Telephone interview with Issar Smith in New York, October 16, 1990; interview with Andrew Zimbalist, professor of economics at Smith College, in Annandale, New York, November 27, 1990.

109. Interview with Manuel Limonta Vidal, director, Center for Genetic Engineering and Biotechnology, Havana, July 12, 1992.

110. *Granma Weekly Review,* January 13, 1991, 3.

111. *Financial Times,* February 17, 1990, survey section, 37. See 1989 and 1990 product catalogs of the Centro de Ingeniería Genética y Biotecnología and *Granma Weekly Review,* November 26, 1989, 12. Cuban economist Miguel Figueras said that the total investment "in 5–6 biotechnology centers" was between 150 million and 200 million pesos. Interview with Figueras, Washington, D.C., April 6, 1991.

112. Interview with Victor R. Jiménez, June 19, 1991.

113. *Granma Weekly Review,* November 26, 1989, 12.

114. Interview with Lorenzo Heredia del Portal, October 25, 1988.

115. Foreign Broadcast Information Service, *Latin America Daily Report,* FBIS-LAT-90-083, April 30, 1990, 7, 8.

116. *Granma Weekly Review,* January 27, 1991, 9.

117. "Cuban-made Interferon," *Newswatch,* March 17, 1986, 4.

118. Centro de Ingeniería Genética y Biotecnología, *Products Catalog, January 1990,* La Habana: CIGB and Heber Biotec, 1990.

119. Interview with Lorenzo Heredia del Portal, November 25, 1988.

120. Interview with Harvey Bialy, September 15, 1990.

121. Telephone interview with Daniel J. Goldstein, October 16, 1990.

122. Foreign Broadcast Information Service, *Latin America Daily Report,* FBIS-LAT-92–112, June 10, 1992, 5.

123. *Granma Weekly Review,* May 31, 1987, 4, and Foreign Broadcast Information Service, *Latin America Daily Report* FBIS–LAT-90–244, December 19, 1990, 2.

124. Pan American Health Organization, internal document HSP/84/242/88, April 6, 1988, 5.

125. Pan American Health Organization, internal document, "Informe de Viaje. Cuba, 24/6–8/7/88," 15.

126. *Pharmaceutical Business News* (London), April 13, 1990.

127. Anonymous source no. 51, July 13, 1990.

128. Foreign Broadcast Information Service, *Latin America Daily Report,* FBIS-LAT-92–104, May 29, 1992, 42.

129. Granda Mir, "La industria de equipos médicos en Cuba," 41.

130. Interviews with vendors from various German and Swiss firms participating in the trade fair at the Biotecnología 92 international conference in Havana, July 10–12, 1992.

131. Technically, the prices and costs are in freely convertible currency with an exchange rate of one dollar to one peso, which means that these prices are in dollars. Less than 2 percent of Cuba's production costs are in nonconvertible pesos, so for simplicity's sake I have used dollars for their entire production cost. Granda Mir, "La industria de equipos médicos en Cuba," 41–42.

132. Ibid.

133. Miguel Alejandro Figueras, *Análisis de las políticas de industrialización en Cuba en el período revolucionario y proyecciones futuras* (La Habana: Universidad de La Habana, Centro de Investigaciones de la Economía Internacional, February 1990), 84.

134. Granda Mir, "La industria de equipos médicos en Cuba," 35, 50.

135. Ibid., anexos 2 and 4, n.p.

136. Interviews with Miguel Figueras, June 14, 1991, and José Luis Rodríguez, June 19, 1991.

137. Granda Mir, "La industria de equipos médicos en Cuba," 54.

138. Ibid., 55.

139. Interview with Miguel Figueras, June 21, 1991.

140. Granda Mir, "La industria de los equipos médicos en Cuba," 58–61.

141. Ibid., 58–61.

142. *Granma,* November 30, 1990, cited in Foreign Broadcast Information Service, *Latin America Daily Report,* FBIS-LAT-91-007, January 10, 1991, 4.

143. Ubell, "Cuba's Great Leap," 746.

144. Miller, "Cuba's Commitment to Genetic Engineering," 22.

145. Foreign Broadcast Information Service, *Latin America Daily Report,* FBIS-LAT-91–007, January 10, 1991, 4.

146. Ibid. According to Rosa Elena Simeón, president of the Cuban Academy of Sciences, Cuba saves U.S. $7 million per year on potato seeds alone. When pressed for a figure, Harvey Bialy estimated that the first CIGB in Havana requires about U.S. $1 million per year for consumables such as reagents and plastics. Interview on February 15, 1991.

147. Interview with Luis Herrera, November 25, 1988.

148. "UNIDO Narrow Choice for Site of Biotechnology Center," *Genetic Technology News* 3, No. 4 (April 1983): 8.

149. "UNIDO World Bio-center Meeting Puts off Decisions," *Biotechnology Newswatch* 5, no. 8 (April 15, 1985): 7.

150. "Five Year Update, 1984–1989," *Biotechnology Newswatch* 9, no. 4 (February 20, 1989): 4.

151. *Financial Times,* February 22, 1989, Sec. I, p. 20.

152. Interview with a North American biotechnology expert who wished to remain anonymous. Source no. 74, 1990.

153. Goldstein, *Biotecnología, universidad y política.* See particularly 211–14. See also Id., "Latin American Pseudobiotechnology"; Id., "The Commercialization of Biotechnology For Food Production," paper presented at the "Workshop on Biotechnology For Food Production in Dry Areas," at the United Nations Centre for Science and Technology African Biosciences Network, Dakar, Senegal, October 8–10, 1990; Id., "A biotechnology agenda for the Third World," *Journal of Agricultural Ethics* 2 (1989): 37–51; Id., "Molecular Biology and National Security," in *Seeds and Sovereignty,* ed. Jack Kloppenburg, Jr., (Durham, N.C.: Duke University Press, 1987). See also Harvey Bialy, "Biotechnology and the Poor: Partnerships or More Poverty," *UNESCO/MIRCEN World Journal of Microbiology and Biotechnology* (1991).

154. David Dembo, Clarence J. Dias, and Ward Morehouse, "The Vital Nexus in Biotechnology: The Relationship Between Research and Production and Its Implications for Latin America," *Interciencia* 14, no. 4 (July–August 1989): 168–180.

155. Ibid., 170, 179–80; and Goldstein, "Molecular Biology and National Security."

156. This has been the case with meningitis B vaccine, for which the Brazilians want the technology. Negotiations have gone on since the beginning of 1990 with occasional announcements of a deal that has not in fact materialized. See criticisms of Cuba on this account by Alceni Guerra, Brazilian minister of health, in *O Estado do São Paulo,* December 11, 1990, cited in Agence France Presse cable of December 11, 1990.

157. Anonymous sources nos. 74 and 78, 1990.

158. Interview by phone with Marta Cehelsky, senior policy officer, Division of International Programs, National Science Foundation, Washington, D.C., October 10, 1990.

159. Interview with Carlos M. Mella, president, Heber Biotec, Havana, June 19, 1991.

160. Interview with Manuel Limonta Vidal, July 13, 1992.

161. Interview with Harvey Bialy, June 17, 1991.

162. Anonymous source no. 74, 1991.

163. Interview with Juan Féliz Amador Pérez, marketing manager, Centro de Inmunología Molecular (CIMAB), Havana, June 19, 1991.

164. Telephone interview with Mark Ratner, patent expert, Immuno-Genetics, Cambridge, Mass., June 18, 1991.

165. Ibid.

166. *Pharmaceutical Business News,* April 13, 1990.

167. Organización Panamericana Sanitaria, Programa de las Naciones Unidas para el Desarrollo, y Sistema Económico Latinoamericano, "Encuentro de cooperación técnica entre paises latinoamericanos y del caribe para el desarrollo tecnológico en salud. Propuesta del trabajo," Santiago, Chile: OPS/OMS-PNUD-SELA, August 24, 1990, 11.

168. There has been a spate of barter agreements involving medical and biotechnology products since 1989 as Cuba has rushed to fill the gap left by

its traditional exports and trade partners. Moreover, Cuba's active participation in UNDP and PAHO regional cooperation projects has led to increased aid for biotechnology and medical technology projects. See Foreign Broadcast Information Service, *Latin America Daily Reports* for 1989, 1990, and 1991, as well as PAHO internal documents.

Chapter 6

1. Peter Bourne, *New Directions in International Health Cooperation* (Washington, D.C.: the White House, Spring 1978), 47.

2. Ministerio de Salud Pública, Dirección de Colaboración Internacional, "Cuba: 25 años de colaboración internacional," La Habana: MINSAP document prepared for the 2nd International Seminar on Primary Health Care, November 1988, 3–4.

3. *Granma Weekly Review,* July 10, 1983, 10.

4. *Granma,* February 25, 1966, 5.

5. *New York Times,* January 22, 1985, A2.

6. *Granma Weekly Review,* supplement, February 24, 1985, 3.

7. *Granma,* December 10, 1981, 1, and July 28, 1982, 3; *Granma Weekly Review,* July 17, 1983, 11; November 18, 1984, 3; and supplement, February 24, 1985, 3; Carlos Martínez Salsamendi, "El papel de Cuba en el Tercer Mundo: América Central, El Caribe y Africa," in Tokatlian (compilador), *Cuba y Estados Unidos,* 144; and interviews with Jaime Davis, head of Colaboración Internacional del MINSAP, Havana, November 15, 1988, and Ydania Balán, Relaciones Internacionales del MINSAP, Havana, November 21, 1988.

8. *Granma Weekly Review,* November 11, 1990, 2; and July 7, 1991, 9.

9. Manuel Yepe Menéndez, "International Economic Cooperation: The Cuban Experience," *Foreign Trade* (April 1990): 43.

10. Cuban figures calculated from the *New York Times,* January 22, 1985, A2 (16,000 civilian internationalists); *Granma Weekly Review,* September 16, 1984, 3 (population 10 million); Yepe Menéndez, "International Economic Cooperation," 43 (46,000 internationalists); and Ministerio de Salud Pública, *Informe anual 1989,* 19 (population estimate for June 1989 of 10.5 million). The U.S. figures are calculated from 1985 Peace Corps and AID personnel figures of 6,250 and 1,454 and a population of 239 million, and 1990 Peace Corps and AID personnel figures of 6,000 and 1,047 with a population of 252 million. It must be noted that AID uses mostly contractors or recipient governments' agencies for project implementation. See U.S. General Accounting Office, *Donor Approaches To Development Assistance: Implications for The United States,* GAO/ID-83–23 (Washington, D.C.: GAO, May 4, 1983), 13, 17, 19. U.S. AID data are from U.S. International Development Agency, Office of Personnel, July 22, 1991, and Peace Corps data for those years are from Peace Corps, Office of Personnel, July 22, 1991. The U.S. population

figure for 1985 and 1990 came from the Bureau of the Census, *Statistical Abstract of the United States, 1990,* 7, 15.

11. Cited in U.S. General Accounting Office, *Donor Approaches to Development Assistance,* 73.

12. Ibid., 38–39, 70.

13. Organization for Economic Co-Operation and Development, *Development Co-Operation 1990 Report* (Paris: OECD, 1990), 135.

14. Calculated from total of 118,760 technicians, of whom 23,075 are Cuban. U.S. Department of State, *Soviet and East European Aid to the Third World, 1981* (Washington, D.C.: U.S. Government Printing Office, February 1983), 20.

15. The USSR and the eastern European countries combined had a population 38.8 times larger than Cuba's. Calculated from Sivard, *World Military and Social Expenditures 1985,* 35.

16. Central Intelligence Agency, *Communist Aid Activities in Non-Communist LDCs, 1979 and 1954–1979* (Washington, D.C.: CIA, April 15, 1980), 8.

17. Ibid., 21; and Central Intelligence Agency, *Communist Aid Activities in Non-Communist LDCs, 1977* (Washington, D.C.: CIA, 1978), 9.

18. *China Daily,* July 19, 1986, 3.

19. Dirección de Colaboración Internacional, "Cuba: 25 años de colaboración internacional," 5–6. For general civilian aid in 1981–1985, see Julio Díaz-Vázquez, "Cuba: colaboración económica y científico-técnica con paises en vías de desarrollo de Africa, Asia, América Latina," *Economía y desarrollo,* no. 68 (May-June, 1982): 29.

20. Ernesto Meléndez, "Colaboración cubana (final) 1981–1985," *Colaboración internacional* (April–June, 1986): 5–6.

21. Grundy and Budetti, "The Distribution and Supply of Cuban Medical Personnel," 718. The seven countries are Cape Verde, Angola, Equatorial Guinea, Guinea-Bissau, Ethiopia, São Tomé, and South Yemen.

22. "Embajadores de la salud," *Verde Olivo* 23, no. 3 (January 21, 1982): 18–19.

23. República Popular de Angola, Misión Médica Cubana, *Balance anual 1987* (Angola: Misión Médica Cubana, n.d. [probably December 1987]), p. 8, table 1.

24. *Jornal de Angola,* April 24, 1991, and May 8, 1991, as cited in Foreign Broadcast Information Service, *Latin America Daily Report,* FBIS-LAT-91–104, May 30, 1991, 4; and *New York Times,* April 9, 1991, A8.

25. *Granma Weekly Review,* October 28, 1984, 9, cited in Domínguez, *To Make A World Safe For Revolution,* 161; and *Granma,* November 10, 1978, 8.

26. "Country's Cooperation with Ethiopia Discussed," *Prisma Latinoamericano,* January 1983, 24–26, reproduced in Foreign Broadcast Information Service, *Latin American Report,* no. 2661 (Springfield, Va.: National Technical Information Service, JPRS 83190, April 4, 1983), 28.

27. Interview with anonymous source no. 36 at the Tanzanian border in Numanga, Kenya, 1989.

28. *Granma Weekly Review,* August 12, 1990, 9.

29. Interview with Francisco Rojas Ochoa, June 17, 1991.

30. *Granma,* January 5, 1978, 5.

31. Pamela S. Falk, "Cuba's Foreign and Domestic Policies, 1968–78: The Effect of International Commitments on Internal Development," (Ph.D. diss., New York University, 1980), 242; and *Granma,* April 14, 1979, 5.

32. Domínguez, *To Make A World Safe For Revolution,* 163.

33. *Granma,* September 7, 1976, 5; and October 19, 1979, 3.

34. *Granma,* May 28, 1981, 5.

35. *Granma Weekly Review,* March 6, 1988, 2.

36. Foreign Broadcast Information Service, *Latin America Daily Report,* FBIS-LAT-91–004, January 7, 1991, 26.

37. Foreign Broadcast Information Service, *Latin America Daily Report,* FBIS-LAT-90–238, December 11, 1990, 1.

38. Foreign Broadcast Information Service, *Latin America Daily Report,* FBIS-LAT-92–102, May 27, 1992, 4.

39. *Colaboración internacional* (January–March 1986): 19

40. *Granma Weekly Review,* August 17, 1986, 10.

41. *Resumen semanal de Granma,* August 21, 1988, 3.

42. *Granma Weekly Review,* April 21, 1991, 2; and Foreign Broadcast Information Service, *Latin America Daily Report,* FBIS-LAT-91–011, January 16, 1991, 6, and FBIS-LAT-91–013, January 18, 1991, 7.

43. Dirección de Colaboración Internacional, "Cuba: 25 años de cooperación médica," 3; and *Granma Weekly Review,* November 11, 1984, p. 10, col. 1.

44. "Cubanos en Lao," *Colaboración internacional* (January–March 1986): 27.

45. Julio Hernández, "Internacionalismo junto al Niger," *Cuba internacional,* 209 (April 1987): 53–54.

46. Ciro Bianchi Ross, "Internacionalismo: De Addis Abeba al desierto de Ogadén," *Cuba internacional,* 184 (March 1985): 41.

47. Comité Estatal de Colaboración Económica (CECE), "Cuba y su economía," internal document, 1988, 6; and *Granma,* February 7, 1989, 4.

48. *Granma,* February 17, 1988, 7, and October 19, 1988, 1.

49. Foreign Broadcast Information Service, *Latin America Daily Report,* FBIS-LAT-91–146, July 30, 1991, 20.

50. *Granma Weekly Review,* March 17, 1991, 9; and Foreign Broadcast Information Service, *Latin America Daily Report,* FBIS-LAT-91–045, March 7, 1991, 3.

51. Foreign Broadcast Information Service, *Latin America Daily Report,* FBIS-LAT-90–198, October 12, 1990, 4; FBIS-LAT-90–235, December 6, 1990, 4; and *Granma Weekly Review,* August 19, 1990, 9.

52. Foreign Broadcast Information Service, *Latin America Daily Report,* FBIS-LAT-91, January 2, 1991, 22–23.

53. Foreign Broadcast Information Service, *Latin America Daily Report,* FBIS-LAT-91–040, February 28, 1991, 2; FBIS-LAT-91–060, March 28, 1991, 2; and FBIS-LAT-91–089, May 8, 1991, 3.

54. *Granma Weekly Review,* May 26, 1991, 4.

55. Foreign Broadcast Information Service, *Latin America Daily Report,* FBIS-LAT-91-085, 9.

56. Interview with Francisco Rojas Ochoa, June 17, 1991.

57. Interview with Miguel Figueras, June 21, 1991.

58. "Guyana, Cuba Agree on Cooperation, Trade," FL281730 Bridgetown, CANA, 2104 GMT March 26, 1983, reproduced in Foreign Broadcast Information Service, *Latin American Report,* no. 2666 (Springfield, Va.: National Technical Information Service, JPRS 83262, April 14, 1983), 23.

59. Foreign Broadcast Information Service, *Latin America Daily Report,* FBIS-LAT-91–103, May 29, 1991, 3.

60. *Granma Weekly Review,* July 12, 1987, 8; and September 20, 1987, 5.

61. Interview with Ramón Casanova, December 1, 1988.

62. Personal observation at the Cardiocentro William Soler, Havana, December 1, 1988.

63. *Granma Weekly Review,* July 14, 1991, 8.

64. Interview with Zenobio González León, November 30, 1988.

65. The information on non-Cubans seeking medical treatment in Cuba is from an interview with Francisco León, CEPAL, Pittsburgh, Pa., April 27, 1992; the information on Andrés Alemán is from an interview with Arturo Valenzuela, director of the Center for Latin American Studies, Georgetown University, Los Angeles, September 26, 1992.

66. Foreign Broadcast Information Service, *Latin America Daily Report,* FBIS-LAT-90–091, 5.

67. Ibid.

68. Foreign Broadcast Information Service, *Latin America Daily Report,* FBIS-LAT-90–063, April 2, 1990, 21.

69. Ibid.

70. Foreign Broadcast Information Service, *Latin America Daily Report,* FBIS-LAT-91–060, March 28, 1991, 2; and *Granma Weekly Review,* April 7, 1991, 3; and April 28, 1991, 3.

71. *Granma Weekly Review,* April 28, 1991, 3.

72. Interview with Osvaldo Castro Miranda, March 19, 1993.

73. Cable News Network, June 29, 1991.

74. Interview with Jaime Davis, November 15, 1988.

75. *Granma Weekly Review,* February 28, 1982, 7; and *Granma,* July 28, 1982, 4.

76. *Granma Weekly Review,* October 22, 1978, 9, cited in Falk, "Cuba's Foreign and Domestic Policies," 245.

77. "Internacionalismo: una sabia iniciativa," *Cuba internacional,* 215 (November 1987): 20–23.

78. *Granma Weekly Review,* October 14, 1984, 5.

79. The report indicated that in 1977 the contingent in rural areas was considerably larger. *Granma Weekly Review,* October 28, 1984, p. 9, col. 1.

80. Vieira, "Informe de Viaje a Cuba," 4.

81. *Granma Weekly Review,* May 26, 1991, 4.

82. *Granma Weekly Review,* Sept. 7, 1986, 3.

83. Ibid.

84. *Granma Weekly Review,* May 10, 1987, 9.

85. *Granma,* July 17, 1986, 6.

86. Dirección de Colaboración Internacional. "Cuba: 25 años de cooperación médica," 3–4.

87. Ibid., 4.

88. *Granma Weekly Review,* November 11, 1984, 5; November 11, 1990, 2.

89. *Granma Weekly Review,* July 22, 1990, 4.

90. *Granma Weekly Review,* Nov. 18, 1984, 3.

91. *Informe del Gobierno de Cuba a la Organización Panamericana de Salud sobre las condiciones de salud,* 6.

92. Interview with Jaime Davis, November 15, 1988; and Ministerio de Salud Pública, Area de Docencia, "Recursos humanos en salud," MINSAP, December 1990, 7 (typescript).

93. Data compiled by María Matilda Serrano, Formación de Recursos Humanos en Colaboración Internacional, MINSAP, November 30, 1988.

94. Ministerio de Salud Pública, "Recursos humanos," 7.

95. Statement by Sen. Charles Mathias, Jr., quoted in *Center for Peace and Conflict Studies/Detroit Council for World Affairs Newsletter,* Spring 1985, 2.

96. U.S. Information Agency, *U.S. Advisory Commission on Public Diplomacy: 1986 Report* (Washington, D.C.: USIA, 1986), 36.

97. Information from the United States Information Agency, Board of Foreign Scholarships, July 22, 1991.

98. Central Intelligence Agency, *Communist Aid Activities, 1954–1979,* 11.

99. *New York Times,* June 9, 1985, 6.

100. Alfonso Mejía, Helena Pizurki, and Erica Royston, *Foreign Medical Graduates: The Case of the United States* (Lexington, Mass.: Lexington Books, 1980), 34.

101. *New York Times,* May 7, 1984, B2; and August 23, 1983, Y1.

102. U.S. Department of Health and Human Services, Public Health Service, Health Resources and Services Administration, Bureau of Health Professions, Office of Data Analysis and Management, *The Impact of Foreign-Trained Doctors on the Supply of Physicians* (Washington, D.C.: U.S. Government Printing Office, DHHS Publication no. HRS–P–OD-83–2, September 1983), I-5.

103. U.S. Department of Commerce, Bureau of the Census, *Statistical Abstract of the United States, 1990,* 101.

104. *New York Times,* August 23, 1983; and May 7, 1984.

105. *Granma Weekly Review,* April 13, 1986, 3; May 25, 1986, 1; November 2, 1986, 11; May 13, 1990, 10; June 3, 1990, 4; August 5, 1990, 12; April 28, 1991, 3; Foreign Broadcast Information Service, *Latin America Daily Report,* FBIS-LAT-85–185, vol. 6, September 24, 1985; and *Granma,* October 11, 1974, 6; and March 25, 1985, 5.

106. Díaz-Vázquez, "Cuba: colaboración económica," 43; and *Granma,* June 10, 1970, 1.

107. *Granma,* May 6, 1986, 1.

108. *Granma,* October 20, 1986, 6.

109. *Granma,* January 8, 1973, 1.

110. *Granma Weekly Review,* September 16, 1990, 4.

111. Interview with Jaime Davis, Havana, November 15, 1988; and with Sergio Arouca (Brazil), Havana, November 16, 1988; and *Granma Weekly Review,* February 17, 1991, 9; and February 17, 1991, 9; and *Granma,* May 2, 1988, 4.

112. *Granma Weekly Review,* February 17, 1991, 9; and April 28, 1991, 3.

113. *Juventud Rebelde,* December 11, 1988, 16; and *Granma,* December 28, 1988, 6.

114. *Granma,* December 9, 1988, 1.

115. *Trabajadores,* June 14, 1989, 1.

116. "Abalkin Views State of Ties With Cuba," Foreign Broadcast Information Service, *Soviet Union Daily Report,* FBIS-SOV-90–090, May 9, 1990, 36.

117. *Granma Weekly Review,* July 8, 1990, 1, 9; July 22, 1990, 4; and August 5, 1990, 13.

118. *Granma Weekly Review,* December 16, 1990, 5.

119. Foreign Broadcast Information Service, *Latin America Daily Report,* FBIS-LAT-91–022, February 1, 1991, 2.

120. Foreign Broadcast Information Service, *Latin America Daily Report,* FBIS-LAT-90–091, May 10, 1990, 4–5.

121. Ibid., 4.

122. *Granma Weekly Review,* June 21, 1987, 1.

123. Interview with Javier Torres Goitia, former minister of health of Bolivia (1982–1985) in the government of Hernán Siles Suazo, and currently director of the Fundación Salud y Sociedad, Instituto Andino de Desarrollo en Salud y Educación in La Paz, Bolivia, Campinas, Brazil, July 4, 1990.

124. *Granma,* April 30, 1986, 6.

125. U.S. Commerce Department, Bureau of the Census, *Statistical Abstract of the United States, 1990,* 835.

126. Information culled from the conference attendence records for 1980 through 1988 at the Oficina de Promociones, Palacio de Convenciones, in Havana, November 25, 1988; and *Calendario de reuniones y exposiciones 1988/92. Palacio de las Convenciones* (La Habana: Palacio de las Convenciones, n.d.), 104–111, 119.

127. Personal communication with various conference participants from a number of Latin American countries, and participant observation at meetings in Cuba, 1980–1981, 1990, and 1992. Travel reports published in a variety of American medical journals substantiate this claim.

128. *Granma,* November 19, 1988, 1; and November 27, 1988, 8.

129. Participant observation at the conference.

130. According to Carlos Medina of the Honduran delegation.

131. *Granma Weekly Review,* March 31, 1991, 3.

132. *Granma Weekly Review,* June 22, 1986, 4.

133. Interview with Victor Jimenez, June 19, 1991.

134. Danilo Salcedo and Eduardo Joly, *Informe de misión para determinar las necesidades de asistencia en materias de población* (New York: United Nations Family Planning Agency, April 5, 1979), 93.

135. *Granma Weekly Review,* November 11, 1990, 2.

136. *Granma Weekly Review,* December 30, 1990, 3.

137. Interview with Mario Pichardo, deputy director of international relations for the Cuban Ministry of Public Health, Havana, June 17, 1991. Pichardo had the PAHO budget in front of him when citing these figures.

138. For a detailed explanation of CTPD see OPS/OMS–PNUD–SELA, "Encuentro de cooperación técnica entre paises latinoamericanos y del caribe para el desarrollo tecnológico en salud: propuesta de trabajo," PAHO internal document, August 24, 1990.

139. Ibid.; and Ministerio de Salud Pública, *Evaluación estrategías de salud para todos,* 16.

140. Foreign Broadcast Information Service, *Latin America Daily Report,* FBIS-LAT-91–051, March 15, 1991, 2.

141. Fidel Castro, *2nd Period of Sessions of the National Assembly,* 39.

142. *Bohemia,* December 22, 1978, 46.

143. Central Intelligence Agency, *Communist Aid Activities, 1977,* 5; and Helen Mathews Smith, "Castro's Medicine: An on-the-Scene Report," *M.D.* 27, no. 5 (May 1983): 163.

144. *Granma Weekly Review,* February 27, 1983, 9.

145. Interview with Jaime Davis, November 15, 1988.

146. *Granma Resumen Semanal,* May 28, 1989, 9.

147. Edith Felipe, "Cuba y la colaboración económica con el mundo subdesarrollado," *Temas de la economía mundial* 15 (1985): 88.

148. Margarita Díaz Ravelo, Olga Isla Bauza, and Teolinda Pérez Abreu Suárez, "Desarrollo de la colaboración económica científica técnica de Cuba con Iraq hasta 1987," Tésis de Grado, Instituto de Colaboración Económica (La Habana), 1988, 33–34, 42–43.

149. Domínguez, *To Make a World Safe for Revolution,* 156.

150. Mireya Galiano Jorda and Maria Elena Noriega Almora, "Colaboración técnica con Tanzania, 1987–1988," Proyecto de Grado, Centro Nacional de Capacitación Técnica (La Habana), 1988, 16–17.

151. Martínez Salsamendi, "El papel de Cuba en el Tercer Mundo," 145; and interview with Dr. Jaime Davis, November 15, 1988.

152. Interview with Miguel Figueras, June 21, 1991.

153. See Susan Eckstein, "Comment: The Global Political Economy and Cuba's African Involvement," *Cuban Studies/Estudios Cubanos* 10, no. 2 (July 1980): 90, and "Structural and Ideological Bases," 107. It is alleged that Ethiopia paid Cuba U.S. $250 for each soldier providing military assistance. However, most analysts argue that Cuban military aid is provided without charge. Ethiopia and Angola did pay for food for Cuban soldiers but not salaries. See "Sterben lassen, damit andere uberleben," *Die Zeit* Overseas Edition, no. 26 (June 29, 1984): 5–6; and Roca, "Economic Aspects," 60.

154. Roca, "Economic Aspects," 66.

155. Calculated from Carlos Martínez Salsamendi, "El papel de Cuba en el Tercer Mundo," 145; and Grundy and Budetti, "The Distribution and Supply of Cuban Medical Personnel," 718.

156. Comité Estatal de Colaboración Económica, "Datos generales de los organismos," CECE internal document (report on a review trip to Angola by CECE officials), March 1982, 2.

157. Ibid.

158. "Turismo de Salud: ¿Vacaciones en un hospital?" *Cuba internacional* 210 (May 1987): 52–57; *Granma Weekly Review,* February 7, 1988, 3; *Granma Weekly Review,* February 28, 1988, 12; and *New York Times,* May 29, 1988, sec. 1, p. 4.

159. Mathews Smith, "Castro's Medicine," 155; and *Granma Weekly Review,* May 25, 1986, 8.

160. External fixators were first developed in Italy and Yugoslavia, but Alvarez Cambras expanded, modified, and further developed them. Personal communication from Peggy Gilpin, Havana, November 16, 1988.

161. Interview with Ricardo E. Martínez Rojas, director of health tourism, Cubanacán, Havana, November 24, 1988.

162. *Granma Weekly Review,* May 31, 1987, 4; and March 1, 1987, 5.

163. Interview with Eduardo Joly, Havana, June 22, 1991.

164. Ibid.

165. *New York Times,* May 29, 1988, sec. 1, p. 4.

166. *Journal do Brasil* article, cited in *Center for Cuban Studies Newsletter,* September 1986, 3.

167. *Granma Weekly Review,* February 1, 1987, 9.

168. *Granma Weekly Review,* December 16, 1990, 3.

169. These associations exist in Venezuela, Costa Rica, Curaçao, Brazil, Panama, Colombia, Trinidad and Tobago, Uruguay, England, India, and Sweden, among others. Interview with Ricardo E. Martínez Rojas, November 24, 1988. See also articles in the *Kölner Stadtarzeiger* (Cologne, West Germany), June 9, 1988; *El Nacional* (Maracay, Venezuela), April 10, 1986; *El Sol de México* (México DF), September 24, 1985; *Jornal do Brasil,* June 8, 1986, 16; *El Carabobeno* (Valencia, Venezuela), May 10, 1986; *Revista Tele-Hogar Cine y T.V.* (Panama), August 1988; and *Granma Weekly Review,* December 16, 1990, 3.

170. Interview with Ricardo Martínez Rojas, November 24, 1988.

171. *Granma Weekly Review,* December 16, 1990, 3.

172. Ibid.

173. *Granma Weekly Review,* November 29, 1987, 3.

174. Interview with Ricardo Martínez Rojas, November 24, 1988.

175. Interview with José Luis Rodríguez, Smith College, February 7, 1991.

176. *Juventud Rebelde,* May 4, 1989, 1–2; and *Granma,* August 6, 1989, 6.

177. Brochure from the Center and *Granma Weekly Review,* December 16, 1990, 3.

178. Ibid.

179. *Granma Weekly Review,* March 31, 1991, 6.

180. *Granma Weekly Review,* July 14, 1991, 3.

181. Gail Reed, "Eyesight to the Blind: Promising Treatment for Retinitis Pigmentosa," *Cuba Update* 12, no. 3 (Summer 1991): 22.

182. Pan American Health Organization, internal document HSP program, May 28, 1991, 9.

183. Interview with Ricardo Martínez Rojas, November 24, 1991, and June 13, 1991.

184. Pan American Health Organization, internal document, May 28, 1991, 9.

185. Daily patient register of the clinic, November 25, 1988.

186. *Granma Weekly Review,* January 10, 1988, 3. The other countries included Angola, Argentina, Benin, Brazil, Cape Verde, Colombia, Congo, Costa Rica, Dominican Republic, Ecuador, Equatorial Guinea, Ethiopia, Guinea, Guinea-Bissau, Guyana, Mexico, Mozambique, Nicaragua, Panama, Peru, São Tomé, Uganda, Uruguay, and Venezuela.

187. *Granma Weekly Review,* April 26, 1987, 1.

188. *Latin American Economic Report,* LAER-90–05, May 31, 1990, 12; and *Latin America Weekly Report,* WR-90–25, July 5, 1990, 12.

189. "The Outlook for Cuban Production and Exports," *F. O. Lichts International Sugar and Sweetener Report* (Germany) 123, no. 32 (October 28, 1991): 532.

190. *Granma,* July 29, 1986, 4; and *Latin America Weekly Report,* WR-86–28, July 24, 1986, 7.

191. *Granma Weekly Review,* April 19, 1987, 10.

192. *Granma Weekly Review,* February 31, 1988, 2.

193. *Latin America Weekly Report,* WR-89–50, December 21, 1989, 10.

194. *Latin America Weekly Report,* WR-92–13, April 2, 1992, 7.

195. *Latin America Regional Report, Caribbean,* RC-86–08, October 2, 1986, 2.

196. *Washington Post,* July 29, 1990, 19A.

197. *Granma International,* November 3, 1991, 19.

198. *Granma International,* November 3, 1991, 20–21.

199. It has been estimated that between 1977 and 1980, Cuba's earnings from international contracts have represented between 6 percent and 18 percent of the island's hard-currency exports. See Susan Eckstein, "Cuban Internationalism," in *Cuba: Twenty-Five Years of Revolution, 1959–1984,* 379–80.

200. Eckstein, "Structural and Ideological Bases," 121.

201. *Bohemia* 70, no. 37 (September 15, 1978): 39.

202. Central Intelligence Agency, *Communist Aid Activities, 1954–1979,* iv, 11.

203. Interview with Miguel Figueras, June 21, 1991.

204. *Granma Weekly Review,* July 20, 1986, 9.

205. *Granma Weekly Review,* March 17, 1991, 9.

206. Central Intelligence Agency, *Communist Aid Activities 1977,* 10.

207. FAO, OMS, PAM, PNUD, UNESCO, "Informe de las agencias de las Naciones Unidas representadas en Cuba," internal document, November

1989; and Organización Panamericana de la Salud, "Lineamientos para la ejecución de la cooperación de OPS/OMS en Cuba 1991," internal document (La Habana: OPS/OMS, January 1991), 22.

208. Comité Estatal de Estadísticas. *Anuario estadístico de Cuba 1989.* La Habana: Comité Estatal de Estadísticas, 1991, 268–69.

Chapter 7

1. "Integran comités de salud en zonas rurales y urbanas," *Novedades de Quintana Roo,* May 13, 1988, 44; *New York Times,* March 13, 1988, 8; John M. Donahue, *The Nicaraguan Revolution in Health* (South Hadley, Mass.: Bergin and Garvey, 1986); Organización Panamericana Sanitaria, "Cooperación Técnica de la OPS/OMS: Desarrollo de Servicios de Salud," internal document URU/DHS/010/P2 (Washington, D.C.: OPS, November 16, 1987), 20–22; Marjorie Woodford Bray and Donald W. Bray, "Cuba, the Soviet Union, and Third World Struggle," in *Cuba: Twenty-Five Years of Revolution, 1959 to 1984,* ed. Halebsky and Kirk, 364; and *Granma Weekly Review,* May 26, 1991, 4.

2. Interviews conducted in various Cuban cities, towns, and rural areas in 1978, 1979, 1980–1981, 1988, 1990, 1991, and 1992. According to Jesus Escandell of the national leadership of the CTC (Confederation of Cuban Trade Unions), the main demand of the workers in 1987 was housing. *Granma Weekly Review,* May 17, 1987, 3.

3. *Boletín Especial: A Public Survey on the Quality of Health Care in the Province of Holguín, Cuba,* A Confidential Report by the Cuban Communist party (Washington, D.C.: Cuban American National Foundation, 1988); *New York Times,* February 15, 1989, 8; and March 5, 1989, 3.

4. Stephen White, "Economic Performance and Communist Legitimacy," *World Politics* 38, no. 3 (April 1986): 463–64.

5. Italics mine. Education was second. *Granma Weekly Review,* November 18, 1984, 3.

6. As in Cuba, education was cited as the other top priority. *New York Times,* February 15, 1989, 8.

7. Some say that Castro is a "médico frustrado," meaning that he should have been a doctor or that his real essence is that of a doctor.

8. Personal observation at the 2nd International Seminar on Primary Health Care, Havana, November 14–18, 1988.

9. The medal was awarded on April 7, 1988. Suárez Lugo, *Actividades antitabáquicas en Cuba,* 31.

10. *Granma Weekly Review,* May 24, 1987, 3.

11. Eckstein, "Structural and Ideological Bases," 104–105; Domínguez, *To Make a World Safe for Revolution,* 236, 238, 241; *Granma Weekly Review,* April 12, 1987, 4; November 22, 1987, 4; July 8, 1990, 4, and December 23, 1990; *Trabajadores,* May 9, 1989, 7; interview with Luis Heredero, No-

vember 22, 1988, Havana, and personal communication from Alberto Pellegrini, Pan American Health Organization, October 1990.

12. *New York Times,* October 19, 1989, A19.

13. *Granma Weekly Review,* August 20, 1989, 1.

14. *Granma,* October 16, 1986.

15. *Granma Weekly Review,* May 10, 1987, 9.

16. *Granma Weekly Review,* June 22, 1986, 3. The Reagan administration tightened the economic embargo against Cuba and curtailed the North American Cuban Scientific Exchange (NACSEX), which organized informal collaboration. Interview with Jon Beckwith, September 26, 1986; and *New York Times,* August 23, 1986, 3.

17. Roca, "Economic Aspects," 70.

18. On primarily military but also general civilian aid, Roca argues that costs seem to outweigh benefits; Pérez López indicates that the data are insufficient to definitively claim anything; Eckstein and Pérez López both point out benefits that Roca fails to mention. Roca, "Economic Aspects," 67–75; Jorge F. Pérez López, "Comments: Economic Costs and Benefits of African Involvement," *Cuban Studies/Estudios Cubanos* 10, no. 2 (July 1980): 80–84; and Eckstein, "Comment: The Global Political Economy," 85–90.

19. Domínguez, "Political and Military Limitations," 28.

20. *Granma Weekly Review,* November 11, 1990, 2.

21. *Granma Weekly Review,* January 25, 1987, 3. It was in fact completed in late 1988.

22. *Granma Weekly Review,* December 14, 1986, supplement, 6; and *Granma Weekly Review,* January 11, 1987, 4.

23. *Boletín Especial.* The Spanish version of this document indicates that it is not a survey, as the English title implies, but a compilation of information received from the suggestions and complaints boxes in all of the health facilities in Holguín province during the second half of 1987. The distribution of this report by an anti-Castro organization does not diminish its credibility, but its deliberately distorting nature does.

24. *Granma Weekly Review,* January 25, 1987, 3–4.

25. Ibid., 3.

26. Ibid.

27. Interviews with numerous Cubans from a range of backgrounds and in both professional positions and less skilled positions, 1978, 1979, 1980–1981, 1988, 1990, 1991, and 1992. As one person asked, "Why should I work harder to become an engineer when I can earn almost the same amount of money and work less as a skilled laborer?" A researcher said that he didn't see why he should work very hard because it wouldn't make his life any better. He claimed that it might be ten years before he and his wife could get their own apartment. He was in his mid thirties at the time of the interview. Observations of people in different work centers over time indicated a great deal of inefficiency, make-work, and chatting. This is not uncommon in many countries, particularly when job security is not an issue.

28. *Granma Weekly Review,* January 17, 1982, 1, 3.

29. Site visit and interview with Luis Herrera, November 25, 1988.

30. The Center for Genetic Engineering and Biotechnology (CIGB) researchers work an average of twelve to fourteen hours per day. Interview with Luis Herrera, November 25, 1988. Such long hours are exceptional and likely a result of both the moral and material incentives awarded to this group of young researchers working on advanced scientific research.

31. Bourne, *New Directions in International Health Cooperation,* 47.

32. Ministerio de Salud Pública, *Informe anual 1991* (La Habana: MINSAP, 1992), 37, 50, 52, 54, 67, 80. Mortality from infectious and parasitic diseases increased slightly to 10.6 per 100,000 inhabitants from 9.4. Deaths caused by diarrhea rose to 3.9 per 100,000 inhabitants from 3.5. Maternal mortality rose to 36.2 per 100,000 live births from 31.6. The percentage of infants born with low birth weight also rose slightly to 7.8 from 7.6.

Appendix

1. Servimex, Turismo de Salud Cubanacán, "Chequeos médicos 1988" (La Habana: Cubanacán, 1988) (typescript).

2. Prices from a list for internal use by Cubanacán and supplied by Ricardo E. Martinez Rojas, November 24, 1988.

3. Approximate prices from Ann Unbehaun, Department of Public Relations, University of Michigan Medical Center, Ann Arbor. Personal communication, January 31, 1989.

Selected Bibliography

Cuban government and Pan American Health Organization documents are listed in the language in which they were written. Cuban documents are listed under "Republic of Cuba" or "República de Cuba" and the name of the issuing agency, and PAHO documents are listed under "Pan American Health Organization" or "Organización Panamericana Sanitaria."

Books, Articles, Addresses, and Government Documents

Abel-Smith, Brian. "The World Economic Crisis. Part 1: Repercussions on Health." *Health Policy and Planning* 1, no. 3 (September 1986): 210–11.

Agresiones de Estados Unidos a Cuba 1787–1976. La Habana: Editorial de Ciencias Sociales, 1978.

Agrupación Católica Universitaria. "Encuesta de trabajadores rurales, 1956–1957." *Economia y desarrollo* 3, no. 12 (July–August 1972): 188–213.

Aldereguía Henriques, Jorge, and Osvaldo J. Castro Miranda. "Lo sviluppo della salute pubblica nell'esperienza cubana." *The Practitioner (Edizione Italiana)* (Milano) 103 (June 1987).

Alexander, Robin, and Pamela K. Anderson. "Pesticide Use, Alternatives and Workers' Health in Cuba." *International Journal of Health Services* 14, no. 1 (1984): 31–41.

Alvarez Alonso, Manuel, Carlos Dotres Martínez, Francisco Valdés Lazo, and Mario Callejo Hernández. "Importancia de la madre acompañante en pacientes hospitalizados." *Revista cubana de pediatría* 54, no. 5 (September–October 1982): 622–34.

Apter, David E. "Ideology and Discontent." In *Ideology and Discontent,* ed. David E. Apter, 15–46. New York: Free Press of Glencoe, 1964.

————. "The New Mytho/Logics and the Specter of Superfluous Man." *Social Research* 52, no. 2 (Summer 1985): 269–70.

Apter, David E., and Nagayo Sawa. *Against the State: Politics and Social Protest in Japan.* Cambridge, Mass.: Harvard University Press, 1984.

Arbona, Guillermo, with Annette B. Ramírez de Arellano. *Regionalization of Health Services: The Puerto Rican Experience.* Santurce, Puerto Rico: Talleres Gráficos, 1977.

Atención primaria de salud. Geneva and New York: Organización Mundial de la Salud y Fondo de las Naciones Unidos para la Infancia, 1978.

Azicri, Max. "The Institutionalization of the Cuban Revolution: A Review of the Literature." *Cuban Studies/Estudios Cubanos* 9, no. 2 (July 1979): 63–78.

Balari, Eugenio R. "Cinco Años de trabajo del Instituto Cubano de Investigaciones y Orientación de la Demanda Interna." In *Investigaciones científicas de la demanda interna en Cuba,* 3–19. Ciudad La Habana: Editorial Orbe, 1979.

Beardsley, Tim. "Cuban Biotechnology: Progress Despite Isolation." *Nature* 320 (March 6, 1986): 8.

Beckwith, Jon. "Cuba Report: Science and Society are Inseparable." *Science for the People* 17, no. 5 (September–October 1985): 20–24.

Bender, Lynn-Darrell. *Cuba vs. United States: The Politics of Hostility.* 2nd Ed. Hato Rey, Puerto Rico: Inter American University Press, 1981.

Benjamin, Jules Robert. *The United States and Cuba: Hegemony and Dependent Development.* Pittsburgh: University of Pittsburgh Press, 1977.

Benjamin, Medea, Joseph Collins, and Michael Scott. *No Free Lunch: Food and Revolution in Cuba Today.* San Francisco: Food First Books, 1984.

Bialy, Harvey. "Cuban Biotechnology: Interferon as a Model." *Bio/Technology* 4, no. 4 (April 1986): 265.

————. "Cuba to Market an Ultra-Microelisa System." *Bio/Technology* 5, no. 7 (July 1987): 663.

————. "Biotechnology and the Poor: Partnerships or More Poverty," *UNESCO/MIRCEN World Journal of Microbiology and Biotechnology* (1991).

"Biotechnology and Economic Development: Introduction," *Economic Bulletin for Europe* (Journal of the United Nations Economic Commission for Europe) 38, no. 1 (March 1986): 7.

Blasier, Cole. *The Hovering Giant: U.S. Responses to Revolutionary Change in Latin America.* Pittsburgh: University of Pittsburgh Press, 1976.

————. "The Cuban–U.S.–Soviet Triangle, Changing Angles." *Cuban Studies/Estudios Cubanos* 8, no. 1 (January 1978): 1–9.

Bohr, David F. "President-Elect's Tour: Changes in Cuba." *The Physiologist* 22, no. 1 (February 1979): 9–11.

————. "Past President's Address: The Health Market and Physiologists." *The Physiologist* 22, no. 6 (December 1979): 15–17.

Boletín Especial: A Public Survey on the Quality of Health Care in the Province of Holguín, Cuba. A confidential report by the Cuban Communist party. Washington, D.C.: Cuban American National Foundation, 1988.

Bourdieu, Pierre. "The Social Space and the Genesis of Groups." *Theory and Society* 14, no. 6 (November 1985): 723–44.

————. *Outline of a Theory of Practice.* Cambridge: Cambridge University Press, 1987.

Bourne, Peter. *New Directions in International Health Cooperation.* Washington, D.C.: the White House, spring 1978.

Boyd, Edmond, "Castro Remodels the System." *Canadian Medical Association Journal* 111 (November 2, 1974): 991–1002.

"Brasil: Ministro de salud critica duramente a Cuba." EFE wire service. December 11, 1990.

Brenner, Phillip. *From Confrontation to Negotiation: U.S. Relations with Cuba.* Boulder, Colo.: Westview Press, 1988.

Brownlie, Ian, comp. *Basic Documents on Human Rights.* Oxford: Clarendon Press, 1971.

Brundenius, Claes. *Revolutionary Cuba: The Challenge of Economic Growth with Equity.* Boulder, Colo.: Westview Press, 1984.

Brundenius, Claes, and Andrew Zimbalist. "Cubanology and Cuban Economic Performance." In *Cuban Political Economy: Controversies in Cubanology,* edited by Andrew Zimbalist, 39–65. Boulder, Colo.: Westview Press, 1988.

Campos-Outcalt, Douglas, and Edward Janoff. "Health Care in Modern Cuba." *The Western Journal of Medicine* 132 (March 1980): 265–71.

Capote Mir, Roberto E. "La evolución de los servicios de salud y la estructura socioeconómica en Cuba." Parts 1, 2. *Revista cubana de administración de salud* 5 (April–June 1979): 107–17; (July–August 1979): 225–53.

————. "La evolución de los servicios de salud y la estructura socioeconómica en Cuba." La Habana: Instituto de Desarrollo de la Salud, 1979 (mimeographed).

————. "La evolución de los servicios de salud y la estructura socioeconómica en Cuba." *Saúde em debate* (Rio de Janeiro), 14 (1982): 53.

Castro Miranda, Osvaldo. "Situación actual y perspectiva de la salud pública en Cuba." *Revista cubana de administración de salud* 7, no. 2 (1981): 101–18.

————. "Recursos humanos en salud en Cuba." *Educación médica y salud* (Washington, D.C.: PAHO) 20, no. 3 (1986): 375–81.

Castro Ruz, Fidel. *History Will Absolve Me.* Havana: Guairas Book Institute, 1967.

————. *2nd Period of Sessions of the National Assembly of People's Power. Closing Speech.* La Habana: Political Publishers, 1978.

Centro de Ingeniería Genética y Biotecnología. *Products Catalog, January 1990.* La Habana: CIGB and Heber Biotec, 1990.

Challenor, Bernard. "Health and Economic Development: The Example of China and Cuba." *Medical Care* 13, no. 1 (January 1975): 79–84.

Christmas-Möller, Wilhelm. "Some Thoughts on the Scientific Applicability of the Small State Concept: A Research History and a Discussion." In *Small States in Europe and Dependence.* The Laxenburg Papers, edited by Otmar Höll, 35–53. Boulder, Colo.: Westview Press, 1983.

"Cifras de médicos de la familia, según el lugar donde prestan sus servicios, desglosadas por provincias. Noviembre de 1987." *Revista cubana de medicina general integral* 4, no. 1 January–March 1988): 78.

Cira García Clinic, Havana. Daily patient register. November 25, 1988.

Clarke, Robin. *The Silent Weapons.* New York: David McKay, 1968.

Cookson, John, and Judith Nottingham. *A Survey of Chemical and Biological Warfare.* London: Sheed and Ward, 1971.

Crain, Irving J. "Psychiatry in Cuba." U.S.–Cuba Health Exchange, occasional paper, 1978.

Cuban Committee for Human Rights. *Political Executions and Human Rights in Cuba. Annual Report, December 10, 1987.* Washington, D.C.: Of Human Rights (Georgetown University), 1988.

"Cuban-made Interferon Reaches Out for World Markets." *Biotechnology Newswatch* 6, no. 6 (March 17, 1986): 3–4.

Danielson, Ross. "Cuban Health Care in Process: Models and Morality in the Early Revolution." In *Topias and Utopias in Health,* edited by Stanley R. Ingman and Anthony E. Thomas, 307–34. The Hague: Mouton, 1975.

———. *Cuban Medicine.* New Brunswick, N.J.: Transaction Books, 1979.

———. "Medicine in the Community: The Ideology and Substance of Community Medicine in Socialist Cuba." *Social Science and Medicine* 15C (1981): 239–47.

Dea, Marilee. "An American PNP in Cuba." *Pediatric Nursing* 6, no. 5 (September–October 1980): 51–53.

Dembo, David, Clarence J. Dias, and Ward Morehouse. "The Vital Nexus in Biotechnology: The Relationship Between Research and Production and Its Implications for Latin America." *Interciencia* 14, no. 4 (July–August 1989): 168–80.

Díaz-Briquets, Sergio. *The Health Revolution in Cuba.* Austin, Tex.: University of Texas Press, 1983.

———. "How To Figure Out Cuba: Development, Ideology and Mortality." *Caribbean Review* 15, no. 2 (Spring 1986): 8–11, 39–42.

Díaz-Briquets, Sergio, and Lisandro Pérez. "Cuba: The Demography of Revolution." *Population Bulletin* 36, no. 1 (April 1981).

Díaz Ravelo, Margarita, Olga Isla Bauza, and Teolinda Pérez Abreu Suárez. "Desarrollo de la colaboración económica científica técnica de Cuba con Iraq hasta 1987," Tésis de grado, Instituto de Colaboración Económica (La Habana), 1988.

Díaz-Vázquez, Julio. "Cuba: colaboración económica y científico-técnica con paises en vías de desarrollo de Africa, Asia, y América Latina." *Economía y desarrollo,* no. 68 (May–June 1982): 27–43.

Domínguez, Jorge I. *Cuba: Order and Revolution*. Cambridge, Mass.: Belknap Press, 1978.

———. "Cuban Foreign Policy." *Foreign Affairs* 57 (Fall 1978): 83–108.

———. "Political and Military Limitations and Consequences of Cuba's Policies in Africa." *Cuban Studies/Estudios Cubanos* 10, no. 2 (July 1980): 1–35.

———. "Cuba: Domestic Bread and Foreign Circuses." In *Cuban Communism*. 5th ed., edited by Irving Louis Horowitz, 475–85. New Brunswick, N.J.: Transaction Books, 1985.

———. "Cuba in the 1980s." *Foreign Affairs* 65, no. 1 (Fall 1986): 118–35.

———. "U.S.–Cuban Relations in the Mid-1980s." In *Cuban Communism*. 6th ed., edited by Irving Louis Horowitz, 473–88. New Brunswick, N.J.: Transaction Books, 1987.

———. *To Make a World Safe for Revolution: Cuban Foreign Policy,* Cambridge Mass.: Harvard University Press, 1989.

Domínguez, Jorge I., and Juan Lindau. "The Primacy of Politics: Comparing the Foreign Policies of Cuba and Mexico." In *How Foreign Policy Decisions Are Made In The Third World,* edited by Bahgat Kornay, 113–37. Boulder, Colo.: Westview Press, 1986.

Donahue, John M. *The Nicaraguan Revolution in Health*. South Hadley, Mass.: Bergin and Garvey, 1986.

Drew, Elizabeth. "Letter from Washington," *New Yorker,* July 4, 1988, 77; October 31, 1988, 102.

Duncan, W. Raymond. *The Soviet Union and Cuba: Interests and Influence*. New York: Praeger, 1985.

Durkheim, Emile. *The Elementary Forms of Religious Life*. New York: Free Press, 1954.

Eberstadt, Nicholas. "Did Fidel Fudge the Figures? Literacy and Health: The Cuba Model." *Caribbean Review* 15, no. 2 (Spring 1986): 5–7, 37–38.

Eckstein, Susan. "Capitalist Constraints on Cuban Socialist Development." *Comparative Politics* 12, no. 3 (April 1980): 253–74.

———. "Comment: The Global Political Economy and Cuba's African Involvement." *Cuban Studies/Estudios Cubanos* 10, no. 2 (July 1980): 85–90.

———. "Structural and Ideological Bases of Cuba's Overseas Programs." *Politics and Society* 11 (1982): 95–121.

———. "Cuban Internationalism." In *Cuba: Twenty-Five Years of Revolution, 1959–1984,* edited by Sandor Halebsky and John M. Kirk, 372–90. New York: Praeger, 1985.

———. "Why Cuban Internationalism?" In *Cuban Political Economy: Controversies in Cubanology,* edited by Andrew Zimbalist, 154–81. Boulder, Colo.: Westview Press, 1988.

———. "The Rectification of Errors or the Errors of the Rectification Process of Cuba?" *Cuban Studies* 20 (1990): 67–86.

"Encuestas de los servicios externos." Clínica Estomatológica "Elpidio Berovides," La Lisa Municipality, Havana, n.d. [In use on March 11, 1981.]

"Entire Cuban Population To Be Tested For AIDS, Official Says." *Cuba Update* 8, nos. 5–6 (Winter 1987): 10.

Erisman, H. Michael. *Cuba's International Relations: The Anatomy of a Nationalistic Foreign Policy.* Boulder, Colo.: Westview Press, 1985.

Escalona Reguera, Mario. "Panel informativo; 'La medicina en la comunidad,' 'El policlínico': presente y futuro." In *Medicina en la comunidad,* 22–34. Havana: MINSAP, 1975.

———. "El policlínico integral." La Habana: Instituto de Desarrollo de la Salud, 1980 (mimeographed).

———. "El sistema nacional de salud en Cuba." In *Teorías y administración de salud,* 100–111. Havana: MINSAP, 1980.

———. "La medicina en la comunidad." In *Teorías y administración de salud,* 112–23. Havana: MINSAP, 1980.

———. *La participación popular en la salud.* La Habana: MINSAP, Instituto de Desarrollo de la Salud, 1980.

Estado Libre Asociado de Puerto Rico. Oficina del Gobernador. Junta de Planificación. *Compendio estadísticas sociales 1981.* San Juan: Junta de Planificación, October 1982.

Fagen, Richard R. *The Transformation of Political Culture in Cuba.* Stanford, Calif.: Stanford University Press, 1969.

Falcoff, Mark. "How to Think about Cuban-American Relations." In *Cuban Communism.* 6th ed., edited by Irving Louis Horowitz, 542–53. New Brunswick, N.J.: Transaction Books, 1987.

Falk, Pamela S. "Cuba's Foreign and Domestic Policies, 1968–78: The Effect of International Commitments on Internal Development." Ph.D. diss., New York University, 1980.

———. *Cuban Foreign Policy: Caribbean Tempest.* Lexington, Mass.: Lexington Books, 1986.

———. "Cuba in Africa." *Foreign Affairs* 65, no. 5 (Summer 1987): 1077–96.

FAO, OMS, PMA, PNUD, UNESCO, "Informe de las agencias de las Naciones Unidas representadas en Cuba," November 1989 (typescript).

"Feeding the People." *Cuba Review,* 6 (December 1976).

Feinsilver, Julie M. "Cuba as a 'World Medical Power': The Politics of Symbolism." *Latin American Research Review* 24, no. 2 (Spring 1989): 1–34.

———. "Symbolic Politics and Health Policy: Cuba as a 'World Medical Power,'" Ph.D. diss., Yale University, 1989.

———. "Will Cuba's Wonder Drugs Lead To Political and Economic Wonders? Capitalizing on Biotechnology and Medical Exports." *Cuban Studies* 22 (1992): 79–111.

Felipe, Edith. "Cuba y la colaboración económica con el mundo subdesarrollado." *Temas de la economía mundial* 15 (1985): 81–106.

Fernández, Damián J. *Cuba's Foreign Policy in the Middle East.* Boulder, Colo.: Westview Press, 1988.

Field, Mark G. *Soviet Socialized Medicine: An Introduction.* New York: Free Press, 1967.

Figueras, Miguel Alejandro. *Análisis de las políticas de industrialización en Cuba en el periodo revolucionario y proyecciones futuras.* La Habana: Universidad de La Habana, Centro de Investigaciones de la Economía Internacional, February 1990.

————. "Cuba en los 80: retos económicos para los 90." Draft manuscript, June 19, 1991.

"Five Year Update, 1984–1989." *Biotechnology Newswatch* 9, no. 4 (February 20, 1989): 4.

Forster, Nancy, and Howard Handelman. "Food Production and Distribution in Cuba: The Impact of the Revolution." In *Food, Politics, and Society in Latin America,* edited by John C. Super and Thomas C. Wright. Lincoln, Nebraska: University of Nebraska Press, 1985.

Foucault, Michel. *The Order of Things: An Archaeology of the Human Sciences.* New York: Vintage Books, 1973.

Fox, Jeffrey L. "Cuba Plans a Century of Biology." *American Society of Microbiology* 52, no. 5 (1986): 243–48.

Franqui, Carlos. *Diary of the Cuban Revolution.* New York: Viking Press, 1980.

Galaz Góngora, Robna R. et. al. "Análisis de las actividades del policlínico integral docente 'Plaza de la Revolución.'" Trabajo en equipo, Asignatura: Administración de Salud del Curso Internacional de Salud Pública. La Habana: Instituto de Desarrollo de la Salud, March 1979.

Galiano Jorda, Mireya, and Maria Elena Noriega Almora. "Colaboración técnica con Tanzania, 1987–1988." Proyecto de grado, Centro Nacional de Capacitación Técnica (La Habana), 1988.

García Rodríguez, José, Raúl Mazorra Zamora, and Omar Morell Rodríguez. "Plan de actividades físicas que debe realizar el médico de la familia." *Revista cubana de medicina integral* 3, no. 1 (1987): 109–12.

Garfield, Richard M., and Giorgio Solimano. "Health and Revolution in Latin America: An Analysis of Historical Experiences in Chile, Cuba, and Nicaragua." New York, n.d. [probably 1986] (typescript).

Gilpin, Margaret, and Helen Rodríguez-Trias. "Looking at Health in a Healthy Way." *Cuba Review* 7, no. 1 (March 1978).

Goldstein, Daniel J. "Molecular Biology and National Security." In *Seeds and Sovereignty,* edited by Jack Kloppenburg, Jr. Durham, N.C.: Duke University Press, 1987.

————. *Biotecnología, universidad y política.* Mexico: Siglo veintiuno editores, 1989.

————. "A biotechnology agenda for the Third World." *Journal of Agricultural Ethics* 2 (1989): 37–51.

————. "Latin American Pseudobiotechnology: A Pathway to Underdevelopment, Misery, and More Trade Deficit." Paper presented at international conference, "Biotechnology and International Trade: 1992 and Beyond." Maastricht, the Netherlands, June 20–22, 1990.

————. "The Strategic Meaning of Structural Molecular Biology in Biotechnology: X-Ray Crystallography, Nuclear Magnetic Resonance and Protein and Nucleic Acid Engineering." 1990.

Golladay, Fredrick, and Bernhard Lierse. *Health Problems and Policies in the Developing Countries.* World Bank Staff working paper no. 412. Washington, D.C.: World Bank, August 1980.

Gómez, Manuel R. "Occupational Health in Cuba." *American Journal of Public Health* 71, no. 5 (May 1981): 520–24.

González, Septimio, et al. "Descripción y análisis del sistema de atención primaria en el policlínico integral docente 'Plaza de la Revolución.'" La Habana: Instituto de Desarrollo de la Salud, práctica-docente en la asignatura de Administración de Servicios de Salud, December 1978.

González Pacheco, Mario. "Informe de viaje 27–31 mayo de 1989." Washington, D.C.: Pan American Health Organization internal document [unnumbered], n.d.

González Trueba, Gerardo. "Política científica y biotecnología en Cuba: 5a curso de planificación de C & T en América Latina." La Habana: March 1991 (unpublished typescript).

Gordon, Antonio M., Jr. "The Nutriture of Cubans: Historical Perspective and Nutritional Analysis." Cuban Studies/Estudios Cubanos 13, no. 2 (Summer 1983): 1–34.

Granda Mir, Ana María. "2a industria de equipos médicos en Cuba. Estado actual y perspectivas." Instituto Superior de Relaciones Internacionales, Trabajo de diploma, La Habana, November 1989.

Grundy, Paul H., and Peter P. Budetti. "The Distribution and Supply of Cuban Medical Personnel in Third World Countries." American Journal of Public Health 70, no. 7 (July 1980): 717–19.

Guerra de Macedo, Carlyle. "Discurso pronunciado en la sesión inaugural de la conferencia Salud Para Todos." La Habana, July 3–9, 1983.

Gutiérrez Muñiz, José, José Camaros Fabián, José Cobas Manríquez, and Rachelle Hertenberg. "The Recent Worldwide Economic Crisis and the Welfare of Children: The Case of Cuba." World Development 12, no. 3 (March 1984): 247–60.

Guttmacher, Sally, and Ross Danielson. "Changes in Cuban Health Care: An Argument Against Technological Pessimism." International Journal of Health Services 7, no. 3 (1977): 383–99.

Guttmacher, Sally, and Lourdes García. "Social Science and Health in Cuba: Ideology, Planning, and Health." In Topias and Utopias in Health, edited by Stanley R. Ingman and Anthony E. Thomas, 507–22. The Hague: Mouton, 1975.

Hamberg, Jill. Under Construction: Housing Policy in Revolutionary Cuba. New York: Center for Cuban Studies, 1986.

Handelman, Howard. "Cuban Food Policy and Popular Nutritional Levels." Cuban Studies/Estudios Cubanos 11, no. 2, 12, no. 1 (July 1981–January 1982): 127–46.

———. "Comment—The Nutriture of Cubans." Cuban Studies/Estudios Cubanos 13, no. 2 (Summer 1983): 35–37.

Harnecker, Marta. Cuba: los protagonistas de un nuevo poder. La Habana: Editorial Ciencias Sociales, 1979.

Hatcher, Gordon, Peter R. Hatcher, and Eleanor C. Hatcher. "Health Services in Canada." In Comparative Health Systems. Descriptive Analyses of Fourteen National Health Systems, edited by Marshall W. Raffel. University Park, Pa.: Pennsylvania State University Press, 1984.

Hernández Elias, Roberto. "Desarrollo de la salud pública en Cuba." In Teoría y administración de salud, 53–69. La Habana: MINSAP, 1980.

————. "Princípios de la salud pública socialista." In *Teoría y administración de salud,* 23–30. La Habana: MINSAP, 1980.

Hersh, Seymour. *Chemical and Biological Warfare: America's Hidden Arsenal.* Indianapolis: Bobbs-Merrill, 1968.

Hicks, Norman, and Paul Streeten. "Indicators of Development: The Search for a Basic Needs Yardstick." *World Development* 7 (1979): 567–80.

Hill, Kenneth. "An Evaluation of Cuban Demographic Statistics, 1938–1980." Quoted in Paula E. Hollerbach and Sergio Díaz-Briquets, *Fertility Determinants in Cuba.* Washington, D.C.: National Academy Press, 1983.

Hinckle, Warren, and William W. Turner. *The Fish Is Red: The Story of the Secret War Against Castro.* New York: Harper and Row, 1981.

Holden, Constance. "Health Care in the Soviet Union." *Science* 213, September 4, 1981, 1090–92.

Höll, Otmar. "Towards a Broadening of the Small States Perspective." In *Small States in Europe and Dependence.* The Laxenburg Papers, edited by Otmar Höll, 13–31. Boulder, Colo.: Westview Press, 1983.

Hollerbach, Paula E. "Recent Trends in Fertility, Abortion, and Contraception in Cuba." New York: The Population Council, Center for Policy Studies, working paper no. 61, August 1980.

————. "Determinants of Fertility Decline in Postrevolutionary Cuba." In *Fertility Decline in 28 Countries,* edited by W. Parker Mauldin for the Population Council, 1981 (unpublished manuscript).

Hollerbach, Paula E., and Sergio Díaz-Briquets. *Fertility Determinants in Cuba.* Washington, D.C.: National Academy Press, 1983.

Horn, Joshua S. *Away with All Pests: An English Surgeon in People's China, 1954–1969.* New York: Monthly Review Press, 1969.

Hu, Teh-wei. "Health Services in the People's Republic of China." In *Comparative Health Systems: Descriptive Analyses of Fourteen National Health Systems,* edited by Marshall W. Raffel, 133–52. University Park, Pa.: Pennsylvania State University Press, 1984.

Huberman, Leo, and Paul M. Sweezy. *Socialism in Cuba.* New York: Monthly Review Press, 1969.

Hyde, Gordon. *The Soviet Health Service: A Historical and Comparative Study.* London: Lawrence and Wishart, 1974.

Illizastigui Dupuy, Fidel. *La educación médica superior y las necesidades de salud de la población.* La Habana: MINSAP, 1988.

Institute for Policy Studies. *Preliminary Report of U.S. Delegation to Cuba. Institute for Policy Studies-National Union of Cuban Jurists. Joint Commission on the Conviction and Treatment of Prisoners in the United States and Cuba. February 26–March 5, 1988.* Washington, D.C.: Institute for Policy Studies, March 1988 (typescript).

Jiménez de la Jara, Jorge, ed. *Medicina social en Chile.* Santiago, Chile: Ediciones Aconcagua, 1977.

Jiménez Fontao, Lilliam, and Mayra Zaldívar Lores. "Experiencia del médico de la familia en un consultorio de Plaza de la Revolución." *Revista cubana de medicina general integral* 3, no. 1 (1987): 135.

Judson, C. Fred. *Cuba and the Revolutionary Myth: The Political Educa-tion of the Cuban Rebel Army, 1953–1963.* Boulder, Colo.: Westview Press, 1984.

———. "Continuity and Evolution of Revolutionary Symbolism in *Verde Olivo.*" In *Cuba: Twenty-Five Years of Revolution,* edited by Sandor Halebsky and John M. Kirk, 233–50. New York: Praeger, 1985.

Kaiser, Irwin. "Obstetrics in Cuba, 1974." *Obstetrics and Gynecology* 49, no. 6 (June 1977): 709–14.

Kaser, Michael. *Health Care in the Soviet Union and Eastern Europe.* Boulder, Colo.: Westview Press, 1976.

Kay, Bonnie J. "Delivery of Health Care Services in Cuba." *Journal of the Medical Association of Georgia* 68 (February 1979): 99–100.

Knudsen, Odin K. *Economics of Supplemental Feeding of Malnourished Children: Leakages, Costs, and Benefits.* World Bank Staff working paper no. 451. Washington, D.C.: World Bank, April 1981.

Lampton, David M. *Health, Conflict, and the Chinese Political System.* Ann Arbor, Mich.: Center for Chinese Studies, University of Michigan, 1974.

"La participación activa de la comunidad en Cuba." Panel Discussion at 2nd International Seminar on Primary Health Care, Havana, November 14–18, 1988.

Ledo Duarte, Sergio R. "Participación popular en salud." *Revista cubana de administración de salud* 10, no. 3 (July–September 1984): 220–25.

LeoGrande, William M. "Cuban-Soviet Relations and Cuban Policy in Africa." *Cuban Studies/Estudios Cubanos* 10, no. 1 (January 1980): 1–37.

———. "Cuba and Nicaragua: From the Somozas to the Sandinistas." In *The New Cuban Presence in the Caribbean,* edited by Barry B. Levine, 43–58. Boulder, Colo.: Westview Press, 1983.

Levesque, Jacques. *The USSR and the Cuban Revolution: Soviet Ideological and Strategic Perspectives, 1959–1977.* New York: Praeger, 1978.

Leyva, Ricardo. "Health and Revolution in Cuba." In *Cuba in Revolution,* edited by Rolando E. Bonachea and Nelson P. Valdés, 456–96. New York: Anchor Books, 1972.

MacDonald, Scott B., and F. Joseph Demetrius. "The Caribbean Sugar Crisis: Consequences and Challenges." *Journal of Interamerican Studies and World Affairs* 28, no. 1 (Spring 1986): 35–58.

Mahler, Halfdan. "Discurso pronunciado en la sesión inaugural de la conferencia Salud para todos: 25 años de experiencia cubana." La Habana, July 3–9, 1983.

Marshall, Alex. "From Cuba: Health Care the Envy of Developing World." *Medical Tribune* 29, no. 27 (September 1988): 2, 22.

Martin, Sarah. "Busman's Holiday in Cuba." *Nursing Mirror* (Surrey, England) 153, no. 20 (November 11, 1981): 36–38.

Martínez Salsamendi, Carlos. "El papel de Cuba en el tercer mundo: América Central, El Caribe y Africa." In *Cuba y Estados Unidos: Un debate para la convivencia,* comp. Juan Gabriel Tokatlian, 125–98. Buenos Aires: Grupo Editor Latinoamericano, 1984.

Marx, Karl. "The German Ideology." In *The Marx-Engels Reader,* edited by Robert C. Tucker, 110–64. New York: Norton, 1972.

———. "Theses on Feuerbach." In *The Marx-Engels Reader,* edited by Robert C. Tucker, 107–9. New York: Norton, 1972.

Mathéy, Kosta. "Recent Trends in Cuban Housing Policies and the Revival of the Microbrigade Movement." *Bulletin of Latin American Research* 8, no. 1 (1989): 68.

Mathias, Sen. Charles, Jr. Quoted in *Center for Peace and Conflict Studies/ Detroit Council for World Affairs Newsletter,* Spring 1985, 2.

McKeown, Thomas. "Determinants of Health." *Human Nature* (April 1978): 60–67.

Mejía, Alfonso, Helena Pizurki, and Erica Royston. *Foreign Medical Graduates: The Case of the United States.* Lexington, Mass.: Lexington Books, 1980.

"Meningitis B Vaccine." *Cuba Business.* London: 4, no. 1 (February 1990).

Mesa-Lago, Carmelo. *Cuba in the 1970s: Pragmatism and Institutionalization.* Revised edition. Albuquerque: University of New Mexico Press, 1978.

———. "Cuban Statistics Revisited." Parts 1, 2. *Cuban Studies/Estudios Cubanos* 9, no. 2 (July 1979): 59–62; 10, 1 (January 1980): 99.

———. *The Economy of Socialist Cuba: A Two-Decade Appraisal.* Albuquerque: University of New Mexico Press, 1981.

———. "Financing Health Care in Latin America and the Caribbean With a Special Study of Costa Rica." World Bank Population, Health and Nutrition Department. Washington, D.C., March 1983 (Typescript).

Mesa-Lago, Carmelo, and June S. Belkin, eds. *Cuba in Africa.* Pittsburgh: University of Pittsburgh Press, 1982.

Millard, L. Frances. "Health Care in Poland: From Crisis to Crisis." *International Journal of Health Services* 12, no. 3 (1982): 497–515.

Miller, C. Arden, E. J. Coulter, A. Fine, S. Adams-Taylor, and L. B. Schorr. "Update on the 1984 World Economic Crisis and Children: A United States Case Study." *International Journal of Health Services* 15, no. 3 (1985): 431–50.

Miller, C., E. J. Coulter, L. B. Schorr, A. Fine, and S. Adams-Taylor. "The World Economic Crisis and the Children: United States Case Study." *International Journal of Health Services* 15, no. 1 (1985): 95–134.

Miller, Julie Ann. "Cuba's Commitment to Genetic Engineering Grows in Size and Scope." *Genetic Engineering News* (May 1986): 22.

———. "For Cuba, the Key Is Bioresearch." *Chemical Week* (May 7, 1986): 71–2.

Montaner, Carlos Alberto. "The Roots of Anti-Americanism in Cuba: Sovereignty in an Age of World Cultural Homogeneity." *Caribbean Review* 13, no. 2 (Spring 1984): 13–16, 42–46.

Morens, David M., John P. Woodall, and Raúl H. López-Correa. "Dengue in American Children of the Caribbean." *Journal of Pediatrics* 93, no. 6 (December 1978): 1049–51.

Moser, Steven Aker. "The Right to Health: A Comparative Study of the Health Care Systems of the United States, Sweden, and Cuba." Ph.D. diss., University of South Carolina, 1980.

Navarro, Vicente. "Health, Health Services, and Health Planning in Cuba." *International Journal of Health Services* 2, no. 3 (August 1972): 397–432.

————. "Health Services in Cuba." *New England Journal of Medicine* 287, no. 19 (November 9, 1972): 954–59.

————. *Social Security and Medicine in the USSR: A Marxist Critique.* Lexington, Mass.: Lexington Books, 1977.

Oppenheimer, Andres. *Castro's Final Hour: The Secret Story behind the Coming Downfall of Communist Cuba.* New York: Simon and Schuster, 1992.

Ordóñez Carceller, Cosme. "La medicina en la comunidad." In *Medicina en la comunidad.* La Habana: MINSAP, 1976.

————. "Organización de la atención médica en la comunidad." *Revista cubana de administración de salud* 2, no. 2 (April–June, 1976): 141–52.

Organización Mundial de la Salud y Fondo de las Naciones Unidas para la Infancia. *Atención primaria de salud. Informe conjunto del director general de la Organización Mundial de la Salud y del director ejecutivo del Fondo de las Naciones Unidas para la Infancia.* Conferencia internacional sobre atención primaria de salud, Alma-Ata (URSS), September 6–12, 1978. Geneva: OMS, 1978.

Organización Panamericana de la Salud. *Informe sobre medicina familiar.* Washington, D.C.: OPS, April 1984.

————. "Lineamientos para la ejecución de la cooperación de OPS/OMS en Cuba 1991." Internal document, La Habana: OPS/OMS, January 1991.

Organización Panamericana de la Salud, Programa Ampliado de Inmunización. *PAI boletín informativo* vol. 2, no. 6 (December 1980), 5; vol. 3, no. 5 (October 1981), 5.

Organización Panamericana Sanitaria. "Cooperación técnica de la OPS/OMS: Desarrollo de servicios de salud." Internal document URU/DHS/010/P2, November 16, 1987.

————. "Reunión operativa interpaises OPS/OMS en cooperación técnica entre paises (CTPD/CTP) en el contexto del presupuesto programa de la OPS/OMS 1990–1991." La Habana: November 1989.

Organización Panamericana Sanitaria, Programa de las Naciones Unidas para el Desarrollo, y Sistema Económico Latinoamericano. "Encuentro de cooperación técnica entre paises latinoamericanos y del caribe para el desarrollo tecnológico en salud. Propuesta del trabajo." Santiago, Chile: OPS/OMS-PNUD-SELA, August 24, 1990.

Organization for Economic Co-Operation and Development. *Development Co-Operation 1990 Report.* Paris: OECD, 1990.

Organization of American States. *The Situation of Human Rights in Cuba.* Seventh report. Washington, D.C.: OAS, 1983.

Orris, Peter. "The Role of the Consumer in the Cuban National Health System." M.P.H. thesis, Yale University, 1978.

O'Shaughnessy, Hugh. *Grenada.* New York: Dodd, Mead, 1984.

"The Outlook for Cuban Production and Exports," *F. O. Lichts International Sugar and Sweetener Report* (Germany) 123, no. 32 (October 28, 1991): 531–36.

Pan American Health Organization. *Health Conditions in the Americas,* annual reports 1957–1990. Washington, D.C.: PAHO, 1962–1991.

———. *Community Participation in Health and Development in the Americas: An Analysis of Selected Case Studies.* Washington, D.C.: PAHO Scientific Publication no. 473, 1984.

———. *Evaluation of the Strategy for Health for All by the Year 2000: Seventh Report on the World Health Situation. Volume 3: Region of the Americas.* Washington, D.C.: Pan American Health Organization, 1986.

———. Internal document HSP/84/242/88, April 6, 1988.

———. Internal document, "Informe de viaje. Cuba, 24/6–8/7/88," July 1988.

———. Internal document DRC/ICP/RPD-020–534–89, May 10, 1989.

———. Internal document, HSD/BIO program, May 1989.

———. Internal document HSD/MGP/92.18, August 17, 1989.

———. Internal document HSP-C/28/2CUB, December 1990.

Pan American Sanitary Bureau. *Summary of Four Year Reports on Health Conditions in the Americas 1953–1956.* Scientific Publication no. 40. Washington, D.C.: PSB, June 1958.

Panisset, Ulysses B. "Health Diplomacy in Latin America: A Case Study of Health Technology Cooperation between Brazil and Cuba." 1989 (manuscript).

———. "Informe de viaje. Cuba, 24/6–8/7/88." Washington, D.C.: Pan American Health Organization, internal document, 1988 (typescript).

Parmelee, Donna E., Gail Henderson, and Myron S. Cohen. "Medicine under Socialism: Some Observations on Yugoslavia and China." *Social Science and Medicine* 16, no. 15 (1982): 1389–96.

Partido Comunista de Cuba. *Programa del partido comunista de Cuba.* La Habana: Editora Política, 1987.

Pastor, Robert A. "Cuba and the Soviet Union: Does Cuba Act Alone?" In *The New Cuban Presence in the Caribbean,* edited by Barry B. Levine, 191–210. Boulder, Colo.: Westview Press, 1983.

Payer, Cheryl. "The World Bank: A New Role in the Debt Crisis?" *Third World Quarterly* 8, no. 2 (April 1986): 658–76.

Pérez, Silvia N. "La participación de Cuba en la comunidad socialista y su ejemplo para el Tercer Mundo." In *Cuba y Estados Unidos: un debate para la convivencia,* comp. Juan Gabriel Tokatlian, 111–26. Buenos Aires: Grupo Editor Latinoamericano, 1984.

Pérez López, Jorge F. "Comments: Economic Costs and Benefits of African Involvement." *Cuban Studies/Estudios Cubanos* 10, no. 2 (July 1980): 80–84.

———. "Nuclear Power in Cuba after Chernobyl." *Journal of Interamerican Studies and World Affairs* 29, no. 2 (Summer 1987): 79–117.

————. "Cuban-Soviet Sugar Trade: Prices and Subsidy Issues." *Bulletin of Latin American Research* 7, no. 1 (1988): 123–47.

————. *The Economics of Cuban Sugar.* Pittsburgh: University of Pittsburgh Press, 1991.

Pfefferman, Guy P. "Some Economic Aspects of Human Development in Latin America (with Special Emphasis on Education)." In *Poverty and the Development of Human Resources: Regional Perspectives,* 175–93. Washington, D.C.: World Bank, July 1980.

Pharmaceutical Business News. The Financial Times. London: April 13, 1990.

A Pyrrhic Military Victory and a Profound Moral Defeat. Havana: Editorial Política, 1983. Cited in C. Fred Judson, "Continuity and Evolution of Revolutionary Symbolism in *Verde Olivo,*" in Sandor Halebsky and John M. Kirk, eds., *Cuba: Twenty-Five Years of Revolution.* New York: Praeger, 1985.

Raffel, Norma K. "Health Services in the Union of Soviet Socialist Republics." In *Comparative Health Systems: Descriptive Analyses of Fourteen National Health Services,* edited by Marshall W. Raffel, 488–519. University Park, Pa.: Pennsylvania State University Press, 1984.

Ramírez, Abelardo. "El médico de la familia: una experiencia cubana." Address by Vice Minister of Health for Medical Care at the 2nd International Seminar on Primary Health Care, Havana, November 15, 1988.

Ramírez López, Estela et al. "Conocimiento de una comunidad urbana a través del Policlínico Comunitario Docente 'Plaza de la Revolución.'" La Habana: Instituto de Desarrollo de la Salud, Trabajo en equipo, October 21, 1978.

"Recombinant alpha-2 IFN Cloned in Havana, Faces Animal Testing, Questions." *Newswatch,* March 17, 1986, 4.

Reed, Gail. "Eyesight to the Blind: Promising Treatment for Retinitis Pigmentosa," *Cuba Update* 12, no. 3 (Summer 1991): 22.

Republic of Cuba, Ministry of Public Health. *Annual Report of the Minister of Public Health 1986.* Havana: MINSAP, 1987.

República de Cuba. *Constitución.* La Habana: Departamento de Orientación Revolucionaria del Comité Central del Partido Comunista de Cuba, 1976.

————. *Informe del Gobierno de Cuba a la Organización Panamericana de Salud sobre las condiciones de salud pública y los adelantos logrados en el intervalo transcurrido entre la XXI y XXII Conferencias Sanitarias Panamericanas.* Washington, D.C.: Organización Panamericana de Salud, September 1986.

República de Cuba, Comité Estatal de Estadísticas. *Guía Estadística 1985.* La Habana: Comité Estatal de Estadísticas, 1986.

————. *Anuario Estadístico de Cuba 1988.* La Habana: Comité Estatal de Estadísticas, 1989.

————. *Anuario estadístico de Cuba 1989.* La Habana: Comité Estatal de Estadísticas, 1991.

República de Cuba, Comité Estatal de Estadísticas, Dirección de Demografía. *Encuesta demográfica nacional de 1979. Metodología y tablas se-*

leccionadas. Parte 1. La Habana: Comité Estatal de Estadísticas, April 1981.

República de Cuba, Comité Estatal de Estadísticas, Dirección de Demografía, Oficina Nacional del Censo. *Censo de población y viviendas de 1981,* vol. 16, tomo 1. La Habana: Comité Estatal de Estadísticas, July 1983.

República de Cuba, Ministerio de Salud Pública. *Subdesarrollo económico principal enemigo de la salud: como lo combate la revolución cubana. 19 meses de labor del MINSAP.* La Habana: Ministerio de Salud Pública, n.d. [probably late 1961].

————. *Diez años de revolución en salud pública.* Havana: Editorial Ciencias Sociales, 1969.

————. *Política de salud período 1974–1980.* La Habana: Ministerio de Salud Pública, 1974.

————. *Cuba. La salud en la revolución.* La Habana: Editorial Orbe, 1975.

————. *Informe anual.* Each year, 1976–1991. La Habana: Ministerio de Salud Pública, 1976–1992.

————. *Fundamentación para un nuevo enfoque de la medicina en la comunidad.* La Habana: Ministerio de Salud Pública, 1977.

————. *Salud para todos: 25 años de experiencia cubana.* La Habana: Ministerio de Salud Pública, July 9, 1983.

————. *Para tu salud, corre o camina, educación para tu salud.* Havana: Editorial Científico-Técnica, 1983.

————. *Programa de desarrollo 2000: Medicina interna.* La Habana: Editorial Ciencias Médicas, 1987.

————. *Programa de trabajo del médico y enfermera de la familia el policlínico y el hospital.* La Habana: Ministerio de Salud Pública, March 1988.

————. *Médico de la familia: Información estadística.* La Habana: Ministerio de Salud Pública, September 1988.

————. *Evaluación estrategias de salud para todos en el año 2000: Informe de Cuba 1990.* La Habana: Ministerio de Salud Pública, January 1991 (typescript).

República de Cuba, Ministerio de Salud Pública, Area de Docencia. "Recursos humanos en salud." La Habana: Ministerio de Salud Pública, December 1990 (typescript).

República de Cuba, Ministerio de Salud Pública, Dirección de Colaboración Internacional. "Cuba: 25 años de colaboración internacional." Havana: Ministerio de Salud Pública document prepared for the 2nd International Seminar on Primary Health Care, November 1988 (typescript).

República de Cuba, Ministerio de Salud Pública, Dirección de Educación para la Salud. *Temas populares de salud.* La Habana: Ministerio de Salud Pública, 1976.

República de Cuba, Ministerio de Salud Pública, Dirección Nacional de Planificación de Salud. *Programas básicos del área de salud y su evaluación.* La Habana: Ministerio de Salud Pública, 1977.

República de Cuba, Ministerio de Salud Pública, Instituto Superior de Ciencias Médicas de La Habana. *La formación del médico general básico como médico de la familia: Plan de estudio de la carrera.* La Habana: Ministerio de Salud Pública, n.d. [probably 1988].

República de Cuba, Minsterio de Salud Pública, Viceministerio de Higiene y Epidemiología. *Cuba: situación nutricional 1991.* La Habana: Comité Estatal de Estadísticas, 1991 (typescript).

República de Cuba, Ministerio de Salud Pública, Vicerrectoría Desarrollo ISCM-H. "Algunas ideas vertidas en diferentes discursos pronunciados por el Comandante en Jefe Fidel Castro que tienen que ver con la formación del médico a egresar de la educación médica superior y con la especialidad de medicina general integral y que sirvieron de base para la elaboración del nuevo plan de estudio de medicina (1981–1984)." La Habana: Instituto Superior de Ciencias Médicas de La Habana, n.d. [probably 1984] (mimeographed).

República de Cuba, Ministerio de Salud Pública y Organización Panamericana de la Salud. *Informe final sobre la evaluación del programa ampliado de inmunización. República de Cuba.* OPS report PAI/81/002. Washington, D.C.: Organización Panamericana Sanitaria, 1981.

República de Cuba, Organo del Poder Popular Ciudad de La Habana, Dirección Provincial de Salud, Dpto. Provincial Educación para la Salud, Dpto. de Nutrición. *Nutrición.* La Habana: Organos de Poder Popular, 1980 (mimeographed).

República Popular de Angola, Misión Médica Cubana. *Balance anual 1987.* Angola: Misión Médica Cubana, n.d. (probably December 1987).

———. *Public Health in Figures 1986.* Havana: MINSAP, 1987.

"Rise in Infant Mortality Rate." *Cuba Update,* 7, nos. 1–2 (Winter–Spring 1986): 7.

Riverón Corteguera, Raúl, José A. Gutiérrez Muñiz, and Francisco Valdés Lazo. "Mortalidad infantil en Cuba, en el decenio 1970–1979." *Boletín de la Oficina Sanitaria Panamericana* 92, no. 5 (May 1982): 379–90.

Robbins, Carla Anne. *The Cuban Threat.* New York: McGraw-Hill, 1983.

Roca, Sergio. "Economic Aspects of Cuban Involvement in Africa." *Cuban Studies/Estudios Cubanos* 10, no. 2 (July 1980): 55–80.

Roche, Marcel. "Cuba: El Centro de Investigaciones Biológicas." *Interciencia* (Buenos Aires, Argentina) 10, no. 6 (November–December 1985): 299–300.

Rodríguez, José Luis. *Estrategia del desarrollo económico en Cuba.* La Habana: Editorial de Ciencias Sociales, 1990.

———. "La economía cubana ante un mundo cambiante." Paper presented at the 16th Congreso de la Asociación Latinoamericana de Sociología, La Habana, May 1991.

Rodríguez, Rodolfo. "Informe de viaje a Cuba." PAHO/WHO interoffice memorandum HSI/84/2.1 (53/90), May 2, 1990.

Roemer, Milton I. *Cuban Health Services and Resources.* Washington, D.C.: Pan American Health Organization, 1976.

————. "Progreso alcanzado por los servicios de salud en Cuba." Organización Panamericana de la Salud, internal document no. 77/WP/CUBA/ 1300, December 1977.

————. "Health Development and Political Policy: The Lesson of Cuba." *Journal of Health Politics, Policy and Law* 4, no. 4 (Winter 1980): 570–80.

Roig de Leuchsenring, Emilio. *Historia de la enmienda Platt.* Cuarta edición. La Habana: Editorial de Ciencias Sociales, 1979.

Rojas Ochoa, Francisco. "El Policlínico." La Habana: Centro Nacional de Información en Ciencias Médicas, 1972.

————. "Estrategias y prioridades en la formación de recursos humanos." *Revista cubana de administración de salud* 7, no. 2 (April–June 1981): 119–27.

————. "El potencial de recursos humanos para la investigación en salud en Cuba." La Habana: Instituto Superior de Ciencias Médicas de La Habana, Vicerrectoría de Investigaciónes, November 1990 (typescript).

————. "Proyecto sistema nacional de vigilancia de la situación dc salud según condiciones de vida en Cuba." La Habana: Instituto Superior de Ciencias Médicas de la Habana, Vicerrectoría de Investigaciones, March 1992 (typescript).

Rose, Steven, ed. *CBW: Chemical and Biological Warfare.* Boston: Beacon Press, 1968.

Ryan, Michael. *The Organization of Soviet Medical Care.* Oxford: Basil Blackwell & Mott, 1978.

Salcedo, Danilo, and Eduardo Joly. *Informe de misión para determinar las necesidades de asistencia en materias de población.* United Nations Family Planning Agency, April 5, 1979.

Santana, Sarah. "The Cuban Health Care System: Responsiveness to Changing Population Needs and Demands." *World Development* 15, no. 1 (January 1987): 113–25.

————. "Some Thoughts on Vital Statistics and Health Status in Cuba." In *Cuban Political Economy: Controversies in Cubanology,* edited by Andrew Zimbalist, 107–18. Boulder, Colo.: Westview Press, 1988.

Science 200, no. 4347 (June 16, 1978): 1246–49.

Segal, Aaron. "Cuba and Africa: Military and Technical Assistance." In *The New Cuban Presence in the Caribbean,* edited by Barry B. Levine, 123–48. Boulder, Colo.: Westview Press, 1983.

Selowsky, Marcelo. *The Economic Dimensions of Malnutrition in Young Children.* World Bank Staff working paper no. 294. Washington, D.C.: World Bank, October 1978.

————. *Nutrition, Health, and Education: The Economic Significance of Complementarities at Early Age.* World Bank Reprint Series no. 218. Washington, D.C.: 1981.

Servimex, Turismo de Salud Cubanacán. "Chequeos médicos 1988." La Habana: Cubanacán, 1988 (typescript).

Shearman, Peter. *The Soviet Union and Cuba.* Chathman House Papers no. 38. London: Routledge & Kegan Paul, 1987.

Sidel, Ruth, and Victor W. Sidel. *The Health Of China.* Boston: Beacon Press, 1982.

Sidel, Victor W., and Ruth Sidel. *Serve the People: Observations on Medicine in the People's Republic of China.* New York: Josiah Macy, Jr., Foundation, 1973.

Simeon Negrín, Rosa Elena. "Science and Technology, Their Role in the Development of Cuba." N.d. [probably 1988 or 1989] (typescript).

Sivard, Ruth Leger. *World Military and Social Expenditures,* annual reports 1985–1991. Washington, D.C.: World Priorities, 1985–1991.

Smith, Helen Mathews. "Castro's Medicine: An On-the-Scene Report." *M.D.* 27, no. 5 (May 1983): 144–66.

Smith, Issar. "Report on NACSEX 1/28–2/7/90 Trip [to Cuba]." NACSEX (North American–Cuban Scientific Exchange) internal document.

Smith, John T. "Sugar Dependency in Cuba: Capitalism versus Socialism." In *The Gap Between the Rich and the Poor: Contending Perspectives on the Political Economy of Development,* edited by Mitchell Seligson. Boulder, Colo.: Westview Press, 1984.

Smith, Lois M. "Teenage Pregnancy and Sex Education in Cuba." Paper presented at the Latin American Studies Association 14th Congress, New Orleans, March 17–19, 1988.

Smith, Wayne S. "U.S.-Cuba Relations: Twenty-Five Years of Hostility." In *Cuba: Twenty-Five Years of Revolution, 1959–1984,* edited by Sandor Halebsky and John M. Kirk, 333–51. New York: Praeger, 1985.

———. *The Closest of Enemies: A Personal and Diplomatic Account of U.S.–Cuban Relations Since 1957.* New York: Norton, 1987.

Sociedad Científica Cubana para el Desarrollo de la Familia (SOCUDEF). *¿Qué es el SIDA?.* La Habana: MINSAP Educación para la Salud, n.d. [obtained in November 1988].

Solimano, Giorgio, José Gutiérrez-Muñiz, Sarah Santana, Eneida Ríos-Massebot, Nigel Paneth, Raúl Riverón-Corteguera, and Mervyn Susser. "Health for All in Cuba: Policies and Strategies." New York, n.d. [probably 1986] (typescript).

Sorel, George. *Reflections on Violence.* London: Allen and Unwin, 1925.

Stark, Evan. "Overcoming the Diseases of Poverty." *Cuba Review* 7, no. 1 (March 1978): 23–28.

Stein, Z., and M. Susser. "The Cuban Health System: A Trial of a Comprehensive Service in a Poor Country." *International Journal of Health Services* 2, no. 4 (1972): 551–56.

Streeten, Paul. "Basic Needs: Some Unsettled Questions." *World Development* 12, no. 9 (September 1984): 973–78.

Suárez Lugo, Nery. "Actividades antitabáquicas en Cuba." La Habana: ICIODI para la Segunda Reunión de Intercambio de Experiencias, Campaña para Desestimular el Hábito de Fumar, November 1988 (mimeographed).

Szulc, Tad. *Fidel: A Critical Portrait.* New York: William Morrow, 1986.

Tesh, Sylvia. "Health Education in Cuba: A Preface." *International Journal of Health Services* 16, no. 1 (1986): 87–104.

Thomas, Hugh. *Cuba: In Pursuit of Freedom.* New York: Harper and Row, 1971.

Tokatlian, Juan Gabriel, comp. *Cuba y Estados Unidos: Un debate para la convivencia.* Buenos Aires: Grupo Editor Latinoamericano, 1984.

Turits, Richard. "Trade, Debt, and the Cuban Economy." *World Development* 15, no. 1 (January 1987): 163–80.

Ubell, Robert N. "Cuba's Great Leap." *Nature* 302 (April 28, 1983): 745–48.

———. "High-Tech Medicine in the Caribbean: 25 Years of Cuban Health Care." *New England Journal of Medicine* 309, no. 23 (December 8, 1983): 1468–72.

UNICEF, UNFPA, OPS/OMS, MINSAP. *El plan del médico de la familia en Cuba.* La Habana: UNICEF, 1991.

"UNIDO Narrow Choice for Site of Biotechnology Center." *Genetic Technology News* 3, no. 4 (April 1983): 8.

"UNIDO World Bio-center Meeting Puts off Decisions." *Biotechnology Newswatch* 5, no. 8 (April 15, 1987): 7.

United Nations. Department of Economic and Social Affairs. *National Experience in the Formulation and Implementation of Population Policy, 1959–1976: Cuba.* New York: United Nations document ST/ESA/SER.R/17, 1977.

———. *Living Conditions in Developing Countries in the Mid-1980s. Supplement to the 1985 Report on the World Social Situation.* New York: United Nations, 1986.

United Nations. Population Studies. *Model Life Tables for Developing Countries.* No. 77. New York: United Nations, 1982.

U.S. Central Intelligence Agency. *Communist Aid Activities in Non-Communist LDCs, 1977.* Washington, D.C.: Central Intelligence Agency, 1978.

———. *Communist Aid Activities in Non-Communist LDCs, 1978.* Washington, D.C.: Central Intelligence Agency, 1979.

———. *Communist Aid Activities in Non-Communist LDCs, 1979 and 1954–1979.* Washington, D.C.: Central Intelligence Agency, April 15, 1980.

U.S. Congress. House. Committee on Foreign Affairs. *Chemical-Biological Warfare: U.S. Policies and International Effects. Hearings before the Subcommittee on National Security Policy and Scientific Developments of the Committee on Foreign Affairs.* 91st Cong., 1st sess., November 18 and 20, December 2, 9, 18, and 19, 1969.

U.S. Congress. Joint Economic Committee. *Cuba Faces the Economic Realities of the 1980s.* By Lawrence Theriot. 97th Cong., 2nd Sess., Washington, D.C.: U.S. Government Printing Office, March 22, 1982.

———. *Soviet Economy in the 1980s: Problems and Prospects.* Part 2. "Issues in Soviet Health Problems," by Murray Feshbach. 97th Cong., 2nd Sess., Washington, D.C.: U.S. Government Printing Office, December 31, 1982.

U.S. Congress. Senate. *Alleged Assassination Plots Involving Foreign Leaders.* 94th Cong., 1st Sess., Washington, D.C.: U.S. Government Printing Office, November 20, 1975.

U.S. Congress. Senate. Committee on Foreign Relations. *Chemical and Biological Warfare. Hearing before the Committee on Foreign Relations.* 91st Cong., 1st sess., April 30, 1969. (Secret hearing held on April 30, 1969; sanitized and printed on June 23, 1969.)

U.S. Congress. Senate. Committee on Foreign Relations, Subcommittee on Disarmament. *Chemical-Biological-Radiological (CBR) Warfare and Its Disarmament Aspects.* Washington, D.C.: U.S. Government Printing Office, 1960.

U.S. Congress. Senate. Committee on Labor and Public Welfare. Special Subcommittee on the National Science Foundation. *Chemical and Biological Weapons. Some Possible Approaches for Lessening the Threat and Danger.* Washington, D.C.: U.S. Government Printing Office, May 1969.

U. S. Department of Commerce. *Economic Study of Puerto Rico.* Washington, D.C.: U.S. Government Printing Office, 1977.

U.S. Department of Commerce. Bureau of the Census. *Statistical Abstract of the United States* (1986–1990). Washington, D.C.: U.S. Government Printing Office, 1985–1990.

U.S. Department of Health and Human Services. Health Resources and Services Administration. Bureau of Health Professions, Office of Data Analysis and Management. *The Impact of Foreign-Trained Doctors on the Supply of Physicians.* Washington, D.C.: U.S. Government Printing Office, DHHS publication no. HRS-P-OD-83-2, September 1983.

U.S. Department of Health and Human Services. Public Health Service. Human Resources Administration, Office of Graduate Medical Education. *Report of the Graduate Medical Education National Advisory Committee to the Secretary, Department of Health and Human Services.* Vol. 2. DHHS publication no. (HRA) 81–652. Washington, D.C.: U.S. Government Printing Office, 1981.

U.S. Department of Health and Human Services. Public Health Service. National Center for Health Statistics. *Vital Statistics of the United States, 1982.* Vol. 2, sec. 6 (Life tables). DHHS publication no. (PHS) 85–1104. Public Health Services. Washington, D.C.: U.S. Government Printing Office, 1985.

U.S. Department of State. *Soviet and East European Aid to the Third World, 1981.* Washington, D.C.: U.S. Government Printing Office, February 1983.

U.S. General Accounting Office. *Donor Approaches To Development Assistance: Implications for The United States.* GAO/ID-83-23, Washington, D.C.: U.S. General Accounting Office, May 4, 1983.

U.S. Information Agency. *U.S. Advisory Commission on Public Diplomacy. 1986 Report.* Washington, D.C.: U.S. Information Agency, 1986.

Valdés, Nelson P. "Cuba's Involvement in the Horn of Africa." *Cuban Studies/Estudios Cubanos* 10, no. 1 (January 1980): 49–80.

Valladares, Armando. *Against All Hope: The Prison Memoirs of Armando Valladares.* New York: Knopf, 1986.

Vayrynen, Raimo. "Small States in Different Theoretical Traditions of International Relations Research." In *Small States in Europe and Dependence.* The Laxenburg Papers, edited by Otmar Höll, 83–106. Boulder, Colo.: Westview Press, 1983.

Vela Valdés, Juan. Untitled paper presented at the Integrated Conference on Latin American Universities and Health of the Population, Havana, June 3–7, 1991.

Vieira, César. PAHO/WHO Interoffice Memorandum HSP/84/242/88, April 6, 1988. Washington, D.C.: PAHO, 1988 (typescript).

Vogel, Hans. "Small States' Efforts in International Relations: Enlarging the Scope." In *Small States in Europe and Dependence.* The Laxenburg Papers, edited by Otmar Höll, 54–68. Boulder, Colo.: Westview Press, 1983.

Weinerman, E. Richard, with Shirley B. Weinerman. *Social Medicine and the Education of Medical Personnel in Czechoslovakia, Hungary, and Poland.* Cambridge: Harvard University Press, 1969.

Weisskoff, Richard. *Factories and Food Stamps: The Puerto Rico Model of Development.* Baltimore: Johns Hopkins University Press, 1985.

Welch, Richard E., Jr. *Response to Revolution: The United States and the Cuban Revolution, 1959–1961.* Chapel Hill, N.C.: University of North Carolina Press, 1985.

Werner, David. "Health Care in Cuba Today: A Model Service or a Means of Social Control?" Palo Alto, Calif.: The Hesperian Foundation, 1978 (typescript).

Wheeler, David. *Human Resource Development and Economic Growth in Developing Countries: A Simultaneous Model.* World Bank Staff working paper no. 407. Washington, D.C.: World Bank, July 1980.

White, Stephen. "Economic Performance and Communist Legitimacy." *World Politics* 38, no. 3 (April 1986): 462–82.

Williams, William Appleman. *The United States, Cuba, and Castro: An Essay on the Dynamics of Revolution and the Dissolution of Empire.* New York: Monthly Review Press, 1962.

Woodford Bray, Marjorie, and Donald W. Bray. "Cuba, the Soviet Union, and Third World Struggle." In *Cuba: Twenty-Five Years of Revolution, 1959 to 1984,* edited by Sandor Halebsky and John M. Kirk, 352–71. New York: Praeger, 1985.

World Bank. *World Development Report 1990.* New York: Oxford University Press, 1990.

World Health Organization. *World Health Statistics Annual 1987.* Geneva: World Health Organization, 1987.

———. Internal memorandum BLG-B3/449/7. Geneva: World Health Organization, July 31, 1989, 1.

———. Internal memorandum HSD/MGP/92.18. Geneva: World Health Organization, August 17, 1989, 1.

Wyden, Peter. *Bay of Pigs: The Untold Story.* New York: Simon and Schuster, 1979.

Zimbalist, Andrew. "Cuban Political Economy and Cubanology: An Overview." In *Cuban Political Economy: Controversies in Cubanology*, ed. Andrew Zimbalist, 1–21. Boulder, Colo.: Westview Press, 1988.
———. "Incentives and Planning in Cuba." *Latin American Research Review* 24, no. 1 (1989): 65–94.

Interviews and Personal Communications

Over the course of fourteen years, I have interviewed hundreds of Cuban health officials, educators, researchers, and practitioners, as well as other Cuban officials and citizens. Of Cuba's fourteen provinces and one special municipality, the only places in which I have not conducted interviews and site visits are Ciego de Avila, Sancti Spíritus, and Villa Clara. I have also interviewed numerous Latin American and some European health officials, as well as representatives of international organizations at the 2nd International Seminar on Primary Care held in Havana in November 1988. Moreover, I held discussions with Latin American and European biotechnology researchers and vendors at the 1992 International Biotechnology Conference held in Havana in July 1992. Thus, the following is not a complete listing of those interviewed.

Alvarez Gómez, Juan Antonio. Specialist in integral general medicine, Policlínico Docente Plaza de la Revolución. Havana, November 1988.
Alzugaray, Carlos. Adviser to Vice Minister of Foreign Affairs Ricardo Alarcón. Halifax, Nova Scotia, October 1989, and Havana, June 11, 1991.
Amador Pérez, Juan Félix. Marketing manager, Center for Molecular Immunology (CIMAB). Havana, June 19, 1991.
Arouca, Sergio. Oswaldo Cruz Foundation (Brazil). Havana, November 16, 1988.
Balán, Ydania. Relaciones Internacionales del MINSAP. Havana, November 21, 1988.
Balari, Eugenio R. President, Instituto Cubano de Investigación y Orientación de la Demanda Interna (ICIODI). Havana, 1978, 1979, 1980, 1981, November 24, 1988, and June 11, 21, and 22, 1991.
Batista Peña, Maria de los Angeles. Family doctor, Cagüeibaje, Baracoa, Guantánamo. November 27, 1988.
Beckwith, Jon. Professor of microbiology and molecular genetics, Harvard Medical School. Boston, September 26, 1986.
Benítez, René. Vice director for Economics, Ministry of Public Health, Province of Pinar del Río. June 18, 1991.

Bialy, Harvey. Research editor, *Bio/Technology.* Red Hook, New York, September 15, 1990, and February 15, 1991.

Bierstock, Richard S. Ophthalmologist. Rhinebeck, New York, January 15, 1991.

Blanco, Juan Antonio. Department of the Americas, Central Committee of the Cuban Communist Party. 1979, 1980, 1988, 1990, and June 13, 14, 16, and 19, 1991.

Bruch, Hans. Director of statistical office, Pan American Health Organization. Washington, D.C., October 1982.

Cabezas, Leonardo. Deputy director, National Center for Laboratory Animal Science (CENPALAB). Havana, June 20, 1991.

Cámara Tejedor, Hugo Rele. Family doctor, Yumurí, Baracoa, Guantánamo. November 27, 1988.

Capetillo, Juan G. Municipal director of health, Baracoa, Guantánamo province. November 27, 1988.

Capote Mir, Roberto. Regional adviser for health systems and hospital administration, Pan American Health Organization. Washington, D.C., April 21, 1987, and Havana, November 1988.

Casanova, Ramón. Director, Cardiocentro William Soler (Pediatric Cardiovascular Surgery Center). Havana, December 1, 1988.

Cash, Richard. Director of international health, Harvard Institute of International Development, and professor, Harvard School of Public Health. Boston, September 24, 1984.

Cassván, Ricardo. Policlínico Elpidio Berovides in San Augustín, La Lisa municipality, City of Havana province. March 12, 1981.

Castellanos Robayo, Jorge. Regional adviser on medical administration and health care, Pan American Health Organization. Washington, D.C., October 21, 1988, and January 19, 1988.

Castro Miranda, Osvaldo. Head of planning department, Vice Ministry of Economics, Ministry of Public Health. Havana, 1978, 1980, 1981, 1991.

Cehelsky, Marta. Senior policy officer, Division of International Programs, National Science Foundation. Washington, D.C., October 10, 1990.

Cordeiro, Hesio. Institute of Social Medicine, University of the State of Rio de Janeiro, and former head of social security. Havana, November 1988.

Curbelo Alfonso, Luis. Director of medical care, Pinar del Río province. Pinar del Río, June 18, 1991.

Davis, Jaime. Director of Colaboración Internacional, Ministerio de Salud Pública. Havana, November 15, 1988.

de la Torre, Rosa Ana. Facultad de Medicina Salvador Allende. Havana, June 22, 1991.

de Quadros, Ciro. Director of the Expanded Program on Immunization in the Americas (Programa Ampliado de Inmunizaciones), Pan American Health Organization. Washington, D.C., April 12, 1984.

Diéguez Dacal, Roberto. Adviser, National Social Welfare Administration. Havana, June 14, 1991.

Domínguez, Jorge I. Professor of government, Harvard University. Personal communication, June 24, 1986.

Domínguez, William. Provincial health director, Guantánamo province. Baracoa, November 28, 1988.

Escalona Reguera, Mario. Instituto de Desarrollo de la Salud. Havana, December 1978, June 1979, March 1980, October 1980, and February and March 1981.

Farina, Ana Teresa. Director, Policlínico Elpidio Berovides, La Lisa municipality, City of Havana province, March 6, 1981.

Feinsilver, Ethel Marcus. Psychiatric social worker. Personal communication, August 1986.

Figueras, Miguel Alejandro. Adviser to the president of the Comité Estatal de Colaboración Económica (CECE). Washington, D.C., April 6, 1991, Havana, June 14 and 21, 1991, and Cancún, July 7, 1992.

Foyo, Luis. Family Doctor Program, Vice Ministry for Medical Care, Ministry of Public Health. Havana, June 17, 1991.

García Arzola, Esteban. Director, Hospital Docente Octavio de la Concepción y de la Pedraja, Baracoa, Guantánamo. November 28, 1988.

Gil, Reinaldo. Vice Ministry of Hygiene and Epidemiology (AIDS), Ministry of Public Health. Havana, June 12, 1991.

Gilpin, Peggy. Medical researcher. Havana, November 16, 1988.

Goldstein, Daniel J. Professor of molecular biology, University of Buenos Aires. Washington, D.C., October 16, 1990, January 7, 1991, and July 21, 1991.

Gómez Cova, David R. Ex-president of the Latin American and Caribbean Public Health Association, and professor, School of Public Health, Universidad Central de Venezuela (Caracas). Campinas, Brazil, July 6, 1990.

González Gotera, Noel. Head of collaboration, National Center for Laboratory Animal Science. Havana, June 20, 1991.

González Lahullier, Rubén D. Director, electromedicine, Ministry of Public Health. Havana, June 12, 1991.

González León, Zenobio. Director of international relations, Hospital Hermanos Ameijeiras. Havana, November 30, 1988.

Grillo, Manuel. Dirección de nutrición, Ministerio de Salud Pública. Havana, June 13, 1991.

Hartmann, Alejandro. Historian of the city of Baracoa and director of the Museo Matachín, Baracoa, Guantánamo. November 26, 1988.

Herédero, Luis. Provincial director of genetics, City of Havana, PAHO consultant, and president of the Latin American Genetics Association. Havana, November 22, 1988.

Heredia del Portal, Lorenzo. Director of immunochemistry, Centro de Inmunoensayos (Immunoassay Center). Havana, November 25, 1988.

Hernández, Rafael. Head of Department of the United States, Center for the Study of America (CEA). Havana, 1988, 1990, 1991.

Herrera, Luis. Assistant director, Centro de Ingeniería Genética y Biotecnología (Center for Genetic Engineering and Biotechnology). Havana, November 25, 1988, and July 12, 1992.

Jacas Joa, Héctor Manuel. Systems programmer, Centro Biotec, Academía de Ciencias de Cuba. Havana, July 1992.

Jiménez, Víctor R. Department head, chemistry, Division of Proteins and Hormones, Center for Genetic Engineering and Biotechnology. Havana, June 19, 1991.

Joly, Daniel. Pan American Health Organization regional representative in Cuba, 1974–1981. Havana, October 18, 1980, November 1988, January and March 1990, June 12 and 22, 1991, and July 1992, and Washington, D.C., October 27, 1982.

Joly, Eduardo. Argentine sociologist and rehabilitation expert. Havana, 1978, 1979, 1980, June 22, 1991, and July 1992, and New York, 1985.

Leal Gómez, Vladimir. Chief of immunodiagnostics production, Centro de Ingeniería Genética y Biotecnología. Havana, July 1992.

León, Francisco. United Nations Economic Commission for Latin America and the Caribbean. Pittsburgh, 1983, and April 27, 1992.

Limonta Vidal, Manuel. Director, Center for Genetic Engineering and Biotechnology. Havana, July 12, 1992.

López Pérez, Manlio. Director, Policlínico Comunitario Docente Monte Carlo, city and province of Camagüey. April 10, 1981.

Lorenzo-Luaces, Luis F. Head of automation processes (computers), Center for Genetic Engineering and Biotechnology. Havana, June 19, 1991.

Machado, Otto. Maternal–Infant Care Department, Vice Ministry for Medical Care, Ministry of Public Health. Havana, June 14, 1991.

Machín, Antonio. Municipal health director, Pinar del Río. June 18, 1991.

Madem, Lázara. Director, Clínica Estomatológica Elpidio Berovides, La Lisa, City of Havana province. March 11, 1981.

Márquez, Miguel. Pan American Health Organization regional representative in Cuba. June 11, 14, 18, and 20, 1991.

Marrero Suárez, Idania. Centro de Inmunología Molecular. Havana, June 19, 1991.

Martínez Rojas, Ricardo E. Director of health tourism, Cubanacán. Havana, November 24, 1988, and June 13, 1991.

Mella, Carlos M. President, Heber Biotec. Havana, June 19, 1991.

Miró, José. Export manager, Heber Biotec. Havana, July 12, 1992.

Montano Díaz, Marco A. Professor of medicine, Pinar del Río Medical School. Pinar del Río, June 18, 1991.

Nit, Igor. Economic adviser to Boris Yeltsin, president of the Russian Republic. Jerome Levy Economics Institute, Bard College, October 27, 1991.

Núñez Jover, Jorge. Director of post-graduate studies, University of Havana. Havana, July 1992.

Ordóñez Carceller, Cosme. Director of the Policlínico "Plaza de la Revolución," Havana. December 28, 1978.

Pantoja Baldoquín, Otto. International Relations Department, Ministry of Public Health. Havana, June 1991.

Pedraza, Rafael O. Head of pulmonary medicine, Hospital Benéfico Jurídico. Havana, 1980, 1981, 1990, and 1991.

Pellegrini, Alberto. Director of research, Pan American Health Organization. Personal communication, October 1990.

Peña Escobar, Manuel. Pan American Health Organization consultant, Havana. Havana, November 17 and December 1, 1988.

Pérez Acosta, Jesús. Vice director, Abel Santamaría Teaching Clinical-Surgical Hospital, Pinar del Río. June 18, 1991.

Pichardo, Mario. Deputy director of international relations, Ministry of Public Health. Havana, June 17, 1991.

Placencia, Delia. Nutrition administration, Vice Ministry of Hygiene and Epidemiology. Havana, June 13, 1991.

Pons Bravet, Pedro. Internist, Policlínico Docente Plaza de la Revolución, 1978.

Ponzoa Periu, Osvaldo. Head of international relations, Pedro Kourí Institute of Tropical Medicine. Havana, June 19, 1991.

Quintana López, Luis. Internist, sector 2, Policlínico Comunitario Docente Monte Carlo, Camagüey. April 10, 1981.

Ratner, Mark. Patent expert, ImmunoGenetics, Cambridge, Mass. June 18, 1991.

Rodríguez, José Luis. Subdirector, Centro de Investigación de la Economía Mundial (CIEM). Smith College, February 8, 1991, Havana, June 19, 1991, and Pittsburgh, April 27, 1992.

Rodríguez, Lidia. Municipal director of genetics for the City of Havana. November 22, 1988.

Rodríguez Morales, Luis. Director, Balneario San Diego, Pinar del Río. June 18, 1991.

Rojas Ochoa, Francisco. Vice rector for research, Higher Institute of Medical Sciences, and former director, Institute for Health Development. Havana, 1978, 1979, 1980, 1981, 1988, 1990, 1991, and 1992.

Rojas Requena, Rogelio. Municipal health director, La Lisa, City of Havana province. February 26, 1981.

Santana, Sarah. Columbia School of Public Health. November 5, 1988.

Selman-Houssein Sosa, Guillermo. Head of Division of Plant Biotechnology, Centro de Ingeniería Genética y Biotecnología. Havana, July 1992.

Serrano, María Matilda. Formación de Recursos Humanos en Colaboración Internacional, Ministerio de Salud Pública. Havana, November 30, 1988.

Sierra Blázquez, Patricia. Centro de Inmunología Molecular. Havana, June 19, 1991.

Silver, George A. Professor emeritus of public health, Yale School of Medicine. New Haven, Connecticut, March 27, 1984.

Simma, Bruno. German delegate to the United Nations Human Rights Commission. Ann Arbor, Michigan, September 10, 1988.

Smith, Issar. North American–Cuban Scientific Exchange. New York, October 16, 1990.

Suárez Lugo, Nery. Coordinator of the anti-smoking campaign, Instituto Cubano de Investigación y Orientación de la Demanda Interna. Havana, June 20, 1991.

Torres, Mercedes. Dirección Nacional de Educación para la Salud, Ministerio de Salud Pública. Havana, June 21, 1991.

Torres Goitia, Javier. Former minister of health of Bolivia (1982–1985), and currently director of the Fundación Salud y Sociedad, Instituto Andino de Desarrollo de Salud y Educación in La Paz, Bolivia. Campinas, Brazil, July 4, 1990.

Unbehaun, Ann. Department of Public Relations, University of Michigan Medical Center. Ann Arbor, January 31, 1989.

Valdés Omedo, Cuahtemoc. Universidad Autónoma de México, Filosofía y Letras. Campinas, Brazil, July 6, 1990.

Vázquez Castillo, Mariela. Marketing, Centro de Investigación y Producción de Vacunas y Sueros Carlos Finlay. Havana, July 12, 1992.

Vela, Osvaldo. Deputy director of MediCuba. Havana, January 16, 1990, and June 13, 1991.

Villafuerte, Rolando. Head of burn unit, Abel Santamaria Provincial Clinical-Surgical Hospital, Pinar del Río. June 18, 1991.

Wald, Karen. Freelance journalist. Havana, 1988, 1990, 1991, and 1992.

Washington, Linda. National Center for Health Statistics. Washington, D.C., January 16, 1991.

Wegman, Myron. Former assistant director of the Pan American Health Organization, and dean emeritus of the University of Michigan School of Public Health. Ann Arbor, March 19, 1984.

Zimbalist, Andrew. Professor of economics at Smith College. Jerome Levy Economics Institute, Bard College, November 27, 1990.

Zunga Aguirre, Loida. Family doctor, Policlínico Comunitario Héroes de Corynthia. Havana, January 22, 1990.

Cuban Medical Journals Consulted

Biotecnología aplicada
Revista cubana de administración de salud
Revista cubana de cirugía
Revista cubana de higiene y epidemiología
Revista cubana de investigaciones biomédicas
Revista cubana de medicina
Revista cubana de medicina general integral
Revista cubana de medicina tropical
Revista cubana de obstetricia y ginecología
Revista cubana de pediatría

Cuban Periodicals Consulted

Bohemia
Colaboración Internacional
Cuba Internacional
Foreign Trade
Granma
Granma International
Granma Weekly Review
Juventud Rebelde
Opina
Trabajadores
Verde Olivo

Selected List of Other Periodicals Consulted

Cuba Update
Economist (London)
Financial Times (London)
Foreign Broadcast Information Service, *Latin America Daily Report*
Latin America Weekly Review
New York Times
Wall Street Journal
Washington Post

Index

Psoriasis treatment, 214
Psychoprophylaxis, 67, 236n.19
Puerto Rico, 10–11, 100, 220n.10, 220–21n.11
Punta Brava, 54

Radio health programs, 69. *See also* Media
Radio Martí, 18
RALCA external fixator, 61, 144
Reagan, Ronald, 56, 98, 169, 266n.16
Recombinant DNA technology, 143
Recombinant streptokinase, 152–53
Rectification of errors, 11, 206, 221n.13
Red book, 37–38, 45
Regionalization, 28, 33, 34–36, 67
Respiratory disease, 78
Retinitis pigmentosa, 60, 189
RETOMED (Fábrica de Equipos Médicos de Santiago de Cuba), 144–45
Revolution: influencing health policy, 31–32, 226n.24; symbolism of, 15–17, 21–22, 202, 223n.36
Rio de Janeiro, 140
Rockefeller Foundation, 119
Rodríguez, Carlos Rafael, 75, 76–77
Rodríguez, José Luis, 128
Romania, 217–18n.3
Rural Health Service, 32
Rural population: guerrillas' contact with, 31, 32, 226n.24; infant mortality of, 101; living conditions of, 50; pre-revolutionary care for, 92; served by family doctors, 42, 46, 104, 109–10, 228n.50
Russian Republic, 128

Sabbaticals, 103–4, 246n.65. *See also* Medical education
SADCC (South African Development Co-operation Council), 163
Sakura Finitechnical, 148
Sancti Spíritus, 101
San Martín, José Francisco de, 10
Sanrizuka airport protest, 20–21
Santiago de Cuba, 107, 108–9
São Paulo, 138, 139–40, 143, 168
Savio, Andrés, 168
Sawa, Nagayo, 20
Schering Plough, 126
Science education, 129–30, 250n.35. *See also* Medical education

SCP ("system of patient control"), 38. *See also* Red book
Secondary health care. *See* Health care
Second International Seminar on Primary Health Care, Family Physicians: A Response to Community Needs, 180
Sedentarism campaign, 71–72
SELA (Pan American Health Organization–Latin American Economic System), 154
Senior citizens, 41, 71
Servimed, 190
Sewerage systems, 111
Siberia, 172
Siles Suazo, Hernán, 174, 176
Silva, Alejandro, 136
Smith, Issar, 132
Smoking: campaign against, 77–80, 238nn.52,62,66
Socialist countries: achieving legitimacy, 200, 202; economic transition in, 11; health care in, 2–3, 28, 30, 32, 217–18n.3, 218n.4
Societies or Associations for the Cure of Vitiligo, 188, 263n.169
Somoza, Anastasio, 171
Soviet Union: aid from, 3, 10, 220n.10; Cuban aid to, 173–74; Cuban relations with, 3, 4, 10, 11–13, 15, 76, 127–28, 142–43, 192, 249n.27; economic aid by, 159; health care in, 3, 4, 28, 30, 47, 200, 217–18n.3, 218n.4, 228n.47, 265n.6; reporting health statistics, 97, 243–44n.28; SUMAs used by, 135–36, 142
Spectrum 32 electroencephalogram equipment, 146
SPF (specific pathogen-free) animals, 124
Spinal cord surgery, 60, 187
Sterilization equipment, 148–49
Stomatologists, 106
Suárez Lugo, Nery, 80
Sugar, 33, 173, 191, 222n.27, 225n.8
SUMA (ultramicro analytic system), 49, 85, 135–36, 142, 152
Sumitomo Pharmaceuticals (Japan), 126
Sweden, 150, 239n.66
Symbolic capital, 2, 6, 198, 208; conversion to material capital, 195; cost of, 203; defined, 24–25; and domestic health care, 46, 49, 56, 70, 89–90, 120–21; long-term benefits of, 199;

8 5 8 5

Compositor: Recorder Typesetting Network
Text: 10/13 Garamond Book
Display: Garamond Book
Printer and Binder: BookCrafters, Inc.